Manual of Definitive Surgical Trauma Care

Manual of Definitive Surgical Trauma Care

FOURTH EDITION

Edited by

Kenneth D Boffard BSc(Hons) FRCS FRCPS FCS(SA) FACS
Professsor Emeritus, Department of Surgery,
Milpark Hospital and University of the Witwatersrand,
South Africa

CRC Press
Taylor & Francis Group
Boca Raton London New York

CRC Press is an imprint of the
Taylor & Francis Group, an **informa** business

CRC Press
Taylor & Francis Group
6000 Broken Sound Parkway NW, Suite 300
Boca Raton, FL 33487-2742

Printed on acid-free paper
Version Date: 20150708

International Standard Book Number-13: 978-1-4987-1487-7 (Pack - Book and DVD)

Visit the Taylor & Francis Web site at
http://www.taylorandfrancis.com

and the CRC Press Web site at
http://www.crcpress.com

Dedication

This manual is dedicated to the six surgeons who in 1993 saw the need for a course in operative trauma surgery and surgical decision making for surgeons who would not routinely be involved in the care of the trauma patient, and from whose foresight the course has been developed.

Howard Champion, Bethesda, Maryland, United States

Stephen Deane, Newcastle, Australia

Abe Fingerhut, Poissy, France

Stenn Lennquist, Linkoping, Sweden

David Mulder, Montreal, Canada

Donald Trunkey, Portland, Oregon, United States

This manual is also dedicated to those who care for the injured patient and whose passion is to do it well.

Contents

Video Contents

A companion DVD is included with this copy of *Manual of Definitive Surgical Trauma Care, Fourth Edition*. To use the DVD:

1 Insert.
2 Open from My Computer.
3 Click in Index.
4 If asked, "allow blocked content."
5 The welcome page will appear, together with a human skeleton.
6 Click on the '+' sign of each area to open files for procedures in that area.

Included on the DVD:

- Access to the neck
- Access to the anterior mediastinum
- Aorta
- Access to the axilla
- Bleeding control
- Craniotomy
- Fasciotomy
- Heart
- Heart and lung
- Iliac shunting
- Kidney
- Laparotomy
- Liver
- Pancreas
- Pelvic packing
- Small bowel
- Spleen
- Sternotomy
- Stomach
- Thoracic
- Ureteric repair

Preface

Unless they deal with major trauma on a particularly frequent basis, few surgeons can attain and sustain the level of skill necessary for decision making in major trauma. This includes both the intellectual decisions and the manual dexterity required to perform all the manoeuvres for surgical access and control. These can be particularly challenging and may be infrequently required, yet rapid access to, and control of, sites of haemorrhage following trauma can be a life-saving surgical intervention. Many situations require specialist trauma expertise, yet often this is simply not available within the time frame in which it is required.

In years past, many surgeons honed their skills in war and translated them into the techniques required in peace. In the twenty-first century, this has changed, so that most surgeons work in an environment of peace, while a few serve in lower-key conflicts. In many countries, the incidence of injury, particularly from vehicle-related trauma, has fallen below the numbers recorded when records were first kept. Many injuries are now treated non-operatively, so operative exposure and the skills required are reduced as well. Occasionally, for this reason, the decision *not* to operate is based on inexperience or insecurity, rather than on good clinical judgement.

It is not enough to be a good operator. The effective practitioner is part of a multidisciplinary team that plans for, and is trained to provide, the essential medical and surgical response required in the management of the injured patient.

Planning the response requires a clear understanding of:

- The causation, including mechanism of injuries occurring within the local population.
- The initial, pre-hospital and emergency department care of the patient.
- The condition in which the patient is delivered to the hospital and subsequently to the operating theatre, which is determined by the initial response, which itself may determine outcome.
- The resources, both physical and intellectual within the hospital, and the ability to anticipate and identify the specific problems associated with patients with multiple injuries.
- The limitations in providing specialist expertise within the time frame required.

In 1993, five surgeons (Howard Champion, United States; Stephen Deane, Australia; Abe Fingerhut, France; David Mulder, Canada; and Don Trunkey, United States), members of the International Society of Surgery – Société Internationale de Chirugie (ISS-SIC) and the International Association for Trauma Surgery and Intensive Care (IATSIC), met in San Francisco, California, during the meeting of the American College of Surgeons. It was apparent that there was a specific need for further surgical training in the technical aspects of surgical care of the trauma patient, and that routine surgical training was too organ- or area-specific to allow the development of appropriate judgement and decision-making skills in traumatized patients with multiple injuries. Particular attention needed to be directed to those who were senior trainees or had completed their training.

It was believed that a short course focussing on life-saving surgical techniques and surgical decision making was required for surgeons, in order to further train the surgeon who dealt with major surgical trauma on an infrequent basis, to deal with major trauma. This course would meet a worldwide need and would supplement the well-recognized and accepted American College of Surgeons Advanced Trauma Life Support (ATLS) course. The experience that Stenn Lennquist had gained offering 5-day courses for surgeons in Sweden was integrated into the programme development, and prototype courses were offered in Paris, Washington DC and Sydney.

At International Surgical Week in Vienna in 1999, IATSIC's members approved a core curriculum and a manual which forms the basis of the Definitive Surgical Trauma Care (DSTC) course. The manual was first published in 2003, subsequently in 2007 and 2011, and this fourth edition in 2015. The manual is updated approximately every 4 years.

Initial DSTC courses were then launched in Austria (Graz), Australia (Melbourne and Sydney) and South Africa (Johannesburg). The material presented in these courses has been refined, a system of training developed using professional education expertise, and the result forms the basis of the standardized DSTC course that now takes place. A unique feature of the course is that while the principles are standardized, once the course has been established nationally in a country, then it can be modified to suit the needs and circumstances of the environment in which the care takes place. The Education Committee of IATSIC has an International DSTC subcommittee that oversees the quality and content of the courses. However, the concept of the DSTC course has remained the same. In addition to the initial 'founding' countries (Australia, Austria and South Africa), courses have been delivered in more than 28 countries across the world, with new participants joining the IATSIC programme each year. The course and its manuals are presented in Portuguese and Spanish, as well as in English.

The DSTC course is designed to support those who, whether through choice or necessity, must deal with major surgical injury, and may not necessarily have the experience or expertise required. The requirements for a DSTC course or the establishment of a DSTC programme can be found in Appendix C of this manual.

A board of contributors, made up of those who have contributed to the DSTC programme, continues to support and update this manual. I would like to thank them for their very great efforts put into the preparation, editing, dissection, re-dissection and assembly of the manual and the course.

This fourth edition had been revised and updated, taking into account new evidence-based information. The increased (and occasionally harmful) role of non-operative management (NOM) has been recognized. With the increased need for peacekeeping, and modern asymmetrical conflicts, each carrying its own spectra of injury, the military module has been substantially updated and broadened to reflect recent conflict experience.

Over the last few years, what has always been obvious has been finally recognized and formalized. The indispensable contribution made by anaesthetic and critical care colleagues has changed the approach to trauma and the concept of a trauma team involving a multidisciplinary team. Anaesthesiology, through the enthusiastic inputs of anaesthetic faculty in the Netherlands, Scandinavia, Switzerland, the United Kingdom, and many other countries, has, in parallel with this course, developed the Definitive Anaesthetic Trauma Care (DATC) course. We are delighted to incorporate these aspects of care in this manual.

The book is divided into sections:

- Trauma system and crew resource management (CRM) communication principles.
- Physiology and the body's response to trauma.
  - Metabolic response.
  - Transfusion.
  - Damage control.
- Each anatomical area or organ system, divided into both an overview of the problems and pitfalls specific to that system, and the surgical techniques required to deal with major injury in that area including burns, brain injury and extremes of age.
- Modern diagnostic and therapeutic technology.
  - Imaging.
  - The role of minimally invasive surgery.
- Specific aspects of specialized care.
  - Anaesthesiology.
  - Austere and military conditions.
  - Critical care.
- Importance of operating room scrub nurses (in a separate appendix).
- Resources for trauma scoring and injury assessment.

Ken Boffard

Introduction

Injury (trauma) remains a major health problem worldwide, and in many countries it continues to grow. The care of the injured patient should ideally be a sequence of events involving education, prevention, acute care and rehabilitation. In addition to improving all aspects of emergency care, improved surgical skills will save further lives and contribute to minimizing disability.

The standard general surgical training received in the management of trauma is often deficient, partly because traditional surgical training is increasingly organ specific, concentrating on 'superspecialties' such as vascular, hepatobiliary or endocrine surgery, and partly because, in most developed training programmes, there is a limited exposure to the range of injured patients.

INJURY PREVENTION

Injury prevention can be divided into three parts:

- *Primary prevention*: education and legislation are used to reduce the incidence of injury (e.g. driving under the influence of alcohol).
- *Secondary prevention*: minimizing the incidence of injury through design (e.g. seatbelts, helmets, etc.).
- *Tertiary prevention*: once the injury has occurred, minimizing the effects of that injury by better and earlier care.

Although primary and secondary prevention of injury will undoubtedly play some of the major roles in the reduction of mortality and morbidity due to trauma, there will also be a need to minimize tertiary injury to patients as a result of inadequate or inappropriate management. This will require training in the techniques of advanced management of physical injury.

SURGICAL SAFETY

The term 'never event' was first introduced in 2001 by Ken Kizer, former chief executive officer of the National Quality Forum. Never events are largely preventable patient safety incidents that should not occur; now recognized on both sides of the Atlantic, the three recognized surgical never events are:

- Wrong site surgery.
- Retained foreign object post-procedure (such as a laparotomy pack or sponge).
- Wrong implant.

Safety checklists (such as the World Health Organization's Safer Surgery Checklist)[1] have been shown to reduce never events, and there is no excuse for skipping routine safety checks within the surgical process of a major trauma patient simply because of perceived urgency in the patient's condition. During damage control laparotomy, packs (sponges) are commonly left within a body cavity at the end of the primary surgery. Documentation of numbers and sizes of the packs must be meticulous, especially if the patient's management will be handed over to a colleague. In military damage control surgery, surgeons will commonly write externally on the dressings exactly what operation has been undertaken.

Missed injury can be considered as an 'unofficial' never event for the trauma surgeon. Missed injuries in adult trauma patients range in frequency from 9 per cent to 28 per cent; many will be minor, but others may be life-threatening or permanently disabling. In one study of paediatric trauma care, a missed injury rate in a series of injured children was 20 per cent. Critically injured patients are at particular risk of missed injury. The injuries may be within a body cavity, alongside a more obvious or compelling injury and overlooked by the surgeon, or anatomically remote from the main region of injury and have been overlooked by the trauma team during the resuscitation phase of treatment and may involve any region of the body. Patient factors predisposing to missed injury include altered level of consciousness or time-critical injuries, perhaps with associated poly-trauma with haemodynamic instability. Inexperience or incompetence on the part of the surgeon may be thought to increase the chances of a missed injury; however, it can happen to even the most experienced and eminent practitioner.

Systematic protocols for the initial assessment of injured patients, such as the primary and secondary surveys of the Advanced Trauma Life Support (ATLS) course, reduce the chance of missing immediately life-threatening injuries in the emergency department. The tertiary survey, a careful re-examination of the trauma patient and review of imaging once the patient is safely in the critical care unit or ward area after primary surgery, is extremely useful in ensuring no injury is missed. During surgery, a systematic, consistent and thorough intraoperative approach must be used in all patients, so that all areas are examined for possible injury, rather than concentrating simply on what is known to be injured. This cautious approach is particularly important in the patient with multiple injuries. In a modern series of military laparotomy, the missed injury rate for visceral injury at first laparotomy was 1.3 per cent[2].

TRAINING IN THE MANAGEMENT OF SEVERE TRAUMA

The IATSIC National Trauma Management Course (NTMC™)

IATSIC has developed the NTMC as part of an initiative toward improving trauma care in resource-challenged countries, where medical expertise may be available, but the area is resource poor. Based on the ATLS course, and modified for local conditions, the course can be offered either as an isolated course organized by IATSIC, or under the banner of a local trauma organization. To date, some 7000 physicians have been trained under the aegis of organizations such as the Academy of Traumatology of India (http://www.indiatrauma.org), the College of Surgeons of Sri Lanka (http://www.lankasurgeons.org), and IATSIC, in some 12 countries worldwide.

The Advanced Trauma Life Support Course

The Advanced Trauma Life Support (ATLS) programme of the American College of Surgeons is probably the most widely accepted trauma programme in the world, with nearly 60 national programmes taking place at present, and more than one million physicians trained.

Surgical Trauma Training beyond ATLS

Trauma in both well-developed and developing countries continues to be a major public health problem and financial burden, both in the pre-hospital setting and within the hospital system. In addition to increasing political and social unrest in many countries, and an increasing use of firearms for interpersonal violence, the car has become a substantial cause of trauma worldwide. These socio-economic determinants have resulted in a large number of injured patients.

In the United States, trauma affects both the young and the elderly. It is the third leading cause of death for all ages, and the leading cause of death from age 1 to 44 years[3]. Persons under the age of 45 account for 61 per cent of all injury fatalities and 65 per cent of hospital admissions. However, persons aged 65 and older are at a higher risk of both fatal injury and a more protracted hospital stay. About 50 per cent of all deaths occur minutes after injury, and most immediate deaths are because of massive haemorrhage or neurological injury. Autopsy data have demonstrated that central nervous system injuries account for 40–50 per cent of all injury deaths, and haemorrhage accounts for 30–35 per cent. Motor vehicles and firearms accounted for 29 per cent and 24 per cent of all injury deaths, respectively, in 1995[4,5].

In South Africa, there is a high murder rate (56 per 100 000 population) and a high motor vehicle accident rate[6].

There are other areas of the world, such as Australia and the United Kingdom, where penetrating trauma is unusual, and sophisticated injury prevention campaigns have significantly reduced the volume of trauma. However, there is a significant amount of trauma from motor vehicles, falls, recreational pursuits and injury affecting the elderly. The relatively limited exposure of surgeons to major trauma has reduced their expertise in this field, mandating a requirement for designated trauma hospitals and specific skill development in the management of major trauma.

Furthermore, there are multiple areas of the developing world in the West Indies, South America, the Asia-Pacific region and Africa where general surgical training may not necessarily include extensive operative education and psychomotor technical expertise in terms of trauma procedures. There are other countries where thoracic surgery is not an essential part of general surgical training. Therefore a general surgeon called upon to definitively control thoracic haemorrhage may not have had the techniques required incorporated into his or her formal surgical training.

With improving pre-hospital care across the world, patients who would have died previously are reaching hospital alive. In many situations, their airway and ventilation are controlled, but the deaths occur in hospital from uncontrollable bleeding. Not only do the various techniques for orthopaedic haemostasis, such as stabilization of fractures, pelvic fixation and the management of major cranial injury, have an important place in the initial management of trauma patients, but also the surgical control of bleeding and a clear understanding of the physiology of trauma are essential.

Military conflicts occur in numerous parts of the world. These conflicts involve not only the superpowers, but also the military forces of a large number of other countries. It is essential that the military surgeon be well prepared to manage any and all penetrating injuries that occur on the battlefield. The increasing dilemma that is faced by the military is that modern conflicts are in general asynchronous, with only one side in uniform, small and well contained, and do not produce casualties in large numbers or on a frequent basis. For this reason, it is difficult to have a large number of military surgeons who can immediately be deployed to perform highly technical surgical procedures in the battlefield arena or under austere conditions.

It is increasingly difficult for career military surgeons to gain adequate exposure to battlefield casualties, or indeed penetrating trauma in general, and, increasingly, many military training programmes are looking to their civilian counterparts for assistance.

These statistics mandate that surgeons responsible for the management of these injured patients, whether military or civilian, are skilled in the assessment, diagnosis and operative management of life-threatening injuries. There remains a poorly developed appreciation among many surgeons of the potential impact that timely and appropriate surgical intervention can have on the outcome of a severely injured patient. Partly through lack of exposure, and partly because of other interests, many surgeons quite simply no longer have the expertise to deal with such life-threatening situations. For these reasons, a course needs to be flexible in order to accommodate the local needs of the country in which it is being taught.

There is thus an increasing need to provide the surgical skills and techniques necessary to resuscitate and manage these patients surgically not only in the emergency department, but also during the period *after* ATLS is complete.

Surgical Training Courses in Trauma

The Advanced Trauma Operative Management (ATOM) course of the American College of Surgeons was developed by Lenworth M. Jacobs about 15 years ago. It is a one-day course including a didactic lecture series followed by exercises on live, anaesthetized animal models. It is an effective method of increasing surgical competence and confidence in the operative management of penetrating injuries to the chest and abdomen.

The Definitive Surgical Trauma Care (DSTC) course was developed on the initiative of six international surgeons in 1993, and it is owned by the International Association for Trauma Surgery and Intensive Care (IATSIC), an integrated society of the International Society of Surgery in Lupsingen, Switzerland. It is a 3-day course with short didactic lectures followed by extensive operative discussion, group discussions, case discussions and operative exercises on live anaesthetized animals. The emphasis is on both the surgical techniques used in trauma and the surgical decision making required to choose the best method of management. The course currently takes place in 24 countries, and in four languages (English, Portuguese, Spanish and Thai).

THE DSTC COURSE

Course Objectives

By the end of the course, the student will have received training to allow:

- Enhanced knowledge of the surgical physiology of the trauma patient.
- Enhanced surgical decision making in trauma.
- Enhanced surgical techniques in the management of major trauma.
- An improved awareness of the treatment possibilities in major trauma and their evidence base.

Description of the Course

A prerequisite of the DSTC course is a complete understanding of all the principles outlined in a general surgical training and also the ATLS course. For this reason, there are no lectures on the basic principles of trauma surgery, or the initial resuscitation of the patient with major injuries.

The course consists of a core curriculum, designed to be an activity lasting two and one-half days. In addition to the core curriculum, there are a number of modules that can be added to the course to allow it to be more suited to local conditions in the area in which it is being taught.

The course consists of a number of components:

- Didactic lectures – which are designed to introduce and cover the key concepts of surgical resuscitation, discuss the endpoints and provide an overview of the best access to organ systems.
- Cadaver sessions – in which use is made of fresh or preserved human cadavers and dissected tissue. These are used to reinforce the vital knowledge of human anatomy related to access in major trauma. Other alternatives are available if local custom or legislation does not permit the use of such laboratories.
- Animal laboratories – where possible, use is made of live, anaesthetized animals, prepared for surgery. The instructor introduces various injuries. The objects of the exercise are to both improve psychomotor skills and teach new techniques for the preservation of organs and the control of haemorrhage. The haemorrhagic insult is such that it is a challenge to both the veterinary anaesthetist and the surgeon to maintain a viable animal. This creates the real-world scenario of managing a severely injured patient in the operating room.
- Case presentations – this component is a strategic thinking session illustrated by case presentations. Different cases are presented that allow free discussion between the students and the instructors. These cases are designed to put the didactic and psychomotor skills that have been learned into the context of real patient management scenarios.

The Tertiary Survey

Approximately 20 per cent of more minor injuries will be missed at the initial assessment. These include facial bone injury, wrist and hand injuries, etc. It is essential, once the patient is fully stable and awake, to do a tertiary survey to exclude these injuries[7].

SUMMARY

The course is therefore designed to prepare the relatively fully trained surgeon to manage difficult surgically created injuries that mimic the injuries that might present to a major trauma centre. The course fulfils the educational, cognitive and psychomotor needs for mature surgeons, surgical trainees and military surgeons, all of whom need to be comfortable in dealing with life-threatening penetrating and blunt injury, irrespective of whether it is in the military or the civilian arena.

REFERENCES

1. World Alliance for Patient Safety. *WHO Surgical Safety Checklist and Implementation Manual.* http://www.who.int/patientsafety/safesurgery/. Accessed January 2015.
2. Smith I, Beech Z, Lundy JB, Bowley DM. A prospective observation study of abdominal injury management in contemporary military operations: damage control laparotomy is associated with high survivability and low rates of fecal diversion. *Ann Surg.* 2015;261(4):765–73.
3. Fingerhut LA, Warner M. *Injury Chartbook. Health, United States. 1996–1997.* Atlanta, GA: National Center for Health Statistics; 1997.
4. Fingerhut LA, Ingram DD, Felman JJ. Firearm homicide among black teenagers in metropolitan counties: comparison of death rates in two periods, 1983 through 1985 and 1987 through 1989. *JAMA.* 1992;267:3054–58.
5. Bonnie RJ, Fulco C, Liverman CT, eds. *Reducing the Burden of Injury, Advancing Prevention and Treatment.* Washington, DC: National Academy Press; 1999:41–59.
6. Brooks AJ, Macnab C, Boffard KD. Trauma care in South Africa. *Trauma Q.* 1999;14:301–10.
7. Enderson BL, Maull KI. Missed injuries. The trauma surgeon's nemesis. *Surg Clin North Am.* 1991;71(2):399–418.

Contributors

EDITOR

Ken Boffard
Professor Emeritus
Department of Surgery
Milpark Hospital and University of the Witwatersrand
Johannesburg
South Africa

BOARD OF CONTRIBUTORS (DSTC)

Philip Barker
Professor Emeritus
Defence Medical Services
Royal College of Surgeons
United Kingdom
Retired
British Columbia

Chris Bleeker
Consultant Anaesthesist
Radboud University Medical Center
Nijmegen
Netherlands

Douglas Bowley
Consultant Surgeon
Centre for Defence Medicine
Birmingham
United Kingdom

Col (ret) Mark W Bowyer
Professor of Surgery and Chief Division of Trauma and Combat Surgery
The Norman M. Rich Department of Surgery
Uniformed Services University of the Health Sciences
Bethesda, Maryland
United States of America

Adam Brooks
Consultant Surgeon
Queens Medical Centre
Nottingham
United Kingdom

Ian Civil
Professor of Surgery
Faculty of Medical and Health Sciences
University of Auckland
Auckland City Hospital
Auckland
New Zealand

Scott D'Amours
Consultant Surgeon and Trauma Surgeon
Trauma Director
Liverpool Hospital
University of New South Wales
Sydney
Australia

Elias Degiannis
Professor of Surgery
Head
Trauma Directorate
Chris Hani Baragwanath Hospital
University of the Witwatersrand
Johannesburg
South Africa

Jesper Dirks
Consultant Anaesthetist
Department of Anaesthesia
Centre for Head and Orthopaedics
Rigshospitalet
Copenhagen University Hospital
Copenhagen
Denmark

Abe Fingerhut
Professor of Surgery
Medical University of Graz
Graz
Austria
Hipokrateon University Hospital
University of Athens
Greece

Megan Fisher
Consultant Urologist
Linksfield Hospital
Johannesburg
South Africa

Sascha Flohé
Consultant Surgeon
Klinikum Solingen
Solingen
Germany

Tina Gaarder
Consultant Surgeon
Ulleval University Hospital
Oslo
Norway

Georgios Gemenetzis
Chief Resident in Surgery
4th Surgical Clinic
Attikon Hospital
University of Athens
Greece

Timothy Hardcastle
Consultant Trauma Surgeon
Inkosi Albert Luthuli Hospital
University of KwaZuluNatal
Durban
South Africa

Catherine Heim
Consultant Anaesthetist
University Hospital of Lausanne
Lausanne
Switzerland

Gareth Hide
Consultant Surgeon
Sunninghiill Hospital
Sandton
Johannesburg
South Africa

Annette Holian
Consultant Orthopaedic Surgeon
National Critical Care and Trauma Response Centre
Royal Darwin Hospital
Darwin
Australia

Lenworth M Jacobs
Professor of Surgery
University of Connecticut School of Medicine
Hartford, CT
United States of America

Rifat Latifi
Professor of Surgery
Co-Director
Trauma Research Institute
University of Arizona
Tucson, AZ
United States of America

Ari Leppaniemi
Consultant Surgeon
Meilahti Hospital
University of Helsinki
Helsinki
Finland

Peter Mahoney
Defence Professor Anaesthesia and Critical Care
Royal Centre for Defence Medicine
Birmingham
Visiting Professor
Centre for Blast Injury Studies
Imperial College
London

Ronald V. Maier
Professor and Vice-Chair, Surgery
University of Washington
Harborview Medical Center
Seattle, WA
United States of America

Ernest E. Moore
Professor and Vice Chairman
Department of Surgery
University of Colorado Health Sciences Centre
Denver, CO
United States of America

Pål Axel Næss
Consultanht Paediatric Surgeon
Ulleval University Hospital
Oslo
Norway

Andrew Nunn
Instructor in Surgery
Division of Traumatology, Surgical Critical Care and
Emergency Surgery
Perelman School of Medicine University of Pennsylvania
Philadelphia, PA
United States of America

Michael Parr
Professor
Director of Intensive Care
Liverpool Hospital
University of New South Wales
Sydney
Australia

Andrew Peitzman
Mark M. Ravitch Professor of Surgery
University of Pittsburgh
Pittsburgh, PA
United States of America

Graeme Pitcher
Consultant Paediatric Surgeon
University Hospital
Iowa City, IA
United States of America

Frank Plani
Trauma Surgery (SA)
Principal Surgeon
Trauma Directorate
Chris Hani Baragwanath Academic Hospital
Adjunct Professor
Department of Surgery
University of Witwatersrand
Johannesburg
South Africa

James Ralph
Consultant Anaesthetist
Centre for Defence Medicine
Birmingham
United Kingdom

Noelle N. Saillant
Instructor in Surgery
Perelman School of Medicine
Hospital of the University of Pennsylvania
Philadelphia, PA
United States of America

Patrick Schoettker
Associate Professor
Head of Neuro, ENT and Trauma Anesthesia
Departement of Anesthesiology
University Hospital of Lausanne
Lausanne
Switzerland

C William Schwab
Professor of Surgery
Chief
Division of Traumatology and Surgical Critical Care
Hospital of the University of Pennsylvania
Philadelphia, PA
United States of America

Jacob Steinmetz
Associate Professor
Consultant Anaethetist
Trauma Centre and Department of Anaesthesia
Centre for Head and Orthopaedics
Rigshospitalet
Copenhagen University Hospital
Copenhagen
Denmark

Jakob Stensballe
Consultant Anaesthetist
Department of Anaesthesiology
Centre for Head and Orthopaedics Trauma
Section for Transfusion Medicine
Capital Region Blood Bank
Rigshospitalet
Copenhagen University Hospital
Copenhagen
Denmark

Elmin Steyn
Consultant Surgeon and Trauma Director
Christiaan Barnard Memorial Hospital
Cape Town
South Africa

Nigel Tai
Consultant Vascular Surgeon
Royal London Hospital
London
United Kingdom

Fernando Turegano
Consultant Surgeon
University Hospital Gregorio Maranon
Madrid
Spain

Selman Uranues
Professor of Surgery
Medical University of Graz
Graz
Austria

Pantelis Vassiliu
Assistant Professor of Surgery
4th Surgical Clinic
Attikon Hospital
University of Athens
Greece

Arie van Vugt
Professor in Traumasurgery
Medisch Spectrum Twente
Enschede
Netherlands

Jonathan White
Consultant Anaesthetist and ICU Physician
Rigshospitalet
Copenhagen University Hospital
Copenhagen
Denmark

Adrian Wilson
Visiting Professor
Medicine
National University of Science and Technology Faculty of Medicine
Ascot, Bulawayo
Zimbabwe

Paul R Wood
Consultant Anaesthetist
University Hospital
Birmingham NHS Foundation Trust
Birmingham
United Kingdom

Mauro Zago
Medical University of Graz
Graz
Austria

David Zonies
Associate Professor of Surgery
Oregon Health & Science University,
Portland, OR
United States of America

About the Editor

Professor Ken Boffard is Professor of Surgery and Trauma Director at Milpark Hospital, Johannesburg, and until recently, Head of the Department of Surgery at Johannesburg Hospital and the University of the Witwatersrand. He was previously Head of the Johannesburg Hospital Trauma Unit. He qualified in Johannesburg, and trained in Surgery at the Birmingham Accident Hospital and Guy's Hospital.

He is past President of the International Society of Surgery (ISS) in Switzerland, the International Association for Trauma Surgery and Intensive Care (IATSIC), and Chair of the IATSIC Education Committee. He is a Fellow of five Surgical Colleges, and has received Honorary Fellowships from the American College of Surgeons, Royal College of Surgeons of Thailand, College of Surgeons of Sri Lanka, and the Association of Surgeons of Great Britain and Ireland.

His passion is surgical education, and various aspects of trauma resuscitation, intensive care, and regional planning of Trauma Systems. His interests include flying (he is a licensed fixed wing and helicopter pilot), scuba diving, and aeromedical care. His research interests include coagulation, haemostasis and critical bleeding.

He is a Colonel in the South African Military Health Service.

He is a Freeman of the City of London by redemption, and an elected Liveryman of the Guild of Air Pilots of London.

He is married with two children.

Part 1

Trauma system and communication principles

Overview 1

1.1 RESUSCITATION IN THE EMERGENCY DEPARTMENT

Patients with life-threatening injuries represent approximately 10–15 per cent of all patients hospitalized for injuries[1]. Some authors have defined severe trauma in a patient as a person who has an injury severity score (ISS) greater than 15[2-4]. For triage purposes, information available in the prehospital phase and primary survey should be used.

A standardized approach, utilizing the 'MIST' handover, should be used (Table 1.1). Deforming and destructive injuries can be obvious, but the surgeon or physician initially treating the patient must promptly conduct a systematic workup, so that all wounds, including occult mortal injuries, can be treated optimally.

Table 1.1 The 'MIST' handover

M	Mechanism of injury
I	Injuries observed
S	Vital signs
T	Therapy instituted

1.2 MANAGEMENT OF MAJOR TRAUMA

The principles of management for patients suffering major trauma are

- Simultaneous assessment and resuscitation.
- Life-saving surgery.
- A complete physical examination.
- Diagnostic studies if the patient becomes haemodynamically stable.

The first physician to treat a severely injured patient must start the resuscitation immediately and collect as much information as possible. In addition to patient symptoms, necessary information includes mechanism of injury and the presence of pre-existing medical conditions that may influence the critical decisions to be made. Time is working against the patient: 62 per cent of all trauma patients who die in hospital die within the first 4 hours of hospitalization[5]. The majority of these patients either bleed to death or die from primary or secondary injuries to the central nervous system. In order to reduce this mortality, the surgeon must promptly restore adequate tissue oxygenation and perfusion, identify and control any haemorrhage, diagnose and evacuate mass intracranial lesions and treat cerebral oedema.

Unfortunately all this requires time. Time is usually not available, and the workup of the critically injured patient often must be rushed. In order to maximize resuscitative efforts and to avoid missing life-threatening injuries, various protocols for resuscitation have been developed, of which the Advanced Trauma Life Support Course (ATLS)[6] is a model. We use the ATLS as a paradigm for assessment, resuscitation and prioritization of the patient's injuries.

Guideline times for the length of stay in the emergency department (ED) should be as follows:

- For the unstable patient, time in the ED should be no longer than 15 minutes.
- The unstable patient should be in either the operating room or the intensive care unit (ICU) within 15 minutes.
- For the stable patient, time in the ED should be no longer than 30 minutes.
- The stable patient should be in the computed tomography (CT) scanner or ICU within 30 minutes.

1.2.1 Resuscitation

Resuscitation is divided into two components:

- Primary survey and initial resuscitation.
- Secondary survey and continuing resuscitation.

All patients undergo the primary survey of airway, breathing and circulation. Only those patients who become haemodynamically stable will progress to the secondary survey, which focuses on a complete physical examination that directs further diagnostic studies. The great majority of patients who remain haemodynamically unstable require immediate operative intervention.

1.2.1.1 PRIMARY SURVEY

The priorities of the primary survey are:

- Establishing a patent airway with cervical spine control.
- Ensuring adequate ventilation.
- Maintaining circulation (including intravascular volume and cardiac function).
- Assessing the global neurological status.

1.2.1.1.1 Airway

Patients with extensive trauma who are unconscious or in shock benefit from immediate endotracheal intubation[7,8]. To prevent spinal cord injury, the cervical spine must not be excessively flexed or extended during intubation. Oral endotracheal intubation is successful in the majority of injured patients. On rare occasions, bleeding, deformity or oedema from maxillofacial injury will require emergency cricothyroidotomy or planned tracheostomy. Patients who may require a surgical airway include those with a laryngeal fracture and those with a penetrating injury of the neck or throat. The airway priorities are to clear the upper airway, to establish high-flow oxygen initially with a bag mask and to proceed immediately to a definitive airway (cuffed tube in the trachea) – an endotracheal tube in the majority and to a surgical airway in a few.

1.2.1.1.2 Breathing

Patients with respiratory compromise are not always easy to detect. Simple parameters such as the respiratory rate (RR) and adequacy of breathing should be examined within the first minute after arrival. One of the most important things is to detect a tension pneumothorax, necessitating direct drainage by needle thoracostomy followed by the insertion of a chest tube. Other major threats to life, for example, massive haemothorax, flail chest and pulmonary contusion, cardiac tamponade and tracheal-bronchial injury, must be identified urgently, and treatment instituted urgently after arrival.

1.2.1.1.3 Circulation

Simultaneous with airway management, a quick assessment of the patient will determine the degree of shock present. Shock is a clinical diagnosis and should be apparent. A quick first step is to feel an extremity. If shock is present, the extremities will be cool and pale, lack venous filling and have poor capillary refill. The pulse will be thready, and consciousness will be diminished. At the same time, the status of the neck veins must be noted. A patient who is in shock with flat neck veins is assumed to have hypovolaemic shock until proven otherwise. If the neck veins are distended, the most likely possibilities are:

- Tension pneumothorax.
- Pericardial tamponade.
- Myocardial contusion (cardiogenic shock).
- Myocardial infarct (cardiogenic shock).
- Air embolism.

1.2.1.1.3.1 *Pitfall*

Note that the absence of distended neck veins does not exclude these diagnoses because the circulating volume may be so depleted that the circulation is too empty.

Tension pneumothorax always should be the number one diagnosis in the physician's differential diagnosis of shock since it is the life-threatening injury that is easiest to treat in the ED. A simple tube thoracostomy is the definitive management.

Pericardial tamponade is most commonly encountered in patients with penetrating injuries to the torso. Approximately 25 per cent of all patients with cardiac injuries will reach the ED alive. The diagnosis is often obvious. The patient has distended neck veins and poor peripheral perfusion, and a few will have pulsus paradoxus. Ultrasonography may establish the diagnosis in those few patients with equivocal findings. Pericardiocentesis is of doubtful diagnostic or therapeutic use; ultrasound is a more reliable diagnostic modality, and a sub-xiphoid pericardial window is preferable therapeutically. However, proper treatment is immediate thoracotomy, preferably in the operating room, although ED thoracotomy can be life saving[9].

Myocardial contusion is a rare cause of cardiac failure in the trauma patient.

Myocardial infarction from coronary occlusion is not uncommon in the elderly.

Air embolism[10,11] is a syndrome that has relatively recently been appreciated as important in injured patients; it represents air in the systemic circulation caused by a bronchopulmonary venous fistula. Air embolism occurs in 4 per cent of all major thoracic injuries. Thirty-five per cent of the time it is due to blunt trauma, usually a laceration of the pulmonary parenchyma by a fractured rib. In 65 per cent of patients, it is due to gunshot wounds or stab wounds. The surgeon must be vigilant when pulmonary injury has occurred. Any patient who has no obvious head injury but has focal or lateralizing neurological signs may have air bubbles occluding the cerebral circulation. The observation of air in the retinal vessels on funduscopic examination confirms cerebral air embolism. Any intubated patient on positive-pressure ventilation who has a sudden cardiovascular collapse is presumed to have either tension pneumothorax or air embolism to the coronary circulation. Doppler monitoring of an artery can be a useful aid in detecting air embolism. Definitive treatment requires immediate thoracotomy followed by clamping of the hilum of the injured lung to prevent further embolism, followed by expansion of the intravascular volume. Open cardiac massage, intravenous adrenaline (epinephrine) and venting the left heart and aorta with a needle to remove residual air may be required. The pulmonary injury is definitively treated by oversewing the laceration or resecting a lobe.

If the patient's primary problem in shock is blood loss, the intention is to stop the bleeding. If this is not possible, the priorities are:

- To gain venous access to the circulation.
- To obtain a blood sample from the patient.
- To determine where the volume loss is occurring.
- To give resuscitation fluids.
- To prevent and treat coagulopathy.
- To prevent hypothermia.

Access is preferably central, via the subclavian route, and an 8 French Gauge (FG) introducer, more commonly used for passing a pulmonary artery catheter, can be used. Alternatively, percutaneous cannulation of the femoral vein can be performed with a large-bore catheter or an 8 FG introducer (the equivalent can be done at elbow level). Alternative ways to gain access to the circulation are by a surgical cut down on the saphenous vein at the ankle.

As soon as the first intravenous line has been established, baseline blood work is obtained that includes haematocrit, toxicology, blood type and cross match, and a screening battery of laboratory tests if the patient is older and has premorbid conditions. Blood gas determinations should be obtained early during resuscitation.

The third priority is to determine where the patient may have occult blood loss. Three sources for hidden blood loss are the pleural cavities, which can be eliminated as a diagnosis by rapid chest X-ray, the thigh and the abdomen, inclusive of the retroperitoneum and pelvis. A fractured femur should be clinically obvious. However, assessment of the abdomen by physical findings can be extremely misleading. Fifty per cent of patients with significant haemoperitoneum have no clinical signs[12,13]. Common sense dictates that if the patient's chest X-ray is normal and the femur is not fractured, the patient who remains in shock must be suspected of having ongoing haemorrhage in the abdomen or pelvis. Most of these unstable patients require immediate laparotomy to avoid death from haemorrhage. An important caveat is not to delay mandated therapeutic interventions to obtain non-critical diagnostic tests.

The fourth priority for the resuscitating physician is to consider activation of the massive bleeding protocol and order resuscitation fluids, starting with crystalloids and adding type-specific whole blood or blood components as soon as possible[14,15].

The fluid used to resuscitate a hypotensive patient will depend on the patient's response to fluid load. The 'rapid responder' may require no more than crystalloids to replace the volume deficit. The 'transient responder' may need the addition of blood. The only practical way to measure atrial filling pressure in the ED and immediately in the operating room is by central venous pressure monitoring. In elderly patients with extensive traumatic injuries, early cardiac flow monitoring is helpful. Resuscitation should be directed to achieve adequate oxygen delivery and oxygen consumption.

Crystalloid, synthetic colloids such as gelatins, as well as blood are available to replace volume in hypotensive patients, but blood is the fluid of choice. It is clear that patients requiring massive transfusion need the oxygen-carrying capacity of red cells. Data suggest that trauma leads to leaky cells in the pulmonary capillary bed, and the use of colloid puts these patients at further risk, and should be avoided wherever possible. The use of starches in the bleeding patient has specific negative effects on coagulation, and is therefore contraindicated.

Bickell and colleagues[16] found that the survival in patients with penetrating torso trauma was improved if fluid replacement was delayed. He suggested that immediate volume replacement in these patients might disrupt blood clots that had obliterated bleeding vessels.

Research continues on the use of haemoglobin oxygen carriers (HBOCs) as effective substitutes for blood.

Although whole blood is preferred, especially in the military situation, it is commonly difficult to obtain whole blood from modern blood banks, forcing the use of blood components. Loss of more than two units of blood and ongoing bleeding which requires blood transfusion should invoke a predefined massive bleeding protocol (most current massive transfusion protocols aim at predefined ratios of packed red blood cells:fresh frozen plasma:platelets mimicking whole blood) and monitored by frequent coagulation tests, conventional laboratory tests – platelet count, international normalized ratio (INR), prothrombin time (PT), partial thromboplastin time (PTT) and fibrinogen, and more functional tests (TEG or RoTEM) when available (see Section 1.3).

The criteria for adequate resuscitation are simple and straightforward:

- Keep the atrial filling pressure at normal levels.
- Give sufficient fluid to achieve adequate urinary output (0.5 mL/kg per hour in the adult, 1 mL/kg per hour in the child).
- Maintain peripheral perfusion.

The only practical way to measure atrial filling pressure in the ED and immediately in the operating room is by central venous pressure monitor. In elderly patients with extensive traumatic injuries, placing a pulmonary artery catheter or utilizing a cardiac computer may be prudent because it will be used to direct a sophisticated multifactorial resuscitation in the operating room or ICU. Resuscitation should be directed to achieve adequate oxygen delivery and oxygen consumption. An important caveat is not to delay mandated therapeutic interventions to obtain non-critical diagnostic test results.

1.2.1.1.4 Neurological Status (Disability)

The next priority during the primary survey is to quickly assess neurological status and to initiate diagnostic and treatment priorities. The key components of a rapid neurological evaluation are

- Determine the level of consciousness.
- Observe the size and reactivity of the pupils.
- Check eye movements and oculovestibular responses.
- Document skeletal muscle motor responses and spontaneous movement of extremities.
- Determine the pattern of breathing.
- Perform a peripheral sensory examination.

A decreasing level of consciousness is the single most reliable indication that the patient may have a serious head injury or secondary insult (usually hypoxic or hypotensive) to the brain. Consciousness has two components:

awareness and arousal. Awareness is manifest by goal-directed or purposeful behaviour. The use of language is an indication of functioning cerebral hemispheres. If the patient attempts to protect himself from a painful insult, this also implies cortical function. Arousal is a crude function that is simple wakefulness. Eye-opening, either spontaneous or in response to stimuli, is indicative of arousal and is a brainstem function. Coma is a pathological state in which both awareness and arousal are absent. Eye-opening does not occur, there is no comprehensible speech detected and the extremities move neither to command nor appropriately to noxious stimuli. By assessing all six components and making sure the four primary reflexes (ankle, knee, biceps and triceps) are assessed, and repeating this examination at frequent intervals, it is possible to both diagnose and monitor the neurological status in the ED. An improving neurological status reassures the physician that resuscitation is improving cerebral blood flow. Neurological deterioration is strong presumptive evidence of either a mass lesion or significant neurological injury. A CT scan of the head is the definitive test for head injury and should be done as soon as possible.

1.2.1.1.5 Environment

The clothes are to be removed in order to examine the whole patient. A logroll must be performed, especially after penetrating injuries, in order to identify all wounds. The patient is at risk of hypothermia, and warming measures should be promptly instituted.

The body temperature of trauma patients decreases rapidly, and if the 'on-scene time' has been prolonged, for example by entrapment, patients arrive in the resuscitation room hypothermic. This is aggravated by the administration of cold fluid, the presence of abdominal or chest wounds and the removal of clothing. Most patients will be expected to drop their core temperature by 1–2° C per hour unless protected. All fluids need to be at body temperature or above, and there are rapid infusor devices available that will warm fluids at high flow rates prior to infusion. Patients can be placed on warming mattresses and their environment kept warm using warm air blankets. Early measurement of the core temperature is important to prevent heat loss that will predispose to problems with coagulation. Hypothermia will shift the oxygen dissociation curve to the left, reduce oxygen delivery, reduce the liver's ability to metabolize citrate and lactic acid and may produce arrhythmias.

The minimum diagnostic studies that should be considered in the haemodynamically unstable patient after the primary survey include:

- Chest X-ray.
- Plain film of the pelvis.

Focussed Abdominal Sonar for Trauma (FAST) examination may be helpful:

- To assess whether there is blood in the chest or abdomen.
- To exclude cardiac tamponade.

It must be emphasized that resuscitation should not cease during these films, and the resuscitating team must wear protective lead aprons. Optimally, the X-ray facilities are juxtaposed to the ED but the essential X-rays can all be obtained with a portable machine.

1.2.1.2 SECONDARY SURVEY

Finally, if the patient stabilizes, a secondary survey and diagnostic studies are carried out. However, if the patient remains unstable, he or she should be taken immediately to the operating room in order to achieve surgical haemostasis, or to the surgical ICU.

The patient must have a full 'top-to-toe' and 'front-to-back' examination. If the patient has been haemodynamically unstable, the site of the bleeding is traditionally:

'Blood on the floor, and four more.'

- External bleeding ('blood on the floor').

  ... and four more.

- Bleeding into the chest (exclude by chest X-ray).
- Bleeding into the abdomen.
- Bleeding into the pelvis (exclude by clinical examination and pelvic X-ray).
- Bleeding into the extremities (exclude by clinical examination and long bone X-ray).

Investigation and assessment of the abdomen can be based on three groups:

- The patient with a normal abdomen.
- An equivocal group requiring further investigation.
- The patient with an obvious injury to the abdomen.

1.2.1.2.1 Haemodynamically Normal Patient

There is ample time for a full evaluation of the patient, and a decision can be made regarding surgery or non-operative management. Computed tomography (CT) scanning is currently the modality of choice.

1.2.1.2.2 Haemodynamically Stable Patient

The stable patient, who is not haemodynamically normal but who is maintaining blood pressure and other parameters with resuscitation, will benefit from investigations aimed at establishing:

- Has the patient bled into the abdomen?
- Has the bleeding stopped?

Thus, serial investigations of a quantitative nature will allow the best assessment of these patients. The CT scan is the modality of choice, provided awareness of the fact that the patient may decompensate.

1.2.1.2.3 Haemodynamically Unstable Patient

Efforts must be made to try to define the cavity where bleeding is taking place (e.g. chest, pelvis or abdominal cavity). Negative chest and pelvic X-rays leave the abdomen as the most likely source. Diagnostic modalities are of necessity limited. The FAST examination is effective for detecting free fluid in the abdomen and pericardium, but is operator dependent – haemodynamic instability caused by intraperitoneal haemorrhage is likely to be readily found but a negative FAST does not exclude intra-abdominal bleeding. Diagnostic peritoneal lavage (DPL) remains one of the most sensitive, cheapest and most readily available modalities to confirm the presence of blood in the abdomen. Importantly, DPL and FAST can be performed without moving the patient from the resuscitation area, since an unstable patient should not have a CT scan, even if it were to be readily available.

During resuscitation, standard ATLS guidelines should be followed. These should include:

- Nasogastric tube or orogastric tube.
- Urinary catheter.

1.2.2 Management of Penetrating Trauma

Many forces can act on the torso to cause injury to the outer protective layers or the contained viscera. Penetrating trauma is most often due to knives, missiles and impalement. Knife wounds and impalement usually involve low-velocity penetration, and mortality is directly related to the organ injured. Secondary effects such as infection are due to the nature of the weapon and the material (i.e. clothing and other foreign material) that the missile carries into the body tissue. Infection is also influenced by spillage of contents from an injury to a hollow viscous organ. In contrast, missile injuries can cause more extensive tissue destruction, related to the kinetic energy (KE) that is expressed as:

$$KE = \frac{1}{2} MV^2$$

where M is mass, and V is velocity.

Perhaps more appropriate is the concept of 'wounding energy' (WE), expressed as:

$$WE = \frac{1}{2} M (V_{EN} - V_{EX})^2$$

where M is mass, V_{EN} is velocity on entry and V_{EX} is velocity on exit.

Velocity is important in determining final kinetic energy. If the exit velocity is high, very little injury is imparted to the tissue. Thus, bullets are designed so that upon impact the missile expands or shatters, imparting all of its energy to the tissue. Other characteristics of the missile may contribute to tissue destruction, including yaw, tumble and pitch. It has been appreciated that tumbling may be particularly important in higher-velocity weapons (>800 m/s). Shotgun blasts can be the most devastating since almost all of the energy is imparted to the tissue.

An equally important component of the physical examination is to describe the penetrating wound. It is imperative that surgeons do not label the entrance or exit wounds unless common sense dictates it. An example is a patient with a single penetrating missile injury with no exit. However, in general, it is best to describe whether the wound is circular or ovoid and whether or not there is surrounding stippling (powder burn) or bruising from the muzzle of a weapon. Similarly, stab wounds should be described as longitudinal, triangular-shaped (hunting knives) or circular depending on the instrument used. Experience has shown that surgeons who describe wounds as entrance or exit may be wrong as often as 50 per cent of the time. Experience with forensic pathology is required to be more accurate.

It is good practice to place metallic objects such as paper clips on the skin pointing to the various wounds on the chest wall, which aid the surgeon in determining the missile track[2]. This also can be useful for stab wounds. Tracking the missile helps the surgeon to determine which visceral organs may be injured and, in particular, whether or not there is potential transgression of the diaphragm and/or mediastinum. It is

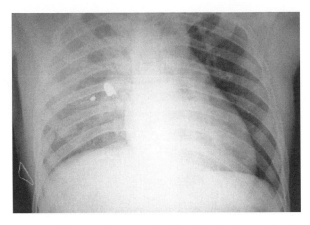

Figure 1.1 Chest X-ray in penetrating injury showing the use of a skin marker to show the wound track.

recommended that an 'unfolded' paper clip be placed on any anterior penetrating injury, and a 'folded' one on any posterior injury[17] (Figure 1.1).

1.3 EMERGENCY DEPARTMENT SURGERY

The emergency management of a critically injured trauma patient continues to be a substantial challenge. It is essential to have a very simple, effective plan that can be put into place to meet the challenges presented by resuscitating the moribund patient. The ATLS principles apply throughout.

As a basic consideration, for all major trauma victims with a systolic blood pressure of less than 90 mm Hg, there is a 50 per cent likelihood of death, which, in one-third of cases, will occur within the next 30 minutes if the bleeding has not been controlled. If death is likely to occur in the next 5 minutes, it is essential to determine in which body cavity the lethal event will occur, as the only chance of survival will be the immediate control of haemorrhage.

If death is likely to occur in the next hour, there is time to proceed with an orderly series of investigations and, time permitting, radiographic or other diagnostic aids, to determine precisely what is injured, and to effect an operative plan for the management of this life-threatening event.

1.3.1 **Craniofacial Injuries**

In the event of severe facial injuries (and often associated severe neck injuries) surgical control of the airway may be necessary, using ATLS described techniques.

It is unusual but possible to exsanguinate from a massive scalp laceration. For this reason, it is essential to gain control of the vascular scalp laceration with rapidly placed surgical clips or primary pressure and immediate suturing.

The more common cause of death is from intracranial mass lesions. Extradural haematomas and subdural haematomas can be rapidly lethal. A rapid diagnosis of an ipsilateral dilated pupil with contralateral hemiplegia is diagnostic of mass lesion with significant enough intracranial pressure to induce coning. This requires immediate decompression. Hyperventilation to produce hypocarbia, and vasoconstriction are no longer routinely employed. The use of mannitol is useful as a temporizing adjunct only.

Attention should be paid to monitoring the end-tidal carbon dioxide, as a proxy for $PaCO_2$, which should not be allowed to fall below 30 mm Hg (4 kPa). This should decrease intracranial volume, and therefore intracranial pressure. There should be an immediate positive effect that usually lasts long enough to obtain a three-cut CT scan to determine a specific site of the mass lesion and the type of haematoma. This will direct the surgeon specifically to the location of the craniotomy for removal of the haematoma.

Intravenous mannitol should be administered as a bolus injection in a dose of 0.5–1 g/kg. This should not delay any other diagnostic or therapeutic procedures.

1.3.2 **Chest Trauma**

Lethal injuries to the chest include tension pneumothorax, cardiac tamponade and transected aorta.

Tension pneumothorax is diagnosed clinically with deviation of the trachea away from the lesion (a late sign), hypertympany on the side of the lesion and decreased breath sounds on the affected side. There is usually associated elevated jugular venous pressure in the neck veins, unless the patient is hypovolaemic. This is a clinical diagnosis, and once made, an immediate needle thoracostomy or tube thoracostomy should be performed to relieve the tension pneumothorax. The tube should then be placed to underwater seal.

The diagnosis of cardiac tamponade is frequently difficult to make clinically. It is usually associated with hypotension and elevated jugular venous pressure. There are usually muffled heart sounds, but this is difficult to hear in a noisy resuscitation suite. Placing a central line with resultant high venous pressures can confirm the diagnosis. If ultrasound is available, this is a helpful diagnostic adjunct. Once the diagnosis is made, the tamponade needs to be relieved if the patient is hypotensive. In the event of a penetrating injury to the heart or blunt rupture of the heart, there is usually a substantial clot in the pericardium. A needle pericardiocentesis may be able to aspirate a few millilitres of blood, and this, along with rapid volume resuscitation to increase preload, can buy enough time to move to the operating room. However, needle pericardiocentesis is unreliable diagnostically and may itself lacerate the ventricle.

It is far better to perform a thoracotomy in the operating room, either through an anterolateral approach or a median sternotomy, with good light and assistance and the potential for autotransfusion and potential bypass, than it is to attempt heroic emergency surgery in the resuscitation suite. However, if the patient is in extremis with blood pressure in the 40 mm Hg or lower range despite volume resuscitation, there is no choice but to proceed immediately with a left anterior thoracotomy in an attempt to relieve the tamponade and control the penetrating injury to the heart. If there is an obvious penetrating injury to either the left or the right ventricle, a Foley catheter can be introduced into the hole and the balloon distended to create tamponade. The end of the Foley should be clamped. Great care should be taken to apply minimal traction on the Foley – just enough to allow sealing. Excessive traction will pull the catheter out and extend the wound by tearing the muscle. Once the bleeding is controlled, the wound can be easily sutured with pledgetted sutures.

Massive haemorrhage from intercostal vessels secondary to multiple rib fractures will frequently stop without operative intervention. This is also true for most bleeding from the lung. It is helpful to collect the shed blood from the hemithorax into an autotransfusion collecting device and return it to the patient.

Aortic transection is usually diagnosed with a widened mediastinum and confirmed with an arteriogram or a CT scan (see Chapter 7). Once the diagnosis has been made, it is useful to maintain control of hypotension in the 100 mm Hg range so as not to precipitate free rupture from the transection, until stenting or operative repair can take place.

Note that abdominal injury generally takes priority over thoracic aortic injury.

1.3.3 **Abdominal Trauma**

Significant intra-abdominal or retroperitoneal haemorrhage can be a reason to go rapidly to the operating room. The abdomen may be distended and dull to percussion. A definitive diagnosis can be made with a grossly positive DPL, ultrasound or CT scan. The decision to operate for bleeding should be based on the haemodynamic status.

Ultrasound (FAST) is a useful tool as it is specific for blood in the peritoneum, but it is operator dependent. A positive FAST result in an unstable patient is an indication for laparotomy. Conversely, a negative FAST result does not exclude intra-abdominal bleeding, and repeat FAST or other investigations need to be considered.

The DPL is easy to perform and gives a highly sensitive but non-specific answer immediately. A volume of 10 mL of grossly positive blood on initial aspiration of the DPL catheter, or a cell count in the lavage fluid of over 10^5 red cells per cubic millimetre mandates immediate laparotomy in the haemodynamically unstable patient. Because of its high sensitivity, a negative DPL excludes the presence of significant blood in the abdominal cavity.

Non-operative management has become the treatment of choice in haemodynamically stable patients with liver and spleen injuries regardless of injury grade (also see the sections on the individual organ systems).

The CT scanner is highly sensitive and very specific for the type, character and severity of injury to a specific organ. However, patients whose condition is unstable should *not* be considered.

1.3.4 **Pelvic Trauma**

Pelvic fractures can be a significant cause of haemorrhage and death. It is essential to return the pelvis to its original configuration as swiftly as possible. As an emergency procedure, a compressing sheet or commercially available pelvic binders can be used. There are also external fixation devices such as the C-clamp and the external fixator, which can be placed in the resuscitation suite and return the pelvis to its normal anatomy. However, their fixation may be time-consuming, requires skill and may not present advantages over the non-invasive binders for initial management. As the pelvis is realigned, it

helps to compress the haematoma in the pelvis. Since approximately 85 per cent of pelvic bleeding is venous, compressing the haematoma usually stops the majority of pelvic bleeding.

If the patient continues to be hypotensive, resuscitation should continue, and an angiogram should be considered. This will identify the presence of significant arterial bleeding in the pelvis, which then can be embolized immediately. If the patient is exsanguinating from the pelvic injury or is haemodynamically unstable, damage control surgery should be performed with extraperitoneal packing of the pelvis combined with a laparotomy before angiography.

1.3.5 **Long Bone Fractures**

Lone bone fractures, particularly of the femur, can bleed significantly. The damage control approach to fractures is external fixation. The immediate treatment for a patient who is hypotensive from haemorrhage from a femoral fracture is to put traction on the distal limb, pulling the femur into alignment. This not only realigns the bones but also reconfigures the cylindrical nature of the thigh. This has an immediate tamponading effect on the bleeding in the muscles of the thigh. It is frequently necessary to maintain traction with a Thomas or Hare traction splint. Attention should be paid to the distal pulses to be sure that there is continued arterial inflow. If the pulses are absent, an arteriogram should be performed to determine whether there are any injuries to major vascular structures. A determination is then made as to the timing of arterial repair and bony fixation. Re-establishing perfusion to the limb takes priority over fracture treatment.

1.3.6 **Peripheral Vascular Injuries**

Peripheral vascular injuries are not in themselves life threatening providing that the bleeding is controlled. However, it is critical to assess whether ischaemia and vascular continuity are present, since this will influence the overall planning.

Every ED should have access to a simple flow Doppler monitor to assess pressures and flow. If there is any doubt over whether the vessel is patent, the ankle-brachial index should be measured, and if it is less than 0.9, an arteriogram is mandatory. Time and availability decide whether the patient can be transported to an angiography suite or should have an angiogram performed in the operating room or ED. Although it is desirable to do this in the angiography suite, that is not always possible, and the necessary equipment may not be available. If there is any doubt, consideration should be given to the use of the ED angiogram[18].

1.4 SUMMARY

The decision of whether to operate in the ED or in the operating room should be made based on an overview of the urgency and the predicted outcome.

It is useful to have a well-thought-out plan for dealing with the critically injured trauma patient so that both clinical diagnosis and relevant investigations can be performed immediately and an operative or non-operative therapeutic approach implemented.

There is no future in altering only the geographical site of death.

REFERENCES AND RECOMMENDED READING

References

1. Committee on Trauma. *Resources for Optimal Care of the Injured Patient 2014.* 6th ed, Chicago, IL: American College of Surgeons (Orange Book), 2014. http://www.facs.org. Accessed December 2014.
2. Coimbra R, Hoyt DB, Bansal V. Trauma systems, triage and transport. In: Mattox KL, Moore EE, Feliciano DV, eds. *Trauma.* 7th ed. New York, NY: McGraw-Hill; 2013:54–76.
3. Baker SP, O'Neill B, Haddon W, Long WB. The Injury Severity Score: a method for describing patients with multiple injuries and evaluating emergency care. *J Trauma.* 1974;14:187–196.
4. American Association for the Advancement of Automotive Medicine. *The Abbreviated Injury Scale: 2005 Revision.* Barrington, IL: American Association for the Advancement of Automotive Medicine; 2005 Update 2008. http://www.AAAM.org. Accessed January 2015.
5. Trunkey DD. Trauma. *Sci Am.* 1983;249:28–35.
6. American College of Surgeons. *Advanced Trauma Life Support Course for Doctors: Student Course Manual.* 8th ed. Chicago, IL: American College of Surgeons; 2008.
7. Jacobs LM, Berrizbeitia LD, Bennett B, Madigan C. Endotracheal intubation in the prehospital phase of emergency medical care. *JAMA.* 1983;250:2175–2177.
8. Taryle DA, Chandler JE, Good JT, Potts DE, Sahn SA. Emergency room intubations – complications and survival. *Chest.* 1979;75:541–543.
9. Baker CC, Thomas AN, Trunkey DD. The role of emergency room thoracotomy in trauma. *J Trauma.* 1980;20:848–855.
10. Thomas AN, Stephens BG. Air embolism: a cause of morbidity and death after penetrating chest trauma. *J Trauma.* 1974;14:633–638.
11. Yee ES, Verrier ED, Thomas AN. Management of air embolism in blunt and penetrating trauma. *J Thorac Cardiovasc Surg.* 1983;85:661–668.
12. Olsen WR, Hildreth DH. Abdominal paracentesis and peritoneal lavage in blunt abdominal trauma. *J Trauma.* 1971;11:824–829.
13. Bivens BA, Sachatello CR, Daugherty ME, Ernst CB, Griffen WD. Diagnostic peritoneal lavage is superior to clinical evaluation in blunt abdominal trauma. *Am Surg.* 1978;44:637–641.
14. Loong ED, Law PR, Healey JN. Fresh blood by direct transfusion for haemostatic failure in massive haemorrhage. *Anaesth Intensive Care.* 1981;9:371–375.
15. Shapiro M. Blood transfusion practice: facts and fallacies. *S Afr Med J.* 1976;50:105–109.
16. Bickell WH. Immediate versus delayed fluid resuscitation for hypotensive patients with penetrating torso injuries. *New Engl J Med.* 1994;331:1105–1108.
17. Brooks A, Bowley DMG, Boffard KD. Bullet markers – a simple technique to assist in the evaluation of penetrating trauma. *J R Army Med Corps.* 2002;148:259–261.
18. MacFarlane C, Saadia R, Boffard KD. Emergency room arteriography: a useful technique in the assessment of peripheral vascular injuries. *J Roy Coll Surg Edin.* 1989;34:310–313.

Recommended Reading

American College of Surgeons. *Advanced Trauma Life Support Course for Doctors: Student Course Manual*, 9th ed. Chicago, IL: American College of Surgeons, 2014.

Jacobs LM, ed. *Advanced Trauma Operative Management.* Chicago/Woodbury, CT: American College of Surgeons/ Ciné-Med Publishing, 2010.

American College of Surgeons. Committee on Trauma. *Resources for Optimal Care of the Injured Patient 2015*, 6th ed. Chicago, IL: American College of Surgeons (Orange Book), 2015. http://www.facs.org. Accessed December 2014.

Communication and Non-technical Skills in Major Trauma **2**

The Role of Crew Resource Management (CRM)

2.1 OVERVIEW

The recognition that human factors, and not mechanical failure, were a recurring theme in many aviation disasters (65 per cent) led to the obligatory training in crew resource management. This is a concept in which effective use is made of all available resources needed to complete a safe and efficient operation.

Other high-risk industries subsequently followed suit, and 30 years ago the medical community started applying this knowledge of crew resource management (CRM) in the training for critical clinical situations. The subsequent years have seen implementation in numerous surgical subspecialties, of which the setting of traumatology has been no exception, and trauma team training based upon the principles of CRM has become an integral part of daily practice in trauma centres worldwide.

What makes trauma care so special is that the decision making has to be done and the interventions have to be executed in a very condensed time period (i.e. minutes or even seconds compared to hours and even days/weeks in other less urgent forms of surgery). This underlines the need for teamwork based on the correct non-technical skills and CRM.

The principles of CRM are built upon a concept of training in human factors with the aim of optimizing communication dynamics in the setting of the multidisciplinary team. The ultimate goal of training is to reduce the occurrence of medical errors, and improve decision making and outcome in trauma care.

The most important aspects of CRM include:

* Having situational awareness.
* Preparing and planning.
* Calling for help early.
* Having effective leadership.

* Allocating attention wisely and using all available resources
* Prioritizing and distributing the workload
* Communicating effectively

It is self-explanatory that when training these principles of CRM the participation of the whole trauma team is mandatory.

2.2 COMMUNICATION IN THE TRAUMA SETTING

The complex task of managing a severely injured trauma patient arriving in the hospital requires both highly specialized surgical and medical skills as well as an ability to master the core concepts of CRM.

In order for damage control surgery and resuscitation to be effective there needs to be open communication between all members of the trauma team. At the centre of this process are the surgeon and the anaesthetist, who in collaboration have the responsibility of prioritizing interventions and management. The team leader, be it a surgeon or an anaesthetist, must keep the entire team aware and involved in the management of a patient whose physiology and subsequent treatment plans are under constant evolution. The deliverance of optimal care in a trauma patient undergoing damage control surgery is a complex process whereby a group of individuals need to function as a unit with all members being heard (listened to) and their individual skills utilized to deliver the most appropriate medical care.

Human factors are vital to the timely assessment and treatment of the complex trauma patient. In the stressful and sometimes highly charged environment of the trauma bay or in theatre, surgeons and anaesthetists can be tempted to focus on immediate tasks with the potential of developing what is commonly termed 'tunnel vision'. This can lead to a situation where management of and focus on single problems are prioritized instead of addressing the patient's problems as a whole hereby leading to loss of control of the situation. The loss of situation or team awareness described above and the evolution of fixation errors may prove fatal to the outcome of the severely injured trauma patient. In trauma care, as in other disciplines, inadequate communication, poor teamwork and lack of leadership have been shown to have a profound impact on patient outcome.

2.3 LEADERSHIP IN TRAUMA CARE

Leadership is key to the management of trauma. A good team leader should possess the ability to make quick decisions under pressure, based on all available information; maintain an overview; plan and execute treatment strategies; and perform regular reviews of the patient's response to treatment. Communication should be performed concisely and be unambiguous, but at the same time the team leader should be open and responsive to the input from all team members. There are several ways of describing successful leadership; one is the Non-Technical Skills for Surgeons (NOTSS) taxonomy identified by University of Aberdeen Industrial Psychology Research, Scotland, and the Royal College of Surgeons

Table 2.1 Non-Technical Skills for Surgeons (NOTSS) Taxonomy

Category	Element
Situation awareness	Gathering information
	Understanding information
	Projecting and anticipating future state
Decision making	Considering options
	Selecting and communicating option
	Implementing and reviewing decisions
Task management	Planning and preparation
	Having flexibility/responding to change
Leadership	Setting and maintaining standards
	Supporting others
	Coping with pressure
Communication and teamwork	Exchanging information
	Establishing a shared understanding
	Coordinating team activities

of Edinburgh, United Kingdom (Table 2.1)[1]. The NOTSS can also be used for behavioural scoring and research.

The aforementioned non-technical skills are not learned from a textbook; they are acquired and reinforced through training in simulated environments with professional instructors who have expertise in both the principles of CRM as well as briefing and debriefing. These skills should then be honed in daily practice.

2.4 COMMUNICATION IN DAMAGE CONTROL

Communication in damage control surgery and during resuscitation efforts, from an operational perspective, can be described in four phases (Table 2.2).

The critical decision-making process is typically started in the emergency department/trauma bay on arrival, and the surgeon together with anaesthetist agree on, and plan for, damage control surgery and resuscitation. At this early start, evaluation of futility of care is also a legitimate consideration.

In the operating room, or shortly before the commencement of surgery, the surgeon states the surgical plan based on the clinical and imaging findings (if present). The anaesthesiologist states the transfusion status, the presence of coagulopathy and any other evolving conditions that should be taken into account. During the damage control surgery and resuscitation re-evaluation is performed every 10 minutes for the entire trauma or theatre team in order to maintain team situational awareness and allow effective anticipation and planning of all aspects of the care of the patient. In the re-evaluation the surgeon states the surgical progress, developing problems and future intentions while the anaesthetist reports the elapsed time, transfusion status, developing coagulopathy, lactate levels, temperature and other relevant developing problems.

Upon completion of surgery, the anaesthetist and surgeon recapitulate the patient's condition and the procedures performed and agree on the plan for the following 24–48 hours. They are responsible for ensuring transfer of relevant information internally in the team and externally with collaborators such as blood bank, ICU, etc. The trauma leader plans the tertiary survey within the following 24 hours.

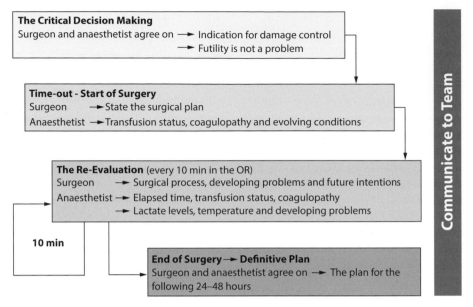

Figure 2.1 Communication in Damage Control

REFERENCES AND RECOMMENDED READING

Reference

1. Non-Technical Skills for Surgeons (NOTSS). *Royal College of Surgeons of Edinburgh*. 2015. http://www.rcsed.ac.uk/education/patient-safety-and-notss/notss.aspx. Accessed January 2015.

Recommended Reading

Arul GS, Pugh HE, Mercer SJ, Midwinter MJ. Optimising communication in the damage control resuscitation: damage control surgery sequence in major trauma management. *J Roy Army Med Corps*. 2012;158(2):82–84.

Catchpole K, Ley E, Wiegmann D, et al. A human factors subsystems approach to trauma care. *JAMA Surg*. 2014;149(9):962–969.

Doumouras AG, Keshet I, Nathens AB, Ahmed N, Hicks CM. Trauma non-technical training (TNT-2): the development, piloting and multilevel assessment of a simulation-based, interprofessional curriculum for team-based trauma resuscitation. *Can J Surg*. 2014;57(5):354–355.

Hughes KM, Benenson RS, Kritchten AE, Clancy KD, Ryan JP, Hammod C. A crew resource management program tailored to trauma resuscitation improves team behaviour and communication. *J Am Coll Surg*. 2014;219:545–551.

McCulloch P, Rathbone J, Cathcpole K. Interventions to improve teamwork and communications among health care staff. *Br J Surg*. 2011;98:469–479.

Yule S, Flin R, Paterson-Brown S, Maran N, Rowley D. Development of a rating system for surgeons' non-technical skills. *Med Educ*. 2006;40:1098–1104.

Ziesmann MT, Widder S, Park J, et al. S.T.A.R.T.T.: development of a national, multidisciplinary trauma crisis resource management curriculum—results from the pilot course. *J Trauma Acute Care Surg*. 2013;75(5):753–758.

Part 2

Physiology and the body's response to trauma

Resuscitation Physiology **3**

3.1 METABOLIC RESPONSE TO TRAUMA

3.1.1 Definition of Trauma

Physical injury is accompanied by systemic as well as local effects. Further stress will initiate the metabolic response to trauma. Following trauma, the body responds locally by inflammation and by a general response which is protective, and which conserves fluid and provides energy for repair. Proper resuscitation may attenuate the response but will not abolish it.

The response is characterized by an acute catabolic reaction, which precedes the metabolic process of recovery and repair. This metabolic response to trauma traditionally was divided into an ebb and flow phase by Cuthbertson in 1932[1].

The ebb phase is relatively short-lived and corresponds to the period of severe shock characterized by depression of enzymatic activity and oxygen consumption.

After effective resuscitation has been accomplished with restoration of adequate oxygen transport, the flow phase comes into play. The flow phase can be divided into two phases:

- A catabolic phase with fat and protein mobilisation associated with increased urinary nitrogen excretion and weight loss.
- An anabolic phase with restoration of fat and protein stores, and weight gain.

The appropriate protective flow phase is characterized by:

- A normal or slightly elevated blood glucose level.
- Increased glucose production.
- Normal or slightly elevated free fatty acid levels, with increased flux.
- A normal or elevated insulin concentration.
- High normal or elevated levels of catecholamine and an elevated glucagon level.

- A normal blood lactate level.
- Elevated oxygen consumption.
- Increased cardiac output.
- Elevated core temperature.

These responses are marked by hyperdynamic circulatory changes, signs of inflammation, glucose intolerance and muscle wasting.

3.1.2 Initiating Factors

The magnitude of the metabolic response depends on the degree of trauma and concomitant contributory factors such as infection, tissue necrosis and pre-existing systemic disease. The response will also depend on the age and sex of the patient, the genetic composition, the underlying nutritional state and the timing of treatment and its effectiveness. In general, the more severe the injury (i.e. the greater the degree of tissue damage), the greater will be the metabolic response.

The metabolic response alterations seem to be less aggressive in children and the elderly and in the premenopausal female. Starvation and nutritional depletion also modify the response. Patients with poor nutritional or immunological status (e.g. those with human immunodeficiency virus [HIV]) have a reduced metabolic response to trauma compared to well-nourished patients, while burns and severe traumatic brain injury cause a relatively greater response than other mechanical injuries.

Wherever possible, efforts should be made to reduce the magnitude and duration of the initial insult, since by doing so it may be possible to reduce the extent of the metabolic changes. Thus, aggressive resuscitation, control of pain and temperature, limiting of acidosis, adequate devitalized tissue débridement, avoidance of unnecessary blood component administration with coagulopathy and nutritional (preferably enteral) support are critical.

The precipitating factors can be broadly divided into the following.

3.1.2.1 HYPOVOLAEMIA

- Decrease in circulating blood volume.
- Increase in alimentary loss of fluid.
- Loss of interstitial volume.
- Extracellular fluid shift.

3.1.2.2 AFFERENT IMPULSES

- Somatic.
- Autonomic.
- Sympathetic ↑.
- Cholinergic ↓.

3.1.2.3 WOUND FACTORS: INFLAMMATORY AND CELLULAR

- Neutrophils – superoxide, elastase.
- Platelets – PF4.
- Macrophages/dendritic cells.
- Endothelial cells.
- Cytokines – interleukins IL1, IL2, IL6, IL10, IL-17, TNF.
- Chemokines – IL8.
- Eicosanoids – LTB4, LTC4, TXA_2, PGE_2.
- Damage associated molecular patterns (DAMPs), $HMGB_1$, HSP_{70}.

3.1.2.4 TOXINS/SEPSIS

- Endotoxins.
- Exotoxins.

3.1.2.5 FREE RADICALS

- Superoxide and derivatives.
- Nitrogen radicals.

3.1.2.6 HYPOVOLAEMIA

Hypovolaemia, specifically tissue hypoperfusion, is the most potent precipitator of the metabolic response. Hypovolaemia can be due to external losses, internal shifts of extracellular fluids and changes in plasma osmolality. However, the most common cause is blood loss. (See Section 3.2.)

The hypovolaemia will stimulate release of catecholamines, which in turn trigger the neuroendocrine response. This plays an important role in volume and electrolyte conservation and protein, fat and carbohydrate catabolism.

3.1.2.7 AFFERENT IMPULSES

Hormonal responses are initiated by pain and anxiety. The metabolic response may be modified by administration of adequate analgesia, which may be parenteral, enteral, regional or local. Somatic blockade may need to be accompanied by autonomic blockade, in order to minimize or abolish the metabolic response.

3.1.2.8 WOUND FACTORS

Endogenous factors may prolong or even exacerbate the systemic trauma insult, despite the fact that the primary cause is treated well. Tissue injury activates a diverse response via release of DAMPs activating toll-like receptors (TLRs), and by release of multiple inflammatory mediators locally at the site of injury and/or infection through two predominant pathways:

- Humoral.
- Cellular.

Uncontrolled activation of endogenous inflammatory mediators and cells may contribute to a syndrome called the systemic inflammatory response syndrome (SIRS). The end result of an excessive SIRS response is diffuse bystander organ injury.

Both humoral- and cell-derived activation products play a role in the pathophysiology of organ dysfunction[2]. It is important, therefore, to monitor post-traumatic biochemical and immunological abnormalities whenever possible as possible guides to direct and confirm the appropriateness of resuscitative interventions.

3.1.3 Immune Response

The immune response is complex and consists of an early enhanced upregulation of the primarily proinflammatory innate system and a concomitant prolonged suppression of the adaptive immune system. The magnitude of these responses is modified by the depth and duration of insult caused by the injury, as well as the patient's genetic composition and pre-existing co-morbidities.

3.1.3.1 INFLAMMATORY PATHWAY

The inflammatory mediators of injury have been implicated in the induction of numerous cellular dysfunctions. While neutrophils have been invoked as primary mediators of inflammatory processes for more than

100 years, we now recognize that these initial responses involve numerous cellular mediators including platelets, macrophages, endothelium and epithelium.

3.1.3.1.1 Cytokines

The term *cytokine* refers to a diverse group of polypeptides and glycoproteins that are important mediators of inflammation. They are produced by a variety of cell types, but predominantly by leucocytes. Cytokines are generally divided into pro-inflammatory, and anti-inflammatory, but some have both properties (e.g. IL-6). Discussion of cytokines is further complicated by confusing nomenclature. Many cytokines were found in different settings (e.g. tumour necrosis factor [TNF], originally termed *cachectin*). Current nomenclature follows a more consistent system. The term *interleukin* (IL) refers to a substance that acts between leucocytes, and is used in conjunction with a number (e.g. IL-6).

3.1.3.1.2 Pro-Inflammatory Cytokines

Certain cytokines, particularly TNF, IL-1 and IL-8, promote the inflammatory response by up-regulating expression of genes that generate the pro-inflammatory mediators. Pro-inflammatory cytokines also mediate inflammation by activating neutrophils, endothelium and epithelium – all of which lead to tissue damage.

The TNF and IL-1 act synergistically to produce the acute innate immune response to ischaemia/reperfusion in many organs. The TNF causes neutrophils to be attracted to injured epithelium, thereby helping to regulate the inflammatory response. It also stimulates endothelial cells to produce a cytokine subset known as chemokines (e.g. IL-8), which produce leukocyte migration into the tissues and IL-1 production. Like TNF, IL-1 is a primary responder in the inflammatory cascade, and its actions are similar to TNF, but it does not induce apoptosis or programmed cell death.

Interferon gamma (IFN-γ) is produced in response to antigens processed by macrophages, an event enhanced by IL-12. The IL-12 is produced by mononuclear phagocytes and dendritic cells in response to intracellular microbes. The IL-6 is produced by mononuclear phagocytes, endothelial cells and fibroblasts, and acts in a pro-inflammatory manner by providing a potent stimulus for hepatocyte synthesis of acute phase proteins.

The IL-2, unlike the above cytokines which exert most of their influence via the innate immune system, stimulates acquired immunity, and has other immunomodulatory functions as well.

3.1.3.1.3 Anti-inflammatory Cytokines

The anti-inflammatory cytokines exert their effects by inhibiting the production of pro-inflammatory cytokines, or countering their action. They reduce gene expression, and mitigate or prevent numerous inflammatory effects.

The IL-10 is important in the control of innate immunity. It can prevent fever, pro-inflammatory cytokine release and clotting cascade activation during endotoxin challenge. Other potent anti-inflammatory modulators include IL-4, IL-13 and transforming growth factor beta (TGF-β).

3.1.3.1.4 Modulation of Cytokine Activity in Sepsis, the Systemic Inflammatory Response Syndrome (SIRS), and Compensatory Inflammatory Response Syndrome (CARS)

Systemic inflammatory activity, which occurs in response to infectious or non-infectious stimuli, is the fundamental overall clinical phenomenon that can provoke whole body Systemic Inflammatory Response Syndrome (SIRS) and can lead ultimately to Multiple Organ Dysfunction Syndrome (MODS) and Multiple Organ Failure (MOF), which is associated with a mortality of up to 50 per cent. It was initially suggested that SIRS and sepsis were attributable to an overwhelming pro-inflammatory innate immune response, mediated by TNF and numerous other cytokines. However, simultaneously, the body also mounts an endogenous counter- or anti-inflammatory reaction in an attempt to restore homeostasis, which can then lead to Compensatory Inflammatory Response Syndrome (CARS). Early, after severe injury or sepsis, the pro-inflammatory response predominates and SIRS and shock result. If the counter-inflammatory response leads to homeostasis the patient does well and recovers. However, if the suppressive response is excessive, it leads to immunosuppression, and greatly increased susceptibility to nosocomial infections that are frequently seen in the severely injured and critically ill patients. The modern view is that, following injury, SIRS and CARS are activated simultaneously.

It is clear that the role of cytokines in sepsis is critical to outcomes and very complex, with both pro-inflammatory and anti-inflammatory factors playing a role, and determining clinical outcome.

3.1.3.1.5 Activated Protein C (Xigris)

Pro-inflammatory mediators have a role in triggering the clotting cascade by stimulating the release of tissue factor from monocytes and the vascular endothelium leading to thrombin formation and a fibrin clot. At the same time thrombin stimulates many inflammatory pathways and suppresses natural anticoagulant responses by activating thrombin-activatable fibrinolysis inhibitor (TAFI). This overall procoagulant response leads to microvascular thrombosis and is implicated in the multiple organ failure associated with sepsis. On the other hand, thrombin binding to endothelial thrombomodulin, generates activated protein C (APC), which is an endogenous anticoagulant. However, previous reports of benefit to providing exogenous APC in the setting of sepsis have subsequently been shown to provide no improvement in survival. While the concepts involved are no doubt important, our ability to appropriately modify their activity to benefit the critically ill patient remains elusive.

3.1.3.1.6 Eicosanoids

These compounds, derived from eicosapolyenoic fatty acids, are subdivided into prostanoids (the precursors of the prostaglandins), and leucotrienes (LT). Eicosanoids are synthesized from arachidonic acid (AA), which has been synthesized from phospholipids of cell walls, by the action of phospholipase A2 (in part, released by activated neutrophils). Cyclo-oxygenase converts arachidonic acid to prostanoids, the precursors of prostaglandins (PG), prostacyclins (PGI) and thromboxanes (TX). The term prostaglandins is used loosely to include all prostanoids. The leucotrienes are produced by the action of 5-lipoxygenase on AA with subsequent by-products produced by LTA4 hydrolase (i.e. LTB4 and LTC4 synthase). Eicosanoids modulate blood flow to organs and tissues by altering local balances between vasodilators and vasoconstricting mediators, and, in addition, directly stimulate certain immune cells.

The prostanoids (prostaglandins of the E and F series), PGI_2 and TX cause not only vasoconstriction (TXA_2 and PGF_1), but also vasodilatation (PGI_2, PGE_1 and PGE_2). The TXA_2 activates and aggregates platelets and white cells, and PGI_2 and PGE_1 inhibit white cells and platelets. The leukotriene LTB4 is a very potent PMN chemo-attractant and activator, while LTC4 causes vasoconstriction, increased capillary permeability and bronchoconstriction.

3.1.3.2 CELLULAR PATHWAY

The classical pathway of complement activation involves an interaction between the specific antibody and the initial trimer of complement components C^1, C^4 and C^2. In the classical pathway, this interaction then cleaves the complement products C^3 and C^5, via proteolysis to produce the very powerful chemotactic factors C^{3a} and C^{5a}.

The so-called alternative pathway appears to be primarily involved following trauma. It is activated by properdin, and proteins D or B, to activate C^3 convertase, which generates the anaphylotoxins C^{3a} and C^{5a}. Its activation appears to be the earliest trigger for activating the innate immune cellular system, and is responsible for aggregation of neutrophils and activation of basophils, mast cells and platelets to secrete histamine and serotonin, which alter vascular permeability and are vasoactive. In trauma patients, the serum C^3 level is inversely correlated with the injury severity score (ISS)[3]. Measurement of C^{3a} is the most useful because the other products are more rapidly cleared from the circulation.

The short-lived fragments of the complement cascade, C^{3a} and C^{5a}, stimulate macrophages to secrete interleukin-1 (IL-1) and proteolysis inducing factor (PIF), an active circulating cleavage product. These mediators cause proteolysis and lipolysis along with fever. The IL-1 activates T_4 helper cells to produce IL-2, which enhances the adaptive cell-mediated immunity. Also, IL-1 and PIF are potent stimulators of the liver, bone marrow, spleen and lymph nodes to produce acute-phase proteins, including complement, fibrinogen, α2-macroglobulin and other proteins required for immune defence mechanisms.

There is also considerable cross-talk between the clotting cascade and inflammation. For example, activation of factor XII (Hageman Factor A) stimulates kallikrein to produce bradykinin from bradykininogen, which affects capillary permeability and vaso-reactivity. Overall, the overlapping combination of these reactions causes the systemic inflammatory response. Kallikrein can activate plasmin to promote fibrinolysis

3.1.3.3 TOXINS

Endotoxin is a lipopolysaccharide component of bacterial cell walls. Endotoxin and other bacterial and viral cell wall components are known to activate many immune cells, along with hepatocytes and myocardiocytes primarily via the TLR receptors. Activated cells release tumour necrosis factor (TNF) and a broad spectrum of potent mediators from macrophages. neutrophils, endothelial cells and many others. Endotoxins cause vascular margination and sequestration of leucocytes, particularly in the capillary bed. At high doses, direct granulocyte destruction is seen.

3.1.3.4 PAMPS AND DAMPS

Injury causes a systemic inflammatory response syndrome (SIRS) clinically much like sepsis. Multicellular animals detect pathogens via a set of pattern recognition receptors (TLRs), which recognize pathogen-associated molecular patterns (PAMPs), which in turn activate innate immunocytes. Evidence is accumulating that trauma and its associated tissue damage are recognized at the cell level by a similar cell receptor-mediated detection of intracellular products released by injured and dying cells. The term 'alarmin' has been used to categorize these endogenous damage associated molecular patterns (DAMPs) that signal tissue and cell damage[4]. A major source of DAMPs is injury-induced release of mitochondrial products, including mitochondrial DNA, coined the 'enemies within'. Endogenous DAMPs and exogenous PAMPS therefore convey a similar message and elicit similar responses. Surgical source control, whether for infection or necrotic tissue, is an attempt to minimize the host exposure to these toxic moieties.

3.1.3.5 FREE RADICALS

Oxygen radical (O_2^-) formation by white cells is a normal host defence mechanism. Diffuse activation after severe injury, however, may lead to excessive production by neutrophils and macrophages, with deleterious cellular effects on diffuse organ function. Nitric oxide (NO) is released by macrophages and endothelial cells, causing vasodilatation and decreased systemic vascular resistance. The NO also combines with O_2^- to form a potent oxidizing agent. Toxic hydroxyl ion (OH^-) and hydrogen peroxide are also increased following sepsis or stress. Protective endogenous antioxidants are rapidly depleted following injury or sepsis leading to an even more enhanced cellular bystander injury.

3.1.4 Hormonal Mediators

In response to trauma, many circulatory hormones are altered. Adrenaline (epinephrine), noradrenaline (norepinephrine), cortisol and glucagon are increased, while certain others are decreased. The sympathetic-adrenal axis is a major system by which the body's response to injury is activated.

3.1.4.1 HYPOTHALAMUS/PITUITARY

The hypothalamus is the highest level of integration of the stress response. The major efferent pathways of the hypothalamus are endocrine via the pituitary, and the efferent sympathetic and parasympathetic systems. In contrast, the cholinergic system is now recognized to have a variety of anti-inflammatory effects. The pituitary gland responds to trauma with increased levels of adrenocorticotrophic hormone (ACTH), prolactin and growth hormone, while the remaining hormones are relatively unchanged.

Pain receptors, osmoreceptors, baroreceptors and chemoreceptors stimulate or inhibit ganglia in the hypothalamus to induce sympathetic nerve activity. The neural endplates and adrenal medulla secrete catecholamines. Pain stimuli via the pain receptors also stimulate secretion of endogenous opiates, β-endorphin and pro-opiomelanocortin (precursor of the ACTH molecule), which modifies the response to pain and reinforces the catecholamine effects. The β-endorphin has little effect, but serves as a marker for anterior pituitary secretion.

Hypotension, hypovolaemia in the form of a decrease in left ventricular pressure and hyponatraemia stimulate secretion of vasopressin, antidiuretic hormone (ADH) from the supra-optic nuclei in the anterior hypothalamus, aldosterone from the adrenal cortex and renin from the juxtaglomerular apparatus of the kidney. The increase in aldosterone secretion results in conservation of sodium, and, thereby, water. As osmolality increases, the secretion of ADH increases, and more water is reabsorbed, thereby decreasing the serum osmolality (negative feedback control system).

Hypovolaemia stimulates receptors in the right atrium, and hypotension stimulates receptors in the carotid artery. This results in activation of paraventricular hypothalamic nuclei, which secrete pituitary releasing hormone from the median eminence into capillary blood, which stimulates the anterior pituitary to secrete adrenocorticotrophin (ACTH). Then ACTH stimulates the adrenal cortex to secrete cortisol and aldosterone. Changes in glucose concentration influence the release of insulin from the β cells of the pancreas, and high amino-acid levels, the release of glucagon from the α cells.

3.1.4.2 ADRENAL HORMONES

Plasma cortisol and glucagon levels rise following trauma. The degree is related to the severity of injury. The function of glucocorticoid secretion in the initial metabolic response is uncertain, since the hormones have little direct action, and primarily they seem to augment the effects of other hormones such as the catecholamines.

With passage into the later phases after injury, a number of metabolic effects take place. Glucocorticoids exert catabolic effects such as gluconeogenesis, lipolysis and amino acid breakdown from muscle. Catecholamines also participate in these effects by mediating insulin and glucose release and the mobilisation of fat.

3.1.4.3 PANCREATIC HORMONES

There is a rise in the blood sugar following trauma. The insulin response to glucose is reduced substantially with alpha-adrenergic stimulation, and enhanced with beta-adrenergic stimulation[6].

3.1.4.4 RENAL HORMONES

Aldosterone secretion is increased by several mechanisms. The renin-angiotensin mechanism is the most important. When the glomerular arteriolar inflow pressure falls, the juxtaglomerular apparatus of the kidney secretes renin, which acts with angiotensinogen to form angiotensin I. This is converted to angiotensin II, a substance that stimulates production of aldosterone by the adrenal cortex. Reduction in sodium concentration stimulates the macula densa, a specialized area in the tubular epithelium adjacent to the juxtaglomerular apparatus, to activate renin release. An increase in plasma potassium concentration also stimulates aldosterone release. Volume losses and a fall in arterial pressure stimulate release of ACTH via receptors in the right atrium and the carotid artery.

3.1.4.5 OTHER HORMONES

Atrial natriuretic factor (ANF) or peptide (ANP) is a hormone produced by the atria, along with brain or B-type natriuretic peptide (BNP) produced by the ventricular muscle cells, in response to an increase in vascular volume and thus distension and pressure[7]. The ANF and BNP produce similar increases in glomerular filtration and pronounced natriuresis and diuresis to decrease intravascular volume by inhibition of aldosterone which also minimizes kaliuresis.

Also, ANF and BNP emphasize the heart's function as an endocrine organ.

3.1.5 Effects of the Various Mediators

3.1.5.1 HYPERDYNAMIC STATE

Following illness or injury, the systemic inflammatory response occurs, in which there is an increase in activity of the cardiovascular system, reflected as tachycardia, widened pulse pressure and a greater cardiac output. There is an increase in the metabolic rate, with an increase in oxygen consumption, increased protein catabolism and hyperglycaemia.

The cardiac index may exceed 4.5 L/min/m² after severe trauma in those patients able to respond. Ideally, decreases in vascular resistance accompany this increased cardiac output, and there is an increase in oxygen delivery to the microcirculation. This hyperdynamic state elevates the resting energy expenditure to more than 20 per cent above normal, total body oxygen consumption (VO_2) is increased and, due to the increase in metabolism, core temperature is increased. With an inadequate response, and a cardiac index of less than 2.5 L/min/m², oxygen consumption may fall to values of less than 100 mL/min/m² (Normal = 120–160 mL/min/m²). Endotoxins and anoxia may also injure cells and limit their ability to utilize oxygen for oxidative phosphorylation.

The amount of ATP synthesized by an adult is considerable. However, there is no reservoir of ATP or creatinine phosphate, and therefore, cellular injury and lack of oxygen result in rapid deterioration of processes requiring energy, and lactate is produced. Because of anaerobic glycolysis, only two ATP equivalents instead of 34 are produced from 1 mol of glucose in the Krebs cycle. Lactate is formed from pyruvate, which is the end product of glycolysis. It is normally reconverted to glucose in the Cori cycle in the liver. However, in shock, the oxidation reduction (redox) potential declines and conversion of pyruvate to acetyl co-enzyme A for entry into the Krebs cycle is inhibited. Lactate therefore accumulates because of impaired hepatic gluconeogenesis, causing a metabolic acidosis.

Lactic acidosis after injury correlates with the ISS, and acute blood loss. Persistent lactic acidosis is indicative of inadequate resuscitation and predictive of the development of multiple organ failure (MOF) and adult respiratory distress syndrome (ARDS)[8].

3.1.5.2 WATER AND SALT RETENTION

Secretion of ADH from the supra-optic nuclei in the anterior hypothalamus is stimulated by volume reduction and increased osmolality of the circulation. The latter is due mainly to increased sodium content of the extracellular fluid. Volume receptors are located in the atria and pulmonary arteries, and osmoreceptors are located near ADH neurones in the hypothalamus. The ADH acts mainly on the connecting tubules of the kidney but also on the distal tubules to promote reabsorption of water.

Aldosterone acts mainly on the distal renal tubules to promote reabsorption of sodium and bicarbonate and increased excretion of potassium and hydrogen ions. Aldosterone also modifies the effects of catecholamines on cells, thus affecting the exchange of sodium and potassium across all cell membranes. The release of large quantities of intracellular potassium into the extracellular fluid may cause a significant rise in serum potassium especially if renal function is impaired. Retention of sodium and bicarbonate may produce metabolic alkalosis with impairment of the delivery of oxygen to the tissues. After injury, urinary sodium excretion may fall to 10–25 mmol/24 h and potassium excretion may rise to 100–200 mmol/24 h.

3.1.5.3 **EFFECTS ON SUBSTRATE METABOLISM**

3.1.5.3.1 Carbohydrates

Critically ill patients develop a glucose intolerance, which resembles that found in diabetic patients. This is a result of both increased mobilisation and decreased uptake of glucose by the tissues. The turnover of glucose is increased, and the serum glucose is higher than normal.

Glucose is mobilized from stored glycogen in the liver by catecholamines, glucocorticoids and glucagon. Glycogen reserves are limited, and glucose can be derived from glycogen for 12–18 hours only. Early on, insulin blood levels are suppressed (usually lower by 8 units/mL) by the effect of adrenergic activity of shock on degranulation of the β cells of the pancreas. Thereafter, gluconeogenesis is stimulated by corticosteroids and glucagon. Suppression of insulin favours the release of amino acids from muscle, which are then available for gluconeogenesis. Growth hormone inhibits the effect of insulin on normal glucose metabolism.

As blood glucose rises during the phase of hepatic gluconeogenesis, blood insulin concentration rises, sometimes to very high levels. Provided that the liver circulation is maintained, gluconeogenesis will not be suppressed by hyperinsulinaemia or hyperglycaemia, because the accelerated rate of glucose production in the liver is required for clearance of lactate and amino acids, which are not able to be used for protein synthesis. This period of breakdown of muscle protein for gluconeogenesis and the resultant hyperglycaemia characterize the catabolic phase of the metabolic response to trauma.

The glucose level following trauma should be monitored carefully in the intensive care unit. The optimum

blood glucose level remains controversial, but the maximum level should be 10 mmol/L. Excessive levels of glucose correlate directly with infectious complications, particularly in surgical or injury wounds. Control of the blood glucose is best achieved by titration with intravenous insulin, based on a sliding scale. However, because of the degree of insulin resistance associated with trauma, the quantities required may be considerably higher than normal.

Enteral nutrition is preferred but parenteral nutrition may be required, and this will exacerbate the problem. However, glucose remains the safest energy substrate following major trauma: 60–75 per cent of the caloric requirements should be supplied by glucose, with the remainder being supplied as a fat emulsion.

3.1.5.3.2 Fat

A major source of energy following trauma is adipose tissue. Lipids stored as triglycerides in adipose tissue are mobilized when insulin falls below 25 units/mL. Initially, because of the suppression of insulin release by the catecholamine spike after trauma, as much as 200–500 g of fat may be broken down early after severe trauma[9]. Tumour necrosis factor (TNF) and possibly IL-1 also play a role in the mobilisation of fat stores.

Catecholamines and glucagon activate adenyl cyclase in the fat cells to produce cyclic adenosine monophosphate (cyclic AMP). This activates lipase, which promptly hydrolyses triglycerides to release glycerol and fatty acids. Growth hormone and cortisol play a minor role in this process as well. Glycerol provides substrate for gluconeogenesis in the liver, which derives energy by β-oxidation of fatty acids, a process inhibited by hyperinsulinaemia.

The free fatty acids provide energy for all tissues and for hepatic gluconeogenesis. Carnitine, synthesized in the liver, is required for the transport of fatty acids into the cells.

3.1.5.3.3 Amino Acids

The intake of protein by a healthy adult is between 80 and 120 g of protein: 1–2 Gm. protein/Kg/day. This is equivalent to 13–20 g of nitrogen per day. In the absence of an exogenous source of protein, amino acids are principally derived from the breakdown of skeletal muscle protein. Following trauma or sepsis, the release rate of amino acids increases by three to four times. The process manifests as marked muscle wasting.

Cortisol, glucagon and catecholamines play a role in this reaction. The mobilized amino acids are utilized for gluconeogenesis or oxidation in the liver and other tissues, but also for synthesis of acute-phase proteins required for immunocompetence, clotting, wound healing and maintenance of cellular function.

Certain amino acids like glutamic acid, asparagine and aspartate can be oxidized to pyruvate, producing alanine, or to α-ketoglutarate, producing glutamine. The others must first be deaminated before they can be utilized. In the muscle, deamination is accomplished by transamination from branched chain amino acids. In the liver, amino acids are deaminated to urea that is excreted in the urine. After severe trauma or sepsis, as much as 20 g/day of urea nitrogen is excreted in the urine. Since 1 g urea nitrogen is derived from 6.25 g degraded amino acids, this protein wastage is up to 125 g/day.

One gram of muscle protein represents 5 g wet muscle mass. The patient in this example would be losing 625 g of muscle mass per day. A loss of 40 per cent of body protein is usually fatal, because failing immunocompetence leads to overwhelming infection. Nitrogen excretion usually peaks several days after injury, returning to normal after several weeks. This is a characteristic feature of the metabolic response to illness. The most profound alterations in metabolic rate and nitrogen loss occur after burns, and may persist for months.

To measure the rates of transfer and utilization of amino acids mobilized from muscle or infused into the circulation, the measurement of central plasma clearance rate of amino acids (CPCR-AA) has been developed. Using this method, a large increase in peripheral production and central uptake of amino acids into the liver have been demonstrated in injured patients, especially if sepsis is also present. The protein-depleted patient can be improved dramatically by parenteral or enteral alimentation provided adequate liver function is present. Amino acid infusions in patients who ultimately die cause plasma amino acid concentration to rise to high levels with only a modest increase in CPCR-AA.

3.1.5.3.4 The Gut

The intestinal mucosa requires rapid synthesis of amino acids. Depletion of amino acids results in atrophy of the mucosa causing failure of the mucosal barrier. This may lead to bacterial translocation from the gut to the portal system. The extent of bacterial translocation in trauma has not been defined[10]. The presence of food in the gut lumen is a major stimulus for mucosal cell growth. Food intake is invariably interrupted after major trauma, and the supply of glutamine may be insufficient for mucosal

cell growth. Early nutrition (within 24–48 h), and early enteral rather than parenteral feeding may prevent or reduce these events.

3.1.6 **Anabolic Phase**

During this phase the patient is in positive nitrogen balance, regains weight and restores fat deposits. The hormones, which contribute to anabolism, are growth hormones, androgens and 17 beta-ketosteroids. The utility of growth hormone, and also more recently, of insulin-like growth factor (IGF-1), in reversing catabolism following injury is critically dependent on adequate caloric intake.

3.1.7 **Clinical and Therapeutic Relevance**

Survival after injury depends on a balance between the extent of cellular damage, the efficacy of the metabolic response and the effectiveness of treatment.

Tissue injury, hypoxia, pain and toxins from invasive infection add to the initiating factor of hypovolaemia. The degree to which the body is able to compensate for injury is astonishing, although sometimes the compensatory mechanisms may work to the patient's disadvantage. Adequate resuscitation to shut off the hypovolaemic stimulus is important. However, once hormonal changes have been initiated, the effects of the hormones will not cease merely because hormonal secretion has been turned off by replacement of blood volume.

Mobilisation and storage of the energy fuel substrates, carbohydrate, fats and protein is regulated by insulin, balanced against catecholamines, cortisol and glucagon. However, infusion of hormones has failed to cause more than a modest response. Rapid resuscitation, maintenance of oxygen delivery to the tissues, removal of devitalized tissue or pus and control of infection are the cornerstones. The best metabolic therapy is excellent surgical care.

3.2 **SHOCK**

3.2.1 **Definition of Shock**

Shock is defined as inadequate delivery of oxygenated blood to the tissues, resulting in cellular hypoxia. This at first leads to reversible ischaemic-induced cellular injury. If the process is sufficiently severe or protracted, it ultimately results in irreversible cellular and organ injury and dysfunction. The precise mechanisms responsible for the transition from reversible to irreversible injury and death of cells are not clearly understood, although the biochemical/morphological sequence in the progression of ischaemic cellular injury has been fairly well elucidated[11]. By understanding the events leading to cell injury and death, we may be able to intervene therapeutically in shock by protecting sublethally injured cells from irreversible injury and death.

3.2.2 **Classification of Shock**

The classification of shock is of practical importance if the pathophysiology is understood in terms that make a fundamental difference in treatment. Although the basic definition of shock, 'insufficient nutrient flow', remains inviolate, six types of shock, based on a distinction not only in the pathophysiology but also in the management of the patients, are recognized:

3.2.2.1   Hypovolaemic.
3.2.2.2   Cardiogenic.
3.2.2.3   Cardiac compressive (e.g. cardiac tamponade).
3.2.2.4   Distributive (previously inflammatory) (e.g. septic shock).
3.2.2.5   Neurogenic.
3.2.2.6   Obstructive (e.g. mediastinal compression).

In principle, the physiological basis of shock is based on the following:

Cardiac Output = Stroke Volume × Heart Rate

Blood Pressure ∝ Cardiac Output × Total Peripheral Resistance

Stroke volume is determined by the pre-load, the contractility of the myocardium and by the afterload.

3.2.2.1 HYPOVOLAEMIC SHOCK

Hypovolaemic shock is caused by a decrease in the intravascular volume. This results in significant degeneration of both pressure and flow. It is characterized by significant decreases in filling pressures with a consequent decrease in stroke volume. Cardiac output is temporarily maintained by a compensatory tachycardia. With continuing hypovolaemia, the blood pressure is maintained by reflex increases in peripheral and, importantly,

splanchnic vascular resistance and myocardial contractility mediated by neurohumoral mechanisms.

Hypovolaemic shock is divided into four classes:

Class	Percentage (%) blood loss	Volume	Pulse Rate	Blood Pressure	Pulse Pressure	Respiratory Rate
Class I	15%	<750 mL	<100	Normal	Normal	14–20
Class II	30%	750–1500 mL	>100	Normal	Increased	20–30
Class III	40%	2000 mL	>120	Decreased	Narrowed	30–40
Class IV	>40%	>2000 mL	>140	Decreased	Narrowed	>35

Initially, the body compensates for shock, and Class I and Class II shock are compensated shock. When the blood volume loss exceeds 30 per cent (Class III and Class IV shock), the compensatory mechanisms are no longer effective and the decrease in cardiac output causes a decreased oxygen transport to peripheral tissues. These tissues attempt to maintain their oxygen consumption by increasing oxygen extraction. Eventually, this compensatory mechanism also fails and tissue hypoxia leads to lactic acidosis, hyperglycaemia and failure of the sodium pump with swelling of the cells from water influx.

3.2.2.1.1 Clinical Presentation

The classic features of hypovolaemic shock are hypotension, tachycardia, pallor secondary to vasoconstriction, sweating, cyanosis, hyperventilation, confusion and an oliguria. Cardiac function can be depressed without gross clinical haemodynamic manifestations. The heart shares in the total body ischaemic insult. Systemic arterial hypotension increases coronary ischaemia, causing rhythm disturbances and decreased myocardial performance. As the heart fails, left ventricular end-diastolic pressure rises, ultimately causing pulmonary oedema.

Hyperventilation may maintain arterial PaO_2 at near normal levels but the $PaCO_2$ falls to 20–30 mm Hg (2.7–4 kPa). Later, pulmonary insufficiency may supervene from alveolar collapse and pulmonary oedema, resulting from damaged pulmonary capillaries, cardiac failure or inappropriate fluid therapy.

Renal function is also critically dependent on renal perfusion. Oliguria is an inevitable feature of hypovolaemia. During volume loss, renal blood flow falls correspondingly with the blood pressure. Anuria sets in when the systolic blood falls to 50 mm Hg. Thus, urine output is a good indicator of peripheral perfusion. Oliguria in the hypovolemic patient is a sign of renal success, not failure.

3.2.2.2 CARDIOGENIC SHOCK

When the heart fails to produce an adequate cardiac output, even though the end diastolic volume is normal, cardiogenic shock is said to be present. Intravascular obstructive shock results when intravascular obstruction, excessive stiffness of the arterial walls or obstruction of the microvasculature imposes an undue burden on the heart. The obstruction to flow can be on either the right or the left side of the heart. Causes include pulmonary embolism, air embolism, acute respiratory distress syndrome (ARDS), aortic stenosis, calcification of the systemic arteries, thickening or stiffening of the arterial walls as a result of the loss of elastin and its replacement with collagen (as occurs in old age) and obstruction of the systemic microcirculation as a result of chronic hypertension or the arteriolar disease of diabetes.

Cardiac function is impaired in shocked patients even if myocardial damage is not the primary cause. Reduced myocardial function in shock includes dysrhythmias, myocardial ischaemia from systemic hypotension and variations in blood flow, and myocardial lesions from high circulatory levels of catecholamines, angiotensin and other myocardial depressant factors, such as DAMPs and other inflammatory mediators.

The reduced cardiac output can be a result of:

- Reduced stroke volume.
- Impaired myocardial contractility due to ischaemia, reperfusion induced oedema, infarction, cardiomyopathy or direct trauma.
- Altered ejection volume.
- Coronary air embolism.
- Mechanical complications of acute myocardial infarction – acute mitral valvular regurgitation, ventricular septal rupture, or trauma.
- Arrhythmias.
- Conduction system disturbances (bradydysrhythmias and tachydysrythmias).

Other forms of cardiogenic shock include those clinical examples in which the patient may have a nearly normal resting cardiac output but cannot raise the cardiac output under circumstances of stress because of poor myocardial reserves or an inability to mobilize those myocardial reserves due to pharmacologic beta adrenergic blockade, for example propranolol for hypertension.

Heart failure and dysrhythmias are discussed in depth elsewhere in this book.

3.2.2.2.1 Clinical Presentation

The clinical picture will depend on the underlying cause. Clinical signs of peripheral vasoconstriction are prominent, pulmonary congestion is frequent and oliguria is almost always present. Pulmonary oedema may cause severe dyspnoea, central cyanosis and crepitations, audible over the lung fields and lung oedema visible on X-rays. A systolic murmur appearing after myocardial infarction suggests mitral regurgitation or septal perforation.

Haemodynamic findings consist of a systolic arterial pressure less than 90 mm Hg, decreased cardiac output, usually less than 1.8 L/min/m², and a pulmonary arterial wedge pressure (PAWP) of greater than 20 mm Hg. However, cardiogenic shock can occur without the PAWP being elevated. This may be a result of excess diuretic therapy, plasma volume depletion by fluid lost into tissues (i.e. third spacing) or blood loss. Patients with relative hypovolaemia below the levels where there is a risk of pulmonary oedema and patients with significant right ventricular failure will also not have elevated PAWP. These patients, although their shock is cardiogenic, will respond dramatically to plasma volume expansion and will deteriorate if diuresis is attempted.

3.2.2.3 CARDIAC COMPRESSIVE SHOCK

The pathophysiology of cardiac compressive shock is very different from cardiogenic shock. External forces compress the thin-walled chambers of the heart (the atria and the right ventricle), the great veins (systemic or pulmonary) or any combination of these. Impaired diastolic filling will result. Clinical conditions capable of causing compressive shock include pericardial tamponade, tension pneumothoraces, positive pressure ventilation with large tidal volumes or high airway pressures (especially in a hypovolaemic patient), an elevated diaphragm (as in pregnancy), displacement of abdominal viscera through a ruptured diaphragm, and the abdominal compartment syndrome (e.g. from ascites, abdominal distension, abdominal or retroperitoneal bleeding, or a stiff abdominal wall, as in a patient with deep burns to the torso).

The consequence of this compression is an increase in right atrial pressure, without an increase in volume, impeding venous return and reducing end diastolic volumes and provoking hypotension.

3.2.2.3.1 Clinical Presentation

Cardiac tamponade follows blunt or penetrating trauma and is a classic example of compressive cardiac shock. As a result of the presence of blood in the pericardial sac, the atria are compressed and cannot fill adequately. The systolic blood pressure is less than 90 mm Hg, and there is a narrowed pulse pressure and a pulsus paradoxus exceeding 10 mm Hg. Distended neck veins may be present, unless the patient is hypovolaemic as well. Heart sounds are muffled. The limited compliance of the pericardial sac means that a very small amount (<25 mL blood) may be sufficient to cause decompensation. Similarly, tension pneumothorax can also produce compressive heart failure. In the patient with chest trauma and hypotension, the problem usually can be identified immediately, from decreased breath sounds, hyperresonance of the affected side and displacement of the trachea to the opposite side. Neck veins also may be distended. Immediate release of the tension, prior to waiting for an X-ray, is required to prevent cardiac arrest.

3.2.2.4 DISTRIBUTIVE (INFLAMMATORY) SHOCK

Dilatation of the capacitance reservoirs in the body occurs with endotoxic shock or prolonged hypovolaemic shock. Endotoxin can have a major effect on this form of peripheral pooling and even though the blood volume is normal, the distribution of that volume is changed so that there is insufficient nutrient flow to meet aerobic metabolism needs.

In the ultimate analysis, all shock leads to cellular defect shock. Aerobic metabolism takes place in the cytochrome system in the cristae of the mitochondria. Oxidative phosphorylation in the cytochrome system produces high-energy phosphate bonds by coupling oxygen and glucose, forming the freely diffusable by-products carbon dioxide and water. Several poisons uncouple oxidative phosphorylation but the most common in clinical practice is endotoxin. Sepsis is frequent in hospitalized patients and endotoxic shock is distressingly common. There is fever, tachycardia may or may not be present, the mean blood pressure is usually below 60 mm Hg, yet the cardiac output varies between 3 and 6 L/m^2/min. This haemodynamic state is indicative of low peripheral vascular resistance.

In addition to maldistribution of blood volume due to increase in capacitance and low peripheral resistance as causes of hypotension in septic shock, other causes inhibiting the cardiovascular system maintenance of cardiac output at a level sufficient to maintain normal blood pressure in sepsis include

- Hypovolaemia due to fluid translocation from the blood into interstitial spaces.
- Elevated pulmonary vascular resistance due to ARDS.
- Bioventricular myocardial depression manifested by reduced contractility and an inability to increase stroke-work.

The ultimate cause of death in septic shock is failure of energy production at the cellular level as reflected by a decline in oxygen consumption. It is not only the circulatory insufficiency that is responsible for this but also the impairment of cellular oxidative phosphorylation by endotoxin or endogenously produced superoxides. There is a narrowing of arterial-mixed venous oxygen difference as an indication of reduced oxygen extraction, which often precedes the fall of cardiac output. Inadequate oxidative phosphorylation leads to anaerobic glycogenolysis and a severe metabolic acidosis due to lactacidaemia.

3.2.2.5 NEUROGENIC SHOCK

Neurogenic shock is a hypotensive syndrome in which there is loss of α-adrenergic tone and dilatation of the arterial and venous vessels. The cardiac output is normal, or may even be elevated, but because the total peripheral resistance is reduced, the patient is hypotensive. The consequence is a reduced perfusion pressure.

A simple example of this type of shock is syncope ('vaso-vagal syncope'). It is caused by a strong vagal discharge resulting in dilatation of the small vessels of the splanchnic bed. The next cycle of the heart has less venous return so that the ventricle will not fill and the next stroke volume does not adequately perfuse the cerebrum, causing a faint. No blood is lost but there is a sudden increase in the amount of blood trapped in one part of the circulation where it is no longer available for perfusion to an obligate aerobic glycolytic metabolic bed – the central nervous system.

3.2.2.5.1 Clinical Presentation

Commonly seen with high spinal cord injury, the patient usually has weakly palpable peripheral pulses, warm extremities, brisk capillary filling and may be anxious. The pulse pressure is wide, with both systolic and diastolic blood pressure being low. Heart rate is below 100 beats per minute, and there may even be a bradycardia. However, the diagnosis of neurogenic shock should only be made once other causes of shock have been ruled out, since the common cause is injury, and there may be other injuries present causing a hypovolaemic shock in parallel.

3.2.2.6 OBSTRUCTIVE SHOCK

Intravascular obstructive shock results when intravascular obstruction, excessive stiffness of the arterial walls or obstruction of the microvasculature imposes an undue burden on the heart. Because of the decreased venous return, the atrial filling is reduced with consequent hypotension. The obstruction to flow can be on either the right or the left side of the heart. Causes include pulmonary embolism, air embolism, acute respiratory distress syndrome (ARDS), aortic stenosis, calcification of the systemic arteries, thickening or stiffening of the arterial walls as a result of the loss of elastin and its replacement with collagen (as occurs in old age) and obstruction of the systemic microcirculation as a result of chronic hypertension or the arteriolar disease of diabetes. The blood pressure in the pulmonary artery or the aorta will be high; the cardiac output will be low.

3.2.3 Measurements in Shock

In physics, flow is directly related to pressure and inversely related to resistance. This universal flow formula is not dependent on the type of fluid and is applied to the flow of electrons. In electricity, it is expressed as Ohm's law. This law applies just as appropriately to blood flow.

$$Flow = \frac{Pressure}{Peripheral\ resistance}$$

From this law it can be deduced that shock is just as much a state of elevated resistance as it is a state of low blood pressure. However, the focus should remain on flow rather than simply on pressure since most drugs that result in a rise in pressure do so by raising the resistance, which in turn decreases flow, while simultaneously increasing work and oxygen consumption by the myocardium.

3.2.3.1 CARDIAC OUTPUT

Blood flow is dependent on cardiac output. Three factors determine cardiac output:

- Pre-load or the volume entering the heart.
- Contractility of the heart.

- After-load or the resistance against which the heart must function to deliver the nutrient flow.

These three factors are interrelated to produce the systolic ejection from the heart. Up to a point, the greater the pre-load, the greater the cardiac output. As myocardial fibres are stretched by the pre-load the contractility increases according to the Frank-Starling principle. However, an excessive increase in pre-load leads to symptoms of pulmonary/systemic venous congestion without further improvement in cardiac performance. The pre-load is a positive factor in cardiac performance up the slope of the Frank-Starling curve but not beyond the point of cardiac decompensation.

Contractility of the heart is improved by inotropic agents. The product of the stroke volume and the heart rate equals the cardiac output. Cardiac output acting against the peripheral resistance generates the blood pressure. Diminished cardiac output in patients with pump failure is associated with a fall in blood pressure. To maintain coronary and cranial blood flow there is a reflex increase in systemic vascular resistance to raise blood pressure. An exaggerated rise in systemic vascular resistance can lead to further depression of cardiac function by increasing ventricular after-load. After-load is defined as the wall tension during left ventricular ejection and is determined by systolic pressure and the radius of the left ventricle. Left ventricular radius is related to end-diastolic volume, and systolic pressure to the impedance to blood flow in the aorta, or total peripheral vascular resistance.

However, the critical emphasis in the definition of shock is on flow, we need to find improved methods to measure flow.

3.2.3.2 INDIRECT MEASUREMENT OF FLOW

In many patients in shock, simply laying a hand upon their extremities will help to determine flow by the cold clammy appearance of hypoperfusion due to increased resistance. Probably the most important clinical observation to indirectly determine adequate nutrient flow to a visceral organ will be the urine output.

The kidney responds to decreased nutrient flow with several compensatory changes to protect its own perfusion. Over a range of blood pressure, the kidneys maintain a nearly constant blood flow. If the blood pressure decreases, the kidney's autoregulation of resistance results in dilatation of the vascular bed. It keeps nutrient flow constant by lowering the resistance even though the pressure has decreased. This allows selective shunting of blood to the renal bed.

If the blood pressure falls further and a true decrease in flow across the glomeruli occurs, then the renin/angiotensin mechanism is triggered. Renin from the juxtaglomerular apparatus acts upon angiotensin from the liver. The peptide is cleaved by renin and a decapeptide results, which in the presence of converting enzyme clips off two additional amino acids to produce the octapeptide angiotensin II, one of the most potent vasopressors known. The third step is that the same octopeptide stimulates the zona glomerulosa of the adrenal cortex to secrete aldosterone, which causes sodium retention and results in volume expansion. The kidney thus has three methods of protecting its perfusion: autoregulation, pressor secretion and volume expansion. When all three compensatory mechanisms have failed, there is a decrease in the quality and quantity of urine as a function of nutrient flow to this organ. Urine flow is such an important measurement of flow in the patient in shock that we can use this to define the presence or absence of shock. For practical purposes, if the patient is producing a normal quantity of normal quality urine, he or she is not in shock.

Another vital perfusion bed that reflects the adequacy of nutrient flow is the brain itself. Since adequate nutrient flow is a necessary, but not the only requirement for cerebration, normal consciousness also can be used to evaluate the adequacy of nutrient flow in the patient with shock.

3.2.3.3 DIRECT MEASUREMENTS

3.2.3.3.1 Central Venous Pressure

Between the groin or axillae and the heart the veins do not have any valves, so measurement of the pressure in this system at the level of the heart will reflect the pressure in the right atrium, and therefore the filling pressure of the heart.

Placement of a central venous line that will allow accurate measurement of the hydrostatic pressure of the right atrium following fluid boluses can help differentiate between the different shock states. The actual measurement, except at the extremes, is frequently inaccurate in determining intravascular volume and less important than the change in value, especially in the acute resuscitation of a patient. Normal is 4–12 cm water. A value below 4 cm indicates that the venous system is empty, and thus the pre-load is reduced, usually as a result of dehydration or hypovolaemia, while a

high value indicates that the pre-load is increased, either as a result of a full circulation or due to pump failure (e.g. cardiogenic shock due to aetiologies such as tension pneumothorax, cardiac tamponade or myocardial contusion).

As a general rule, if a patient in shock has both systemic arterial hypotension and central venous hypotension, the shock is due to volume depletion. On the other hand, if central venous pressure is high though arterial pressure is low, shock is not due to volume depletion and is more likely due to pump failure.

Cannulation of the central venous system is generally achieved using the subclavian, jugular or femoral route.

The subclavian route is the preferred one in the trauma patient, particularly when the status of the cervical spine is unclear. It is ideal for the intensive care setting, where occlusion of the access site against infection is required. The safest technique is that recommended by the Advanced Trauma Life Support (ATLS) programme[13].

The internal jugular route or, occasionally, the external jugular route is the one most commonly utilized by anaesthesiologists, preferably under ultrasonic guidance. It provides ease of access, especially under operative conditions. However, there are significant dangers in the trauma patient, especially where the cervical spine has not yet been cleared, and other routes may be preferable. The ability to occlude the jugular site, especially in the awake patient in the ICU, is, however, more limited, and there is greater discomfort for the patient.

3.2.3.3.1.1 *Subclavian Line Insertion*

The subclavian route is reliable, easy to maintain and relatively safe. Pitfalls include arterial puncture and pneumothorax. The following technique is used for subclavian line insertion[14]:

1. Place the patient in a supine position, at least 15° head down to distend the neck veins and prevent an air embolism. Do not move the patient's head.
2. Cleanse the skin and drape the area.
3. Use lignocaine (lidocaine) 1 per cent at the injection site including the periosteal surface to effect local anaesthesia.
4. Introduce a large calibre needle, attached to a 10-mL syringe with 1 ml of saline in it, 1 cm below the junction of the middle and medial thirds of the clavicle.
5. After the needle has been introduced, with the bevel of the needle upward, expel the skin plug that may occlude the needle.

6. The needle and syringe are held parallel to the frontal plane.
7. Direct the needle medially, slightly cephalad, and posteriorly, behind the clavicle, in the direction of the posterior, superior angle to the sternal end of the clavicle. (Aim at a finger placed in the suprasternal notch.)
8. Advance the needle while gently withdrawing the plunger of the syringe.
9. When a free flow of blood appears on the syringe, rotate the bevel so that it faces caudally, and remove the syringe. Occlude the needle to avoid any chance of air embolism.
10. Introduce the guide wire while monitoring the electrocardiogram (ECG) for abnormalities.
11. Insert the catheter over the guide wire to a pre-determined length. The tip of the catheter should be at the entrance to the right atrium. In an adult, this is approximately 18 cm.
12. Connect the catheter to intravenous tubing.
13. Affix securely to the skin and cover with an occlusive dressing.
14. Obtain a chest X-ray to confirm position.

3.2.3.3.1.2 *Femoral Line Insertion*

The femoral route is easy to access, especially when the line also will be used for venous transfusion. However, the incidence of femoral vein thrombosis is high, and the line should not be left beyond 48 hours because of the risk of infection. Pitfalls include placing the cannula inside the abdominal cavity. This can be particularly misleading if blood is present inside the abdominal cavity, since aspiration of the cannula will yield blood and a false sense of security.

The following technique is used for femoral line insertion[15]:

1. Place the patient in a supine position.
2. Cleanse the skin.
3. Locate the femoral vein by locating the femoral artery. The vein lies immediately medial to the artery.
4. If the patient is awake, infiltrate the puncture site with lignocaine (lidocaine) 1 per cent.
5. Introduce a large calibre needle, attached to a 10-mL syringe containing 1 mL of saline. The needle, directed toward the patient's head, should enter the skin directly over the femoral vein.
6. The needle and syringe are held parallel to the frontal plane.

7. Direct the needle cephalad and posteriorly at 45° to the skin, and slowly advance the needle, while withdrawing the plunger of the syringe.
8. When a free flow of blood appears on the syringe, remove the syringe. Occlude the needle to avoid any chance of air embolism.
9. Insert the catheter over the guide wire to a pre-determined length. The tip of the catheter should be at the entrance to the right atrium. In an adult, this is approximately 30 cm.
10. Connect the catheter to intravenous tubing.
11. Affix securely to the skin and cover with an occlusive dressing.
12. Obtain a chest X-ray to confirm position.

3.2.3.3.2 Systemic Arterial Pressure

Systemic arterial pressure reflects the product of the peripheral resistance and the cardiac output. Measurement can be indirect or direct.

Indirect measurement involves the use of a blood pressure cuff with auscultation of the artery to determine systolic and diastolic blood pressure.

Direct measurement involves placement of a catheter into the lumen of the artery, with direct measurement of the pressure.

In patients in shock, with an elevated systemic vascular resistance, there is often a significant difference obtained between the two measurements. In patients with increased vascular resistance, low cuff pressure does not necessarily indicate hypotension. Failure to recognize this may lead to dangerous errors in therapy.

The arterial Doppler can be used for measuring arterial blood pressure. Only measurement of the systolic blood pressure is possible. However, the Doppler correlates well with the direct measurement pressure.

The radial artery is the most common site for arterial cannulation. It is usually safe to use, provided adequate ulnar collateral flow is present. It is important both medically and legally to do an Allen test, compressing both radial and ulnar arteries, and releasing the ulnar artery to check for collateral flow. Thrombosis of the radial artery is quite common, although ischaemia of the hand is rare, due to collaterals from the ulnar artery.

The femoral artery is generally more unsafe in the emergency situation, and the cannula should be removed as soon as possible.

Cannulation of the brachial artery is not recommended because of the potential for thrombosis and for ischaemia of the lower arm and hand.

3.2.3.3.3 Pulmonary Arterial Pressure

The right-sided circulation is a valveless system through which flows the entire cardiac output from the right side of the heart.

Catheterization can be performed easily and rapidly at the bedside, using a balloon-tipped flow-directed thermodilution catheter. In its passage from the superior vena cava through the right atrium, from which it migrates into the right ventricle on a myocardial contraction, the balloon tip enters the pulmonary valve exactly like a pulmonary embolus, until the balloon-tipped catheter wedges in the pulmonary artery. Additional side holes are provided in the catheter, allowing measurement of pressure in each right-sided chamber, including right atrial pressure, right ventricular pressure, pulmonary artery and pulmonary wedge pressure.

The tip of the catheter is placed in the pulmonary artery, and then the occlusive balloon is inflated. This has the effect of occluding the lumen. As a result, the pressure transmitted via the catheter represents pulmonary venous pressure, and thus, left atrial pressure. The wedged pulmonary atrial pressure is the closest approximation of left ventricular end diastolic pressure (LVEDP). The LVEDP usually correlates with left ventricular end-diastolic volume (LVEDV).

In addition to direct measurement of pressures, a pulmonary artery catheter allows the following:

- Measurement of cardiac output by thermodilution.
- Sampling of pulmonary arterial (mixed venous) blood.

The Swann-Ganz catheter is no longer generally used, and has been superseded by less invasive methods such as ultrasonic computers (e.g. Hemosonic [HemoSonics LLC, Charlottesville, VA], and radial artery catheters e.g. Vigileo Monitor [Edwards Lifesciences, Irvine, CA]). The following equipment is used:

1. Lignocaine (lidocaine) 1 per cent
2. Calibrated pressure transducer with continuous heparin flush and connecting tubing
3. Visible oscilloscope screen showing both ECG and pressure tracings
4. A dedicated assistant (e.g. a nurse)

The following is the technique used for insertion of a pulmonary artery catheter using the internal jugular route[16]:

1. Prepare all supplies at the bedside.
2. Calibrate the transducer for a pressure range of 0–50 mm Hg.

3. Remove all pillows from behind the patient, and turn the patient's head to the left.
4. Make sure airway and breathing are acceptable. The patient should be on oxygen, and preferably also monitored on pulse oximetry.
5. Tilt the bed head down to distend the jugular vein.
6. Prepare and drape the skin, allowing access from below the clavicle to the mastoid process.
7. Locate the right carotid pulse, and infiltrate over the area with local anaesthetic at the apex of the triangle between the sternal and clavicular heads of sternomastoid muscle.
8. Insert a 16-gauge needle beneath the anterior border of sternomastoid, aiming towards the right nipple, to place the needle behind the medial end of the clavicle, and to enter the right internal jugular vein.
9. Pass the J-wire through the needle and advance the wire until well into the vein.
10. Remove the needle, and enlarge the skin site with a No. 11 scalpel blade, followed with the dilator provided in the set.
11. Attach an intravenous solution to the introducer, and suture the introducer to the skin.
12. Connect and flush the catheter to clear all air and to test all balloons, ports, etc. Move the catheter to confirm that the trace is recorded.
13. Insert the catheter into the introducer. If it has a curve, ensure that this is directed anteriorly and to the left. Insert to the 20-cm mark. This should place the tip in the right atrium.
14. Inflate the balloon.
15. Advance the catheter through the right ventricle to the occlusion pressure position. In most adults, this is at the 45–55 cm mark.
16. Deflate the balloon. The pulmonary artery waveform should appear, and with slow inflation the occlusion waveform should return. If this does not occur, advance and then withdraw the catheter slightly.
17. Attach the sheath to the introducer.
18. Apply a sterile dressing.
19. Confirm correct placement with a chest X-ray.

Figure 3.1 shows a recording of pressures showing the passage of the pulmonary artery catheter through the right side of the heart until it is wedged in the pulmonary artery. Note that the wedge pressure is less than the diastolic pulmonary artery pressure.

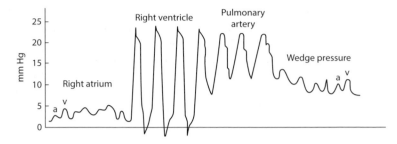

Figure 3.1 A recording of pressures showing the passage of the pulmonary artery catheter through the right side of the heart until it is wedged in the pulmonary artery (a, atrial activity; v, ventricular activity).

3.2.3.3.4 Cardiac Output

Cardiac output can be measured with the thermodilution technique[17]. A thermodilution pulmonary artery catheter has a thermistor at the distal tip. When a given volume of a solution that is cooler than the body temperature is injected into the right atrium, it is carried by the blood past the thermistor, resulting in a transient fall in temperature. The temperature curve so created is analysed, and the rate of blood flow past the thermistor (i.e. cardiac output) can be calculated. By measuring the mixed oxygen saturation in the pulmonary artery, blood oxygen extraction across the circulation can be determined.

3.2.4 Endpoints in Shock Resuscitation

The ultimate measurement of the impact of shock must be at the cellular level[18]. The most convenient measurement is a determination of the blood gases. Measurement of PaO_2, $PaCO_2$, pH, base deficit (BD) and arterial lactate will supply information on oxygen delivery and utilisation of energy substrates. Both PaO_2 and $PaCO_2$ are concentrations – partial pressure of oxygen and carbon dioxide in arterial blood. If the $PaCO_2$ is normal, there is adequate alveolar ventilation. CO_2 is one of the most freely diffusable gases in the body and is not overproduced or under-diffused. Consequently, its partial pressure in the blood is a measure of its excretion through the lung, which is a direct result of alveolar ventilation. The PaO_2 is a similar concentration, but it is the partial pressure of oxygen in the blood and not the oxygen content. A concentration measure in the blood does not tell us the delivery rate of oxygen to the tissues per unit of time without knowing something of the blood flow that carries this concentration.

For evaluation of oxygen utilisation, however, data are obtainable from arterial blood gases that can indicate what the cells are doing metabolically, which is the most important reflection of the adequacy of their nutrient flow. The pH is the hydrogen ion concentration, which can be determined easily and quickly. Loss of buffering by base excess also mirrors excess acid load. The lactate and pyruvate concentrations also can be measured, but this is more time-consuming and can lag metabolic changes due to cellular metabolism or clearance of lactate and other metabolic by-products. Nevertheless, the pH, BD and the two carbon fragment metabolites are very important indicators of cellular function in shock.

In shock, there is a fundamental shift in metabolism. When there is adequate nutrient flow, glucose and oxygen are coupled to produce in glycolysis the high-energy phosphate bonds necessary for energy exchange. This process of aerobic metabolism also produces two freely diffusable by-products – carbon dioxide and water – both of which leave the body by excretion through the lung and the kidney. Aerobic metabolism is efficient, therefore, there is no accumulation of any products of this catabolism, and a high yield of ATP is obtained from this complete combustion of metabolites.

When there is inadequate delivery of nutrients and oxygen, as occurs in shock, the cells shift to anaerobic metabolism within 3–5 minutes. There are immediate consequences of anaerobic metabolism in addition to its inefficient yield of energy. In the absence of aerobic metabolism, energy extraction takes place at the expense of accumulating hydrogen ion, lactate, and pyruvate, which have toxic effects on normal physiology. These products of anaerobic metabolism can be seen as the 'oxygen debt'. There is some buffer capacity in the body that allows this debt to accumulate within limits but it must ultimately be shut off by adequate oxygen and nutrient delivery.

Acidosis has significant consequences in compensatory physiology. In the first instance, oxyhaemoglobin dissociates more readily as hydrogen ions increase. However, there is a significant toxicity of hydrogen ions as well. Despite the salutary effect on oxyhaemoglobin dissociation, the hydrogen ion has a negative effect on oxygen delivery. Catecholamines speed up the heart's rate and increase its contractile force, and the product of this inotropic and chronotropic effect is an increase in cardiac output. Catecholamines, however, are physiologically effective at alkaline or neutral pH. Therefore, an acid pH inactivates this catecholamine method of compensation for decreased nutrient flow. For example, if a catecholamine like isoproterenol is administered to a patient in shock, it would increase myocardial contractility and heart rate and also dilate the periphery to increase nutrient flow to these ischaemic circulation areas. However, the ischaemic areas have shifted to anaerobic metabolism, accumulating hydrogen ion, lactate and pyruvate. When the circulation dilates, this sequestered oxygen debt is dumped into the central circulation, and the drop in pH inactivates the catecholamines circulatory improvement as effectively as if the infusion of the agent had been interrupted.

inadequate circulation. Terminally, the lactacidaemia cannot be corrected by improvement of circulation and oxygen delivery once the cells are irreparably damaged.

In the low-output shock state, plasma concentrations of free fatty acids and triglycerides rise to high levels because ketone production by beta-oxidation of fatty acids in the liver is reduced, suppressing the acetoacetate-to-betahydroxybutarate ratio in the plasma.

The post-shock sequel of inadequate nutrient flow, therefore, is progressive loss of function. The rate at which this loss occurs depends upon the cell's ability to switch metabolism, the cell's ability to convert alternate fuels to energy, the increased extraction of oxygen from haemoglobin, and the compensatory collaboration of failing cells and organs whereby nutrients may be shunted selectively to more critical systems. Not all cells are equally sensitive to shock or similarly refractory to restoration of function when adequate nutrient flow is restored. As cells lose function, the reserves of the organ composed of those cells are depleted until impaired function of the organ results. These organs function in systems and a 'system failure' results. Multiple systems failure occurring in sequence leads to the collapse of the organism.

3.2.5 **Post-shock and Multiple Organ Failure Syndromes**

Although the primary consequence of sepsis following trauma and shock is the development of multiple organ failure as discussed elsewhere in this book, it is important to briefly reiterate the usual sequence of events following shock to enable logical discussion of the management of shock.

The ultimate cause of death in shock is failure of energy production as reflected by a decline in oxygen consumption (VO_2) to less than 100 mL/min/m². Circulatory insufficiency is responsible for this fall in energy, compounded by impairment of cellular oxidative phosphorylation by endotoxin and endogenously produced substances, such as toxic oxides.

In shock, whether hypovolaemic or septic, energy production is insufficient to satisfy cellular requirements. In the presence of oxygen deprivation and cellular injury, the conversion of pyruvate to acetyl-COA for entry into the Krebs cycle is inhibited. Lactic acid accumulates and the oxidation-reduction potential falls. Although lactate is normally used by the liver via the Cori cycle to synthesize glucose, hepatic gluconeogenesis may fail in hypovolaemic or septic shock because of hepatocyte injury and

3.2.6 **Management of the Shocked Patient**

The primary goal of shock resuscitation is the early establishment of adequate oxygen delivery (DO_2). The calculated variable of DO_2 is the product of cardiac output and arterial oxygen content (CaO_2).

By convention, CO is indexed to body surface area and expressed as a cardiac index (CI), and when multiplied by CaO_2, yields an oxygen delivery index (DO_2I). Normal DO_2I is roughly 450 mL/min/m².

CaO_2 and DO_2I are calculated as follows:

$$CaO_2 \text{ (mL. } O_2/dL = [Hb](g/dL) \times 1.38 \text{ mL } O_2/g \text{ Hb} \times SaO_2 \text{ (\%)} + [PaO_2 \text{ (mm Hg)} \times 0.003 \text{ mL } O_2/mm \text{ Hg}]$$

$$DO_2I \text{ (mL/min/m}^2) = CI \text{ (L/min/m}^2) \times CaO_2 \text{ (mL/dL)} \times 10 \text{ dL/L}$$

where Hb is haemoglobin concentration, SaO_2 is haemoglobin oxygen saturation, PaO_2 is arterial oxygen tension and 0.003 is the solubility of O_2 in blood.

Early work demonstrated that the 'survivor' response to traumatic stress is to become hyperdynamic. Supranormal resuscitation based on the DO_2I was therefore proposed. Subsequent randomized controlled trials have failed to demonstrate improved outcomes with goal-directed supranormal therapy, and, in fact, this strategy increased ACS, MOF and death. The 'Glue Grant' study for shock resuscitation[19] suggests using a CI >3.8 L/min/m^2 as the resuscitation goal.

The purpose for distinguishing the different pathophysiologic mechanisms of shock becomes important when treatment has to be initiated. The final aim of treatment is to restore aerobic cellular metabolism. This requires restoration of adequate flow of oxygenated blood (which is dependent on optimal oxygenation of sufficient red blood cells, i.e. haematocrit, and adequate cardiac output). The initial focus is securing a patent airway and controlling ventilation to prevent inadequate alveolar ventilation and oxygenation.

Restoration of optimal circulating blood volume, enhancing cardiac output through the use of inotropic agents and/or MAP through the use of vasopressors, the correction of acid-base disturbances and metabolic deficits and the combating of sepsis are all vital in the management of the shocked patient.

Best practice guidelines for shock resuscitation are summarized by the large-scale collaborative project called Glue Grant that provides standard operating procedures for clinical care. (See recommended reading below.)

3.2.6.1 OXYGENATION

The severely traumatized, hypovolaemic or septic patient has an oxygen demand that may exceed twice the normal. However, the traumatized shocked patient usually cannot generate the additional respiratory effort required, and therefore often develops respiratory failure followed by a lactic acidosis due to tissue hypoxaemia.

In some patients, an oxygen mask may be enough to maintain sufficient oxygen delivery to the lungs. In more severe cases, endotracheal intubation and ventilatory assistance may be necessary. It is important to distinguish between the need for *intubation* and the need for *ventilation*. And early intubation is preferable to cardiac collapse.

3.2.6.1.1 Airway Indications for Intubation

- Obstructed airway.
- Inadequate gag reflex.

3.2.6.1.2 Breathing Indications for Intubation

- Inability to breathe (e.g. paralysis, either spinal or drug induced).
- Tidal volume less than 5 mL/kg.

3.2.6.1.3 Breathing Indications for Ventilation

- Inability to oxygenate adequately.
- PaO$_2$ less than 60 mm Hg (7.9 kPa) on 40% O$_2$.
- SpO$_2$ of less than 90 per cent on oxygen.
- Respiration rate of 30 breaths or more per minute.
- Excessive ventilatory effort.
- PaCO$_2$ of greater than 45 (6 kPa) mm Hg with metabolic acidosis, or greater than 50 mm Hg (6.6 kPa) with normal bicarbonate levels.

3.2.6.1.4 Circulation Indication for Intubation

- Systolic blood pressure less than 75 mm Hg despite resuscitation.

3.2.6.1.5 Disability Indications for Intubation

- High spinal injury with inability to breathe.
- Coma (GCS <8/15).

3.2.6.1.6 Environmental Indication for Intubation

- Core temperature of <32°C.

If ventilatory support is instituted the goals are relatively specific.

The respiratory rate should be adjusted to ensure a PaCO$_2$ of between 35 and 40 mm Hg (4.6–5.3 kPa). This will avoid respiratory alkalosis and a consequential shift of the oxyhaemoglobin dissociation curve to the left, which results in an increased haemoglobin affinity for oxygen and significantly decreases oxygen availability to tissues, which will require increased cardiac output to maintain tissue oxygenation. Respiratory alkalosis also causes vasoconstriction of cerebral vessels and a further decrease in oxygen delivery to the central nervous system (CNS).

The arterial PaO$_2$ should be maintained between 80 and 100 mm Hg (10.6 and 13.2 kPa) with the lowest possible inspired oxygen concentration.

It has also been shown that increased respiratory effort requires a disproportionate share of the total cardiac output for the respiratory muscles and, therefore, other organs are deprived of necessary blood flow and lactic acidosis is potentiated. Mechanical ventilation tends to reverse this lactic acidosis.

3.2.6.2 FLUID THERAPY FOR VOLUME EXPANSION

Considerable controversy exists regarding the type of fluid to be administered for volume expansion in hypovolaemic shock. Despite many studies, minimal convincing evidence exists that favours any specific fluid regimen. Balanced salt solutions (BSSs) are effective volume expanders for the initial resuscitation of patients with shock. For most patients, Ringer lactate solution is the preferred crystalloid solution. The lactate acts as a buffer and is eventually metabolized by the liver to carbon dioxide and water. However, septic patients with significant hepatic dysfunction do not metabolize lactate well and for these patients, other balanced salt solutions are preferred. Also, since Ringer lactate contains potassium, patients in shock with potential acute kidney injury should not be given Ringer lactate during acute resuscitation until adequate renal function is confirmed.

To reverse hypovolaemic shock, a volume of solution in excess of measured losses is generally required. In principle, three times the volume of BSS is given per unit of blood lost. A bolus dose of 2000 mL of BSS (e.g. Ringer lactate) in adults is given and the response of pulse rate, blood pressure and urinary output monitored. If this fails to correct haemodynamic abnormalities, additional crystalloid solution plus blood is indicated, because crystalloids in large quantities will ultimately cause a dilutional effect that can decrease the blood's oxygen-carrying capacity and enhance any ongoing coagulopathy. While increased cardiac output may maintain tissue oxygenation, which can be sustained by the normal heart, in the diseased heart or the elderly patient, it is safer to give blood earlier to obviate the possibility of cardiac failure. In many countries, packed red blood cells with crystalloid solutions, instead of whole blood, are given because the blood banking industry in those countries utilizes component therapy to such an extent that whole blood is not readily available for large volume transfusion.

3.2.6.2.1 Crystalloids or Colloids?

Crystalloids are cheaper, with fewer side effects. Colloids are more expensive, and have more side effects[20]. However, their rate of loss in non-shocked patients is much slower than that of crystalloids, so that the volume remains in the circulation for longer. Balanced salt solutions are said to have a half-life in the circulation of 20 min, while a colloid such as Gelufusine has a half-life of 4–6 hours. However, additional considerations relate to rate of colloid loss from the intravascular space following severe shock and resuscitation-induced capillary leak, which may negate any presumed benefit. A recent Cochrane review of the available trial data comparing crystalloids and colloids for resuscitation after trauma showed no improvement in survival with colloids; in fact, there was a worse outcome, and therefore the preferential use of colloids cannot be supported at present[10]. Lactated Ringer is the currently preferred crystalloid. Similarly, no advantages have been demonstrated in the use of newer formulations utilizing pyruvate or acetate. Normal saline can be used but results in an increased risk of hyperchloraemic acidosis.

3.2.6.2.2 Hypotensive Resuscitation

In 1994, Bickell et al.[21] concluded that patients with penetrating torso trauma in hypovolaemic shock who were not given intravenous fluids during transport and emergency department evaluation had a better chance of survival than those who received conventional volume resuscitation. However, the only difference in survival was in the subgroup with pericardial tamponade. In animal studies, intravenous fluids have been shown to inhibit platelet aggregation, dilute clotting factors, modulate the physical properties of thrombus and cause increases in blood pressure that can mechanically disrupt clot[22]. Thus, the benefit of restricted resuscitation volumes was possibly because the reduced blood pressure limited the amount of blood loss. However, in the typical civilian trauma centre, blunt trauma is the most common form of injury and inadequate resuscitation leads to further organ injury due to inadequate oxygen delivery, particularly with traumatic brain injury (TBI). Thus, while the ideal approach is not known, the optimum systolic blood pressure for a patient with uncontrolled haemorrhage appears to be approximately 90 mm Hg (mean arterial pressure [MAP] approximately 70 mm Hg), for both the military environment, and, likely, the civilian setting also.

3.2.6.2.3 Hypertonic Saline

Hypertonic saline[2,13,14] solutions containing up to 7.5 per cent sodium chloride (compared with 0.9 per cent for normal saline) show promise for resuscitating patients in situations where large-volume resuscitation with isotonic solutions is impossible (e.g. combat, events involving mass casualties and prehospital trauma care). Hypertonic solutions provide far more blood volume expansion than isotonic solutions and result in less cellular oedema. Several randomized controlled trials have evaluated the use of hypertonic saline in the resuscitation of hypovolaemia. In some of these trials, patients resuscitated with saline survived longer than those resuscitated in the conventional fashion. The patients did best when the hypertonic saline was given as the initial therapy and those patients most likely to benefit were those with head injuries. In addition, hypertonic saline may be more effective when mixed with a small amount of an oncotically active molecule such as dextran. However, a recent trial by Bulger et al., with the Resuscitations Outcome Consortium (ROC) showed an increased mortality in patients in whom hypertonic saline had been used[25]. No adequately powered trial to date has demonstrated any survival benefits, and in view of the costs, these solutions cannot be recommended.

3.2.6.2.4 Blood Substitutes

Blood substitutes, including haemoglobin-based preparations and perfluorocarbons, have several potential advantages. No cross-matching is necessary, disease transmission is not an issue, and shelf life is extended. Several haemoglobin substitutes are being evaluated, but at present remain experimental and are not approved for human use in trauma.

3.2.6.3 ROUTE OF ADMINISTRATION

3.2.6.3.1 Intravenous Devices

In principle, with all intravenous lines, the shorter the line and the wider the diameter of the cannula, the faster will be the flow. For the same bore of line, flow rates are reduced:

- 14-Gauge (14G) via peripheral cannula: full flow.
- 14-Gauge via 30-cm central line: 33 per cent reduction in flow.
- 14-Gauge via 70-cm central line: 50 per cent reduction in flow.

Cannula Size	Flow Rates (mL/min)	
	Crystalloid	Colloid
8.5 FG (French gauge)	1000	600
14 G	125	90
16 G	85	65
18 G	60	35
20 G	40	17

A minimum of two lines is required in the severely injured or hypotensive patient. In all cases of hypovolaemic

shock, two large-bore peripheral lines are essential. A central line is most useful for monitoring, but can be used for transfusion as well. The monitoring line should be a central venous line, inserted via the subclavian, jugular or femoral route. In blunt polytrauma, the subclavian route is preferable, since this approach avoids any movement of the head in a patient whose neck has not yet been cleared. The jugular route is less preferable because of issues in securing the lines and earlier sepsis at the insertion site due to movement.

3.2.6.3.2 Intraosseus Devices

Intraosseous infusion is the process of injecting directly into the marrow of a bone to provide a non-collapsible entry point into the venous system. This technique is used in emergency and military situations to provide fluids and medication when intravenous access is not feasible. A comparison of intravenous, intramuscular and intraosseous routes of administration concluded that in children, the intraosseous route is demonstrably superior to the intramuscular route, and comparable to the intravenous route[26].

Insertion in adults requires less than a minute, and flow rates of up to 125 mL/min have been achieved. The devices are for emergency resuscitation and should be removed within 24 hours.

Suitable devices include the BIG gun (WaisMed, Houston, TX) and the EZ-IO (Vidacare Corp., San Antonio, TX).

3.2.6.4 PHARMACOLOGIC SUPPORT OF BLOOD PRESSURE

Stroke volume is controlled by ventricular pre-load, after-load and contractility. Ventricular pre-load is influenced primarily by the volume of circulating blood, but after-load and contractility can be enhanced by pharmacological agents. Reducing the systemic vascular resistance with vasodilators can be a very effective means of improving cardiac output when systemic pressures or cardiac filling pressures are normal or elevated, but is not currently recommended for acute trauma.

3.2.6.4.1 Noradrenaline (Norepinephrine)

The preferred inotropic agent for acute trauma is noradrenaline (norepinephrine). It is a sympathetic neurotransmitter with potent inotropic effects. It activates myocardial β-adrenergic receptors and vascular α-adrenergic receptors. It is used in the treatment of shock and hypotension characterized by low systemic vascular resistance and unresponsiveness to fluid resuscitation.

3.2.6.4.2 Adrenaline (Epinephrine)

Adrenaline is a natural catecholamine with both α- and β-adrenergic agonist activity. The pharmacological actions are complex, and it can produce the following cardiovascular responses:

- Increased systemic vascular resistance.
- Increased systolic and diastolic blood pressure.
- Increased electrical activity in the myocardium.
- Increased coronary and cerebral blood flow.
- Increased strength of myocardial contraction.
- Increased myocardial oxygen requirement.

The primary beneficial effect of adrenaline is peripheral vasoconstriction, with improved coronary and cerebral blood flow. It works as chronotropic and inotropic agents. The initial dose is 0.03 µg/Kg/min, titrated upward until the desired effect is achieved. In trauma patients, it is often used in conjunction with dobutamine.

3.2.6.4.3 Dopamine

Dopamine hydrochloride is a chemical precursor of noradrenaline that stimulates dopaminergic, β_1-adrenergic and α-adrenergic receptors in a dose-dependent fashion. Low doses of dopamine (<3 µg/Kg/min) produce cerebral, renal and mesenteric vasodilatation, and venous tone is increased. Urine output is increased, but there is no evidence to show that this is in any way protective to the kidneys.

At doses above 10 µg/Kg/min, however, the α-adrenergic effects predominate. This results in marked increases in systemic vascular resistance, pulmonary resistance and increases in pre-load due to marked arterial, splanchnic and venous constriction. It increases systolic blood pressure without increasing diastolic blood pressure or heart rate.

Dopamine is used for haemodynamically significant hypotension in the absence of hypovolaemia.

3.2.6.4.4 Dobutamine

Dobutamine is a synthetic sympathomimetic amine that has potent inotropic effects by stimulating β_1- and α_1-adrenergic receptors in the myocardium. Dobutamine-mediated increases in cardiac output also lead to a decrease in peripheral vascular resistance. At a dose of 10 µg/Kg/min, dobutamine is less likely to induce tachycardia than either adrenaline or isoproterenol. Higher doses may produce a tachycardia. Dobutamine increases cardiac output and its lack of induction of noradrenaline release means that there is a minimal effect on myocardial oxygen demand. There is also increased coronary blood flow. Dobutamine in low doses has also been used as a renal protective agent. There is little evidence to support its use on its own, but it may be helpful in improving renal perfusion as an adjunct to the administration of high-dose adrenaline.

Dobutamine and dopamine have been used together. The combination of moderate doses of both (7.5 µg/Kg/min) maintains arterial pressure with less increase in pulmonary wedge pressure than dopamine alone.

3.2.6.4.5 Isoproterenol

Isoproterenol hydrochloride is a synthetic sympathomimetic amine with a particularly strong chronotropic effect. Newer inotropic drugs such as dobutamine have largely superseded isoproterenol in most settings.

3.2.6.4.6 Nitroprusside

Sodium nitroprusside is a potent peripheral vasodilator with effects on both venous and arterial smooth muscle, and has balanced vasodilating effects on both circulations, thus minimizing adverse effects on arterial blood pressure. It has a very short half-life.

3.2.6.4.7 Digoxin

Digoxin enhances cardiac contractility but its use in shock is limited because it takes considerable time to act. In the intensive-care situation, digoxin is usually reserved for the treatment of atrial flutter and supraventricular tachycardias.

3.2.6.5 CORTISOL

The role of relative adrenal insufficiency in the management of the critically injured patient remains controversial.

3.2.6.6 METABOLIC MANIPULATIONS

The endogenous opiate beta-endorphin appears to be involved in the hypotension and impaired tissue perfusion that occur in both hypovolaemic and septic shock states. Elevations in this substance can be demonstrated at the time that these physiological changes take place. Naloxone, an opiate antagonist, has been shown to elevate blood pressure and cardiac output, and to potentially improve survival in septic and haemorrhagic shock.

Prostaglandins also have been implicated in shock. They may play a role in the pathophysiology of shock by vasodilatation or vasoconstriction of the microcirculation with shunting of blood. Experimental evidence suggests cyclo-oxygenase inhibitors like indomethacin and ibuprofen can improve the haemodynamic state in experimental shock.

3.2.7 Prognosis in Shock

The prognosis of the shocked patient depends on the duration of the shock, the underlying cause and the pre-existing vital organ function. The prognosis is best when the duration is kept short by early recognition and aggressive correction of the circulatory disturbance and when the underlying cause is known and corrected.

Occasionally, shock does not respond to standard therapeutic measures. Unresponsive shock requires an understanding of the potential occult causes of persistent physiologic disturbances.

These correctable causes include:

- Underappreciated volume losses with inadequate fluid resuscitation and a failure to assess the response to a fluid challenge.
- Erroneous presumption of overload when cardiac disease is also present.
- Hypoxia caused by inadequate ventilation, barotrauma to the lung, pneumothorax or cardiac tamponade.
- Undiagnosed or inadequately treated sepsis.
- Uncorrected acid-base or electrolyte abnormalities.
- Endocrine failure like adrenal insufficiency or hypothyroidism.
- Drug toxicity.

3.2.8 Recommended Protocol for Shock

3.2.8.1 MILITARY EXPERIENCE

Recent military experience from the Iraq war has shown the value of 'damage control resuscitation'[18,27]. This implies that damage control techniques are used from the time of injury, minimizing the time between injury and care, controlling the bleeding and the contamination, through use of minimal clear fluids, early fresh whole blood, early resuscitation and early damage control surgery. The military use of whole blood has minimized some of the risks of component therapy, and has also shown that survival is improved. From this philosophy has come the change in protocol in civilian practice towards minimizing crystalloid resuscitation (restrictive or limited resuscitation; not hypotensive) and early use of blood and blood products to maintain the normal coagulation profile as much as possible.

3.2.8.2 INITIAL RESUSCITATION

1. Major trauma patients arriving in shock (SBP <90 mm Hg and/or HR >130 bpm) are managed using ATLS protocols.
2. Major torso trauma patients requiring ongoing resuscitation should have a central venous line placed in the emergency department.
3. Early CVP >15 mm Hg (before extensive volume loading) suggests cardiogenic or cardiac compressive shock.
4. CVP <10 mm Hg despite volume loading suggests ongoing bleeding. Endpoints are currently vague. At present the rational compromise is volume limited resuscitation (SBP = 90 mm Hg and HR <130 bpm) with moderate volume loading until haemorrhage is controlled.
5. Boluses of Ringer lactate should be continued, and when the amount exceeds 30 mL/kg, blood should be administered.
6. Patients at risk for trauma-induced coagulopathy (TIC) should have a massive infusion protocol initiated. (See Section 4.7)

3.2.8.3 INTENSIVE CARE UNIT (ICU) RESUSCITATION

1. On arrival, a decision is made on continuing resuscitation using serial vital signs.
2. For patients not responding to ongoing volume loading or transfusion, cardiac output monitoring or pulmonary artery catheterization is warranted.
3. Intubation should be considered if not already performed.
4. If CI >3.8 L/min/m² the patient should be monitored appropriately.
5. Haemoglobin should be maintained at between 8 and 10 g/dL for the acute resuscitation phase.

6. Pulmonary capillary wedge pressure (PCWP) greater than 15 mm Hg may enhance cardiac performance.

7. After obtaining an optimal PCWP, if CI <3.8 L/min/m^2 then infusion of a vasodilating inotropic agent should be considered. Dobutamine is recommended as the preferred agent, commencing at a dose of 5 μg/kg/min. If the patient does not tolerate the vasodilatation, then an agent such as dopamine should be considered.

8. Occasionally an inotropic agent with vasoconstrictive effects such as noradrenaline (norepinephrine), alone or in combination with vasopressin and/or adrenaline (epinephrine), may be required.

REFERENCES AND RECOMMENDED READING

References

1. Cuthbertson D. Observations on disturbance of metabolism produced by injury of the limbs. *Q J Med.* 1932;25:233–236.

2. Lilly MP, Gann DS. The hypothalamic-pituitary-adrenal immune axis. *Arch Surg.* 1992;12712):1463–1474.

3 Kapur MM, Jain P, Gidh M. The effect of trauma on serum C3 activation, and its correlation with Injury Severity Score in man. *J Trauma.* 1986;26(5):464–466.

4. Bianchi ME. DAMPS, PAMPS and alarmins: all we need to know about danger. *J Leukocyte Biol.* 2007;81:1–5.

5. Zhang Q, Raoof M, Chen Y, et al. Circulating mitochondrial DAMPS cause inflammatory responses to injury. *Nature.* 2010;464:104–107.

6. Porte D, Robertson RP. Control of insulin by catecholamines, stress, and the sympathetic nervous system. *Federal Proc.* 1973;32:1792–1796.

7. Needleman P, Greenwald JF. Atriopeptin: a cardiac hormone intimately involved in fluid, electrolyte and blood pressure homeostasis. *New Engl J Med.* 1986;314:828–834.

8. Roumen RMH, Redl H, Schlag G, et al. Scoring systems and blood lactate concentrations in relationship to the development of adult respiratory distress syndrome and multiple organ failure in severely traumatized patients. *J Trauma.* 1993;35(3):349–355.

9. Shaw JHF, Wolfe RR. An integrated analysis of glucose, fat and protein metabolism in severely traumatized patients: studies in the basal state and the response to total parenteral nutrition. *Ann Surg.* 1989;209(1):63–72.

10. Moore FA, Moore EE, Poggetti R, et al. Gut bacterial translocation via the portal vein: a clinical perspective with major torso trauma. *J Trauma.* 1991;31:629–638.

11. Teplitz C. The pathology and ultrastructure of cellular injury and inflammation in the progression and outcome of trauma, sepsis and shock. In: Clowes GHA, ed. *Trauma Sepsis and Shock.* New York, NY: Marcel Dekker Inc.; 1988:71–120.

12. Sillesen M, Rasmussen LS, Jin G, et al. Assessment of coagulopathy, endothelial injury, and inflammation after traumatic brain injury and haemorrhage in a porcine model. *J Trauma.* 2014;76(1):12–19.

13. Central venipuncture. Advanced Trauma Life Support Course. Chicago, IL: American College of Surgeons; 2008:73–81.

14. Subclavian venipuncture. Advanced Trauma Life Support Course. Chicago, IL: American College of Surgeons; 2008:76.

15. Femoral venipuncture. Advanced Trauma Life Support Course. Chicago, IL: American College of Surgeons; 2008:76.

16. Ramsay JG, Bevan DR. Cardiac emergencies. In: Ellis BW, ed. *Hamilton Bailey's Emergency Surgery.* 13th ed. London: Arnold; 2000:48–57.

17. Elkayam U, Berkley R, Asen S, et al. Cardiac output by thermodilution technique. *Chest.* 1983;84:418–422.

18. Gump FE. Whole body metabolism. In: Altura BM, Lefer AM, Shumer W, eds. *Handbook of Shock and Trauma. Vol. I. Basic Sciences.* New York, NY: Raven Press; 1983:89–113.

19. Moore FA, McKinley BA, Moore EE, et al. Inflammation and the Host Response to Injury Large Scale Collaborative Research Program III. Guidelines for shock resuscitation. *J Trauma.* 2006;61(1):82–89.

20. Alderson P, Schierhout G, Roberts I, Bunn F. Colloids versus crystalloids for fluid resuscitation in critically ill patients. *Cochrane Database Syst Rev.* 2000;2:CD000567.

21. Bickell WH, Wall MJ, Pepe PE. Immediate versus delayed resuscitation for hypotensive patients with penetrating torso injuries. *N Engl J Med.* 1994;331:1105–1107.

22. Roberts I, Evans P, Bunn F, Kwan I, Crowhurst E. Is the normalisation of blood pressure in bleeding trauma patients harmful? *Lancet.* 2001;357:385–387.

23 Younes RN, Aun F, Accioly CQ. Hypertonic saline in the treatment of hypovolaemic shock: a prospective controlled randomized trial in patients admitted to the emergency room. *Surgery.* 1992;111:380–385.

24. Wisner DH, Schuster L, Quinn C. Hypertonic saline resuscitation of head injury: effects on cerebral water content. *J Trauma.* 1990;30:75–78.

25. Bulger EM, May S, Kerby JD, et al. Out of hospital hypertonic resuscitation after traumatic hypovolaemic shock: A randomised placebo controlled trial. *Ann Surg.* 2011;253(3):431–441.

26. Moore GP, Pace SA, Busby W. Comparison of intraosseus, intramuscular, and intravenous administration of succinyl choline. *Pediatr Emerg Care.* 1989;5(4):209–210.

27. Holcomb JB, Jenkins D, Rhee P, et al. Damage control resuscitation: directly addressing the early coagulopathy of trauma. *J Trauma.* 2007;62(2):307–310.

28. Hess JR, Holcomb JB, Hoyt DB. Damage control resuscitation: the need for specific blood products to treat the coagulopathy of trauma. *Transfusion.* 2006;46(5):685–686.

Recommended Reading

Advanced Cardiovascular Life Support Provider Manual. Dallas, TX: American Heart Association; 2010.

Dellinger RP, Levy MM, Rhodes A, et al. Surviving Sepsis Campaign: International Guidelines for Management of Severe Sepsis and Septic Shock (2012). *Crit Care Med.,* 2013;41(2):580–637.

Holcroft JT, Anderson JT, Sena MJ. *Shock.* In: *Surgery: Principles and Practice* (Section 8, Chapter 3). New York, NY: Web MD Publishing; 2007.

Moore FA, McKinley BA, Moore EE, et al. Inflammation and the Host Response to Injury Large Scale Collaborative Research Program III. Guidelines for shock resuscitation. *J Trauma.* 2006;61(1):81–89.

Transfusion in Trauma 4

Transfusion of blood and blood components is a fundamental part of our treatment of injured patients. Approximately 40 per cent of 11 million units of blood transfused in the United States each year are used in emergency resuscitation. Despite this, there is little level I evidence to provide a rationale for administration of packed red blood cells (pRBCs) to trauma patients.

4.1 INDICATIONS FOR TRANSFUSION

Anaemia is a decrease in the O_2-carrying capacity of blood, and is defined by a decrease in circulating red cell mass (to below 24 mL/kg in females and 26 mL/kg in males). Anaemia will result in an increase in cardiac output at a haemoglobin (Hb) level of <7 g/dL (4 mmol/L). Oxygen extraction increases as O_2 delivery falls, ensuring a constant O_2 uptake by the tissues. The threshold for O_2 delivery is at a haematocrit of 10 per cent and an Hb level of 3 g/dL (1.8 mmol/L) when breathing 100 per cent O_2 and with a normal metabolic rate.

4.2 TRANSFUSION FLUIDS

Normal humans can survive an 80 per cent loss of red cell mass if they are normovolaemic. Volume-dependent markers such as packed cell volume and Hb are poor indicators of anaemia because of the effect of dilution after fluid transfusion on their values (i.e. they are relative values).

4.2.1 Colloids

4.2.1.1 STARCHES

The use of starches is contraindicated in the actively bleeding patient, since all starches deplete the von Willebrand/factor VIII complex[1], and may make the actively bleeding patient more coagulopathic from both factor depletion and dilution coagulopathy. Hydroxyethyl starch is an independent risk factor for acute kidney injury and death after blunt trauma[2].

4.2.1.2 ALBUMIN

Human albumin is produced from blood donors but is also contraindicated in trauma patients. The Saline versus Albumin Fluid Evaluation (SAFE) study in 2007 tested saline versus albumin and demonstrated an increased mortality in trauma patients and in particular in patients with traumatic brain injury (TBI). Albumin is no longer used in the acute resuscitation of a patient with trauma or burns.

4.2.2 Fresh Whole Blood

The human being is an O_2-dependent organism, and O_2 depletion causes major damage within minutes. Thus, in the exsanguinating patient, blood is transfused, in order to improve O_2 transport. Evidence from the Iraq and Afghan wars and recent studies in civilian trauma have highlighted the advantage of fresh whole blood (FWB) in the resuscitation and survival of the exsanguinating patient[3]. The rationale is that FWB has more function than purely that of an O_2 carrier, providing:

- Oncotic pressure (from plasma and stored fresh frozen plasma [FFP]).
- Coagulation function (clotting factors in FFP and platelets [PLT]).
- Temperature homeostasis (from warm circulating fluid).
- Fresh whole blood offers blood at close to 37°C, RBCs, plasma and platelets in natural proportions, to cover the need of the exsanguinating patient for

O_2 and oncotic pressure, and to minimize the acute coagulopathy of trauma shock (ACoTS). A 500-mL unit of FWB has a haematocrit of 38–50 per cent, 150 000–400 000 fully functional platelets/mm³ and 100 per cent activity of clotting factors diluted only by the 70 mL of anticoagulant. In addition, the viability and flow characteristics of fresh RBCs are better than their stored counterparts that have metabolic depletion and membrane dysfunction[3]. However, FWB, unless in a military environment with a large number of healthy, screened, young blood carriers, is generally not available.

4.2.3 Packed Red Blood Cells

Previous haemorrhage management transfused excessive amounts of crystalloids and packed red blood cells (pRBCs), which diluted native clotting factors, causing hypocoagulation[4]. This additional fluid aggravated the coagulopathy initiated from the moment of injury due to:

- The injury itself, and in proportion to its extent (hypoperfusion resulted in increased activated protein C levels, leading to increased tissue plasminogen activator and increased fibrinolysis).
- Loss of warm blood and replacement with cooler fluid, resulting in decreased body temperature.
- Hypoperfusion, resulting in anaerobic metabolism, increased lactic acid production and a decrease in pH.

Biochemical reactions within the body require a specific and narrow temperature and pH range to proceed. The coagulation cascade does not proceed, even in the presence of all the clotting factors, when the tissue pH is below 7.2 and temperature below 34°C. This is defined as acute coagulopathy of trauma-shock (ACoTS)[5] (also known as trauma-induced coagulopathy [TIC]), and differs from disseminated intravascular coagulopathy, which may develop after hours or days, when the septic component adds its consequences to trauma.

Fresh whole blood can, if warmed, be transfused within 24 hours. It is, however, considered still fresh if stored at 4°C for 48 hours[3]. If it is less than 8 hours old, it can be refrigerated for 3 weeks[2], remaining transfusable but not fresh.

The levels of clotting factors V and VIII decline quickly for 24 hours after collection. The rate of decline then slows until clinically subnormal levels are reached within 7–14 days. It is because FWB contains these factors that it is recommended for massive transfusion and is so effective in the correction of coagulopathy. The other clotting factors remain stable in stored blood. Fresh whole blood has lost most of its platelets after 3 days of storage.

4.2.4 Component Therapy (Platelets, Fresh Frozen Plasma, Cryoprecipitate)

4.2.4.1 PLATELETS

A fall in platelet count occurs somewhat later than the loss of clotting factors. Unfortunately, a platelet count is not helpful, unless very low levels are documented, since it is a poor clinical indicator of the function of the remaining platelets. Hypothermia affects platelet adhesion more than enzymes, above 33°C, while hypothermia affects all aspects of coagulation below 33°C. There is some evidence in which there appears to be a survival advantage of receiving approximately 0.8 units of platelets per unit of RBCs during massive transfusion[6]:

- Prophylaxis: if the platelet count <15 000/mm.
- Pre-surgery: platelet count <50 000/mm³.
- Active bleeding: platelet count <100 000/mm³.
- One unit increases the platelet count by 10 000/mm³ platelets.
- One mega-unit (five units) of apheresis platelets increases the platelet count by 50 000/mm³.

4.2.4.2 FRESH FROZEN PLASMA

Most massively bleeding trauma patients will need FFP early. This is different from most recommendations, which are based on more controlled circumstances, and is founded on computer simulation of the amount of FFP required to avoid excessive plasma dilution compromising haemostasis. Current evidence suggests that most patients will require one unit of FFP for every unit of blood transfused. A unit of FFP also contains most of the citrate anticoagulant from the unit of blood from which it was originally derived. It contains about 0.5 g fibrinogen, and normal levels of pro- and anticoagulants. Solvent-detergent-related/freeze-dried plasma carries about 20 per cent less of the above per unit given. Potential advantages are:

- It contains all coagulation factors, but not all in equal concentrations.
- It is preferred to cryoprecipitate, which contains 50 per cent of coagulation factors (especially of fibrinogen, factor VIII and von Willebrand factor).

4.2.4.3 CRYOPRECIPITATE

Cryoprecipitate contains fibrinogen, von Willebrand factor/factor VIII complex and fibrin stabilising factor/factor XIII. Cryoprecipitate may not be required in all cases of trauma. One unit (250 mL) of FFP contains 0.5 g fibrinogen; one unit of cryoprecipitate contains 0.25 g fibrinogen, but in 10 mL (rather than 250 mL). Therefore, in most cases, FFP will meet the needs required. However, if a rapid increase in the amount of fibrinogen is required, cryoprecipitate is a useful adjunct.

4.2.4.4 FIBRINOGEN CONCENTRATE

Fibrinogen concentrate can be used to correct acquired hypofibrinogenaemia in trauma. There are several guidelines, but evidence is lacking regarding the treatment efficacy and safety in trauma. So far no level I evidence supports the use in trauma.

4.3 EFFECTS OF TRANSFUSING BLOOD AND BLOOD PRODUCTS

Stored pRBCs (stored for a maximum of 42 days with current US Food and Drug Administration [FDA]-approved storage solutions) develop defects proportionate to the duration of storage that assume greater clinical significance when transfused rapidly, or in large quantities, such as in critically ill patients[4].

4.3.1 Metabolic Effects

Stored packed red blood cells (pRBC) (stored for a maximum of 42 days with current FDA-approved storage solutions) develop defects proportionate to the duration of storage that assume greater clinical significance when transfused rapidly.

- There is a storage-related decreased ATP which precedes red blood cell membrane deformability and its survival during storage.
- Degradation of 2,3-diphosphoglycerate (2,3-DPG) occurs after 7–10 days in storage. 2,3-Diphosphoglycerate is an enzyme affecting the affinity of Hb for O_2. After 7 days of storage, the O_2-transporting ability of Hb drops by two-thirds. Adenine added to pRBCs may restore levels of 2,3-DPG *in vivo* after transfusion, although there is limited level I evidence in this respect.

- Increased ammonia release occurs due to the release of intracellular protein after disruption of the red cell membrane during storage.

4.3.2 Effects of Microaggregates

This remains controversial; however, microfilters are no longer used.

- Red cell membrane instability leads to cell rupture.
- Increased amounts of microaggregates (platelets/leukocytes/fibrin debris) are found in the buffy coat.
- Impaired pulmonary gas exchange and adult respiratory distress syndrome (ARDS) and transfusion-related lung injury (TRALI) can occur.
- Reticuloendothelial system (RES) depression can occur.
- Activation of complement and coagulation cascades may occur.
- Vasoactive substances may be produced.
- Antigenic stimulation may occur.
- Acute-phase response may be seen.

4.3.3 Hyperkalaemia

Serum potassium levels rise in stored blood as the efficiency of the Na^+/K^+ pump decreases. Transfused blood may have a potassium concentration of >40 mmol/L. Transient hyperkalaemia may occur as a result but often does not need correction.

4.3.4 Coagulation Abnormalities

Fresh frozen plasma contains all the clotting factors of the coagulation cascade. Thawed plasma is FFP brought to 4°C and stored for 5 days, this timeline being based on the lifetime of factors V and VIII. Recent studies have shown that thawed plasma stored at this temperature retains significant clotting function for up to 14 days[1]. More recent evidence promotes the use of liquid (never frozen) plasma, retaining the clotting factors' efficacy for even longer.

- Thrombocytopenia and a loss of factors V and VIII in stored blood may contribute to the coagulopathy. Platelets have a short half-life, and their functioning is usually minimal after 3–5 days of storage.
- Levels of clotting factors V and VIII decline quickly for 24 hours after collection. The rate of decline

slows until clinically subnormal levels are reached at 7–14 days. It is because FWB contains these factors that it is recommended for massive transfusion, although it is generally not available outside the military for cost and legal reasons. The other clotting factors remain stable in stored blood.

- Packed red cells do not contain platelets as these are generally spun off, and whole blood has lost most of its platelets after 3 days of storage. Spontaneous bleeding rarely occurs if the platelet count is greater than 30 000/mm^3. Levels as low as this are seen after the replacement of one to two times the total blood volume, and may result from dilution. Despite this, the body has large reserves of platelets, sequestrated in the spleen, liver and endothelium, that are mobilized when there is a need.
- In whole blood, platelets may contribute to microaggregates that find their way to the lungs. Their presence is less evident in packed red cells. Transfusion of pooled platelets carries a greater risk of infection, as several donors have contributed to a single pack of platelets.

Ideally, the transfusion of blood components should be guided by viscoelastic laboratory tests of clotting function, such as thromboelastography (TEG). This is most relevant where surgical bleeding is controlled. However, in the face of continued bleeding, despite surgical control, blood products may need to be given empirically.

It is important to detect trauma-induced coagulopathy as early as possible. Conventional coagulation tests, such as prothrombin time/international ratio (PT/INR), activated partial thromboplastin time (APTT), fibrinogen concentration and platelet counts, have traditionally been used. However, there is a striking lack of evidence to support the use of conventional coagulation tests (CCTs) to monitor resuscitation, although thresholds based on CCTs have been suggested.

On the other hand, the enthusiasm and literature around viscoelastic haemostatic assays (VHAs) like rotational thromboelastometry (ROTEM) and TEG in the trauma setting are increasing. The VHA may be performed bedside and provide results within minutes. Over the last years various papers have been published trying to identify VHA patterns and thresholds characterizing ATC and need for massive transfusion in trauma patients. However, the evidence to prove its superiority and practical use in identifying ATC or predicting the need for transfusions in the acute setting is still not conclusive. (See Section 4.4.6.2.)

4.3.5 Other Risks of Transfusion

4.3.5.1 TRANSFUSION-TRANSMITTED INFECTIONS

- Hepatitis A, B, C and D.
- Human immunodeficiency virus 'window period'.
- Cytomegalovirus.
- Atypical mononucleosis and a swinging temperature that can be present for 7–10 days post-transfusion.
- Malaria.
- Brucellosis.
- Yersinia.
- Syphilis.

4.3.5.2 HAEMOLYTIC TRANSFUSION REACTIONS

- Incompatibility: ABO, rhesus (type the blood) and 26 other surface antigens (screen for these).
- To very cold blood, overheated blood or pressurized blood.
- Immediate generalized reaction (plasma).

4.3.5.3 IMMUNOLOGICAL COMPLICATIONS

- Major incompatibility reaction (usually caused by 'wrong blood' due to administrative errors).
- Graft-versus-host disease: Transfusion-related acute lung injury (TRALI).
- Immunomodulation: Reports on transplant and oncology patients have provided evidence that transfusion induces a regulatory immune response in the recipient that increases the ratio of suppressor to helper T cells. These changes may render the trauma patient more susceptible to infection.

4.3.5.4 FACTORS IMPLICATED IN HAEMOSTATIC FAILURE

- Hypothermia: Blood is stored at 4°C but body temperature is 37°C, so the body needs to provide 1255 kJ of energy to heat each unit of blood to body temperature.
- Acidosis (from citrate and lactate).
- Dilution, depletion and decreased production of red cells and platelets.
- Diffuse intravascular coagulation: There is a consumption of clotting factors and platelets within the circulation, which are trapped in the microvascular thrombi created due to fibrin disposition.

- Extrinsic: Tissue thromboplastins, for example blunt trauma and surgery, and burns.
- Intrinsic: Endothelial injury, endotoxin, hypothermia, hypoxia, acidosis and platelet activation.
- Fibrinolysis.
- Consumption of red cells and platelets.
- Protein C activation.

Despite the extensive list quoted above, there is no level I evidence regarding the risks of pRBC transfusion. There is level II evidence that pRBC transfusion is an independent risk factor for:

- Increased nosocomial infections (wound infection, pneumonia, sepsis).
- Multiple organ failure and systemic inflammatory response syndrome.
- Longer length of intensive care unit (ICU) and hospital stay, increased complications and increased mortality.

Additionally, there is level II evidence that

- Pre-storage leucocyte depletion of RBC transfusion reduces complication rates, some studies showing a reduction in infectious complications.
- There is a relationship between transfusion and TRALI and ARDS.

So blood has effects and side effects, some of which are 'bad', and we should use it in a rational and restrictive way in most patients. In trauma haemorrhage, there is no good alternative so far and prioritizing balanced transfusion as part of haemostatic resuscitation secures clotting and oxygenation. The less 'bad' blood may be FWB, and its surrogate components transfusion (which amounts to a reconstitution of whole blood). However, FWB is not generally available outside the military context and may be logistically difficult to obtain in civilian practice.

4.4 CURRENT BEST TRANSFUSION PRACTICE

4.4.1 Initial Response

1. Aggressively pursue the diagnosis and treatment of haemorrhage.
2. Titrate administered fluids to maintain a lower than normal blood pressure (hypotensive resuscitation), until control of haemorrhage.

3. Measure and closely follow serum lactate and arterial pH as indicators of the state of systemic perfusion.
   - If normal, attempt to maintain perfusion.
   - If abnormal, attempt a gradual improvement without elevating the blood pressure and aggravating the haemorrhage.
4. Maintain normothermia.
5. Control ventilation to achieve O_2 saturation of 99–100 per cent and a normal end-tidal carbon dioxide level.
6. Aim for a target Hb of 7–9 g/dL (4–5.5 mmol/L) and a normal prothrombin time at the time that haemorrhage is controlled. Consider maintaining a higher Hb concentration in older patients and in those with known ischaemic disease.
7. If massive transfusion is likely, attempt from the outset to maintain intravascular composition. Use early RBC, plasma and platelet transfusion.

Blood pressure and heart rate are the current standard-of-care monitors of shock resuscitation in the field and in the emergency department when associated with serum lactate or base excess (base deficit). Both, however, are insensitive markers of early compensated shock; alternative monitors are needed for assessing the adequacy of tissue perfusion, with a view to avoiding both under-resuscitation and over-resuscitation. The challenge is to identify as early as possible those patients who are not responding to early interventions. Blind and aggressive volume loading in the hope of normalizing blood pressure and heart rate, without appropriate emphasis on the control of haemorrhage, sets the stage for the so-called bloody vicious cycle, the abdominal compartment syndrome or multiple organ failure (MOF).

4.4.2 Reduction in the Need for Transfusion

Blood is a scarce (and expensive) resource and is also not universally safe. Reducing the need for transfusion[4] is the best way to limit the complications:

- Treat the cause, i.e. undertake urgent surgery to stop bleeding, and avoid hypothermia and acidosis.
- Treat deficiencies and complications as they arise. There is no evidence to support prophylactic therapy with FFP, platelets, etc.[7], however, replacement of components becomes of great importance in massive transfusion. (See Section 4.7.)

- Follow a restrictive transfusion policy in ICU. One large multicentre trial[5] documented a significantly lower mortality rate for critically ill patients managed with a restrictive transfusion strategy and a transfusion threshold of 7 g/dL (5 mmol/L) Hb[8]. However, this assumes normovolaemia, absence of ongoing bleeding and an absence of pre-existing cardiovascular disease or severe brain injury.
- Develop a capacity for cell salvage.

4.4.3 Transfusion Thresholds

There is no level I evidence indicating the ideal trigger for transfusion in trauma patients. In general, the following guidelines apply[9]:

1. Identify the critically ill patient with a Hb less than 7 g/dL (5 mmol/L) or a haematocrit below 21 per cent.
2. If the Hb is less than 7 g/dL, transfusion with pRBCs is appropriate. For patients with severe cardiovascular disease, and trauma patients with ongoing bleeding or haemodynamic instability, a higher threshold of 8–10 g/dL (6–7 mmol/L) is appropriate.
3. If the Hb is less than 7 g/dL, assess the patient for hypovolaemia. If this is found, administer intravenous fluids to achieve normovolaemia, and reassess the Hb level.
4. If the patient is not hypovolaemic, determine whether there is evidence of impaired O_2 delivery.
5. If impaired O_2 delivery is present, consider cardiac output monitoring.
6. If impaired O_2 delivery is not present, monitor Hb as appropriate.

4.4.4 Transfusion Ratios

While principle largely favours fresh whole blood, blood component transfusion is the best feasible alternative in most civilian situations.

Military clinical research[3] and newer studies on civil trauma[9] suggest transfusing pRBC:FFP:platelets in a proportion of 1:1:1, with life-threatening bleeding.

Volumes and content of blood products vary between countries.

Consider an example of a combination of blood products: the mixture of one pRBC unit (335 mL) with a haematocrit of 55 per cent, one unit of platelets (50 mL) with 5.5×10 platelets[10], and one unit of FFP (275 mL) with 80 per cent coagulation factor activity. This combination results in 660 mL of fluid with a haematocrit of 29 per cent, 88000 platelets per mm[3] and 65 per cent coagulation factor activity.

The optimal ratio of RBCs to FFP remains, however, controversial. Currently, an initial two units pRBCs followed by a 1:1:1 ratio of RBC:FFP:platelets appears to be reasonable. If apheresis platelets (usually containing five or six units of platelets) are supplied, this ratio will become 5:5:1 or 6:6:1.

4.4.5 Adjuncts to Enhance Clotting

There has been extensive interest in the provision of adjuncts to enhance clotting as part of the resuscitation of the trauma patient. These include the following.

4.4.5.1 RECOMBINANT ACTIVATED FACTOR VII

Interest has focused on recombinant activated factor VIIa (NovoSeven). This was initially developed as an adjunct for the treatment of haemophilia. However, following its successful use in controlling the bleeding in a trauma patient, there was considerable interest in its use. A large multicentre trial in 2005[11] showed a reduction in red cell transfusion requirements in blunt trauma patients, and the drug has been used extensively 'off-label'. A further large multicentre trial in 2008 showed a reduction in blood product usage of 3.6 units in blunt injury, but there was no significant effect on mortality or for penetrating injury[12]. Although not widely used in the era of better understanding and assessment of the clotting process, it is still utilized in certain countries and in some military situations. A suitable protocol appears in Table 4.5.

4.4.5.2 TRANEXAMIC ACID

Tranexamic acid is indicated for prolonged bleeding (empirically) or when there is evidence of hyperfibrinolysis (measured using TEG or ROTEM). It is given at a dose of 10–20 mg/kg every 6 hours.

The CRASH-2 trial showed a significant reduction in mortality with the use of tranexamic acid[13]; however, although the trial involved very large numbers of subjects, fewer than half the patients require red cell transfusion, and in those who were transfused, the two arms utilized the same amount of blood, and the mortality rate for either arm did not correlate with that in other studies. In addition, no injury severity comparisons were included. Therefore, further studies are in progress. However, a recent study indicated that the majority of severely injured patients have a fibrinolysis shutdown, and therefore tranexamic acid may have no effect[14].

Tranexamic acid's greatest use may be where increased clot lysis is shown to be present (e.g. using thromboelastography).

4.4.5.3 DESMOPRESSIN

Desmopressin potentiates the function of platelets and is indicated only for functional platelet disorders, secondary to platelet inhibitors such as aspirin, clopidogrel, ticagrelor, prasugrel, etc., renal or hepatic failure, haemophilia-A and von Willebrand disease.

4.4.5.4 APROTININ

Aprotinin has no indication in trauma, and was withdrawn from the market in 2008.

4.4.6 Monitoring the Coagulation Status

Ideally, the use of blood components should be guided by laboratory tests of clotting function[5]. This is part of the concept of personalized medicine or in trauma is part of the concept of goal-directed therapy giving the patient only what is needed and avoiding transfusions not needed. Haemostasis according to the cell-based model is described in the phases of initiation, amplification and propagation, from clot formation to clot lysis, with participation of all circulating plasmatic and cellular components. Thrombin generation is central for clot development and strength. It primarily occurs on the surface of activated platelets and, hence, platelets and thrombin generation are closely related to the development of coagulopathy.

4.4.6.1 TRADITIONAL ASSAYS

- Fibrinogen degradation products.
- International normalized ratio (INR) – extrinsic.
- Partial thromboplastin time (PTT) – intrinsic.
- D-dimer values (fibrin deposition).

All of the above are cost effective if frequently done, but specimens are heated to the normal *in vivo* temperature of 37°C. All are time-consuming. Therefore, the conventional approach is inappropriate for the hypothermic trauma patient, whose coagulation status is altered. The TEG/ROTEM therefore is more effective at covering the assessment need in the trauma patient.

4.4.6.2 VISCOELASTIC HAEMOSTATIC ASSAYS (VHAS): THROMBOELASTOGRAPHY (TEG)/ROTATIONAL THROMBOELASTOMETRY (ROTEM)

The VHA technology results in a visual profile, or trace, and variables with a reference value (Figure 4.2)[15,16]. Briefly, the collected whole blood sample is placed in a special designed small cup (approximately 1 cc). Inside the cup is suspended a pin connected to a detector system (a torsion wire in TEG, an optical detector in ROTEM), and the cup and pin are oscillated relative to each other with movement initiated from either the cup (TEG) or the pin (ROTEM). As fibrin strings form between the cup and pin, the transmitted rotation from the cup to pin (TEG) or the impedance of the rotation of the pin (ROTEM) are detected at the pin, and a trace is generated as seen in Figure 4.2. The standard assays are with kaolin activation in TEG, kaolin + tissue factor in

Table 4.1 Interpretation of the Parameters of the TEG and ROTEM

TEG Parameter (Normal Range)	ROTEM Parameter (Normal Range)	Measurement
R time (3–8 min)	CT$_{EXTEM}$ (38–79 sec) CT$_{INTEM}$ (100–240 sec)	Clotting factor activity
α (alpha) angle (55–69 degrees)	A10$_{EXTEM}$ (43–65 mm)	Rate of increase in clot strength
K time (1–3 mm)		Kinetics to maximum clot strength
MA (51–69 mm)	MCF$_{EXTEM}$ (50–72 mm)	Maximum strength of the clot
Ly30 (<4%)	LI30 (94–100%)	Fibrinolysis at 30 minutes
FF$_{MA}$ (14–24 mm)	FibTEM MCF (9–16 mm)	Fibrinogen activity (level)

Note: Thromboelastograph (TEG): *R*, reaction time; MA, maximum amplitude; Ly30, hyperfibrinolysis after 30 min; FFMA, functional fibrinogen. Rotational thromboelastometry (ROTEM): CT, clotting time; A10, amplitude after 10 min; MCF, maximum clot firmness; Li30, hyperfibrinolysis after 30 min.

RapidTEG and tissue factor or kaolin activation, respectively, in the ExTEM and InTEM assays in ROTEM, and several other dedicated assays are available from both technologies. The contribution of fibrinogen to clot strength can be evaluated in the Functional Fibrinogen assay in TEG and the FibTEM assay in ROTEM. The VHAs are portable bedside devices, but there are several advantages in running these in a standardized lab by skilled technicians.

The result is available within 3–10 minutes, in the form of a curve (Figure 4.1a or 4.1b). A number of parameters can be measured (Table 4.2):

- *R* time (reaction time)/clotting time – the latency from the time at which the blood is placed in the cup until the clot begins to form.
- Alpha angle – the progressive increase in clot strength.
- *K* time (kinetic time) – the *K* time starts where the *R* time ends, and ends when the curve is at 20-mm amplitude.

- MA (maximum amplitude) – the maximal clot strength.
- Ly30 – lysis at 30 minutes; thrombolysis in 30 minutes.

The VHAs allow for goal-directed haemostatic therapy, thereby only treating with what is needed. See Table 4.2 for one of several international validated algorithms. Furthermore, it is possible to decide if the bleeding is surgical or coagulopathic/pathological, which clotting factors are missing, the function of platelets and whether fibrinolysis is evolving normally. Transfusion of blood components, coagulation factors and additional medication can be administered rationally, based on the results.

The TEG offers substantial support to decision making during the resuscitation, as it gives real-time accurate information on the coagulation status of the trauma patient and facilitates the differentiation between pathological abnormality and surgically correctable bleeding.

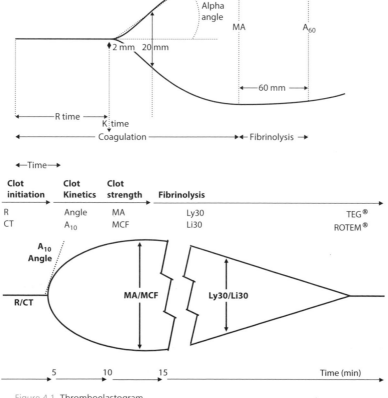

Figure 4.1 Thromboelastogram.

Table 4.2 Goal-Directed Administration of Haemostatic Products and Medication, Based on TEG and ROTEM

TEG	ROTEM	Coagulopathy	Treatment Options
R 10–14 min	ExTEM CT 80–100 sec InTEM CT 200–240 sec	Coagulation factors ↓	FFP 20 mL/kg
R >14 min	ExTEM CT >100 sec InTEM CT >240 sec	Coagulation factors ↓↓	FFP 30 mL/kg rFVIIA (see Table 4.5)
FF_{MA} 7–14 mm	FibTEM MCF 6–9 mm	Fibrinogen ↓	FFP 20 mL/kg or cryoprecipitate 3 mL/kg or fibrinogen concentrate 20 mg/kg
FF_{MA} 0–7 mm	FibTEM MCF 0–6 mm	Fibrinogen ↓↓	FFP 30 mL/kg or cryoprecipitate 5 mL/kg or fibrinogen concentrate 30 g/kg
K (kinetic) time	>4 min		cryoprecipitate 5 mL/kg or fibrinogen concentrate 30 mg/kg or rFVIIA (see Table 4.5)
α angle	<65°		Cryoprecipitate 5 mL/kg or fibrinogen concentrate 30 mg/kg or rFVIIA (see Table 4.5)
MA 45–49 mm and FF_{MA} >14 mm	ExTEM A_{10} 35–42 mm and FibTEM ≥10 mm ExTEM MCF <50 mm and FibTEM ≥10 mm	Platelets ↓	Platelets 5 mL/kg
MA <45 mm and FF_{MA} >14 mm	ExTEM A_{10} <35 mm and FibTEM ≥10 mm	Platelets ↓↓	Platelets 10 mL/kg
Ly30 >3 (− 8)%	ExTEM Li 30 <94%	Hyperfibrinolysis	TXA 1–2 g IV or 10–20 mg/kg
Difference in R Hep TEG versus standard TEG R >2 min	InTEM CT/HepTEM CT >1.25	Heparinization	Protamine 50–100 mg or FFP 10–20 mL/kg

Note: TXA, tranexamic acid; FFP, fresh frozen plasma; rFVIIA: recombinant factor VIIa; sec, seconds.

Normal
R/K/MA/angle = normal

Fibrinolysis (UK SK or TPA)
R = normal, MA = continuous decrease

Heparin
R/K = prolonged; MA/angle = decreased

Hypercoagulation
R/K = decreased, MA/angle = increased

Thrombocytopenia
R = normal, K = prolonged, MA = decreased

No platelet function (DIC)
R = prolonged, MA/angle = decreased

Figure 4.2 Abnormal appearances of the ROTEM.

4.5 AUTOTRANSFUSION

Intra-operative and post-operative blood salvage and alternative methods for decreasing transfusion may lead to a significant reduction in allogenic blood usage.

Autotransfusion eliminates the risk of incompatibility and the need for cross-matching; the risk of transmission of disease from the donor is also eliminated. Autotransfusion is a safe and cost-effective method of sustaining RBC mass while decreasing demands on the blood bank. However, cell salvage in trauma patients is fraught with difficulty as, in the trauma patient, autotransfusion typically involves the collection of blood shed into wounds, body cavities and drains.

Modern autotransfusion devices are basically of two types:

- Collection of blood that is mixed with an anticoagulant, filtered and returned. The blood is collected, anticoagulated with heparin or citrate and then run through a system in which it is washed and centrifuged, before being retransfused.
- Reinfusion after filtration is less labour intensive and provides blood for transfusion quickly. Whole blood is returned to the patient with platelets and proteins intact, but free Hb and procoagulants are also reinfused. A high proportion of the salvaged blood is returned to the patient, and the most recent devices do not require mixing of the blood with an anticoagulant solution. In-line filters are absolutely essential when autotransfusion devices are used. These filters remove gross particles and macroaggregates during collection and reinfusion, thus minimizing microembolization[17].

Cell washing and centrifugation techniques require a machine and (usually) a technician to be the sole operator. This latter requirement can limit the utility of the devices in everyday practice. The cell washing cycle produces red cells suspended in saline with a haematocrit of 55–60 per cent. This solution is relatively free of free Hb, procoagulants and bacteria. However, bacteria have been shown to adhere to the iron in the Hb molecule, and washing therefore does not eliminate the risk of infection.

To a degree, the simpler the system, the less likely it is that problems will occur. In elective situations, nurses, technicians or anaesthesia personnel can participate in the autotransfusion process. In emergency situations without additional personnel, such participation may not be possible. Systems that process reclaimed RBCs may require trained technicians, particularly if the procedure is used infrequently.

In practical terms, bleeding from the chest seems ideal for immediate autotransfusion as the contents of thoracic cavity are sterile, in contrast with abdominal bleeding, where visceral injury and contamination may coexist. The simplest effective method is to use the sterile chest drain container. Use saline to create the fluid valve at the end of a chest drainage tube, to which is added 1000 IU fractionated heparin. The contents of the bottle may be hung and (using a microfilter to collect microaggregates) immediately reintroduced intravenously.

Autotransfusion is generally contraindicated in the presence of bacterial or malignant cell contamination (e.g. an open bowel, infected vascular prostheses, etc.) unless no other RBC source is available and the patient is in a life-threatening situation. However, there are several studies showing the practice may not be as unreasonable as previously thought[18].

Cell salvage techniques have been shown to be cost-effective and useful in some trauma patients (e.g. in splenic trauma with significant blood loss), but further studies are indicated to clarify the indications.

4.6 **RED BLOOD CELL SUBSTITUTES**

The ideal pRBC substitute is cheap, has a long shelf life, is universally compatible and well tolerated and has an O_2 delivery profile identical to that of blood. Significant effort has been made to find a suitable substitute that could, essentially, be treated as an artificial O_2 carrier.

Artificial O_2 carriers can be grouped into perfluorocarbon (PFC) emulsions and modified Hb solutions. The native Hb molecule needs to be modified in order to decrease its O_2 affinity and to prevent rapid dissociation of the native $alpha_2$–$beta_2$ tetramer into $alpha_2$–$beta_2$ dimers.

4.6.1 **Perfluorocarbons**

Perfluorocarbons are carbon–fluorine compounds that are completely inert and have low viscosity, but dissolve large amounts of gas. They do not mix with water and therefore need to be produced as emulsions. Unlike the sigmoid relationship of Hb, they exhibit a linear relationship with O_2, therefore their efficacy relies on maintaining a high PaO_2; however, PFCs unload O_2 well. They do not expand the intravascular volume and can only be given in small volumes as they overload the reticuloendothelial system. Once thought to hold potential, they have so far not been found to confer additional benefit compared with crystalloid solutions, especially as there is a significant incidence of side effects.

4.6.2 **Haemoglobin Solutions**

Although free haemoglobin can transport O_2 outside of the red cell membrane, it is too toxic to be clinically useful. Techniques have been developed to remove the need for the red cell membrane and create haemoglobin-based oxygen carriers (HBOCs).

4.6.2.1 LIPOSOMAL HAEMOGLOBIN SOLUTIONS

These are based on the encapsulation of Hb in liposomes. The mixing of phospholipid and cholesterol in the presence of Hb yields a sphere with Hb at its centre. These liposomes have O_2 dissociation curves similar to red cells, with low viscosity, and their administration can transiently produce high circulating levels of Hb.

Problems associated with HBOCs relate to effects on vasomotor tone, which appears to be modulated by the carriers' interaction with nitric oxide, causing significant vasoconstriction.

4.6.2.2 POLYMERIZED HAEMOGLOBIN SOLUTIONS (HUMAN-OUTDATED/BOVINE RBCS)

Techniques have been developed for cross-linking the haemoglobin molecules, initially with a di-aspirin link and recently as a haemoglobin polymer. Both human and bovine Hb have been used.

Considerable research has taken place in the past decade with regard to the development of synthesized Hb solutions. Bovine-derived Hb (Hemopure) is approved for clinical use in South Africa. Currently, the products have not been licensed for use in the trauma patient.

No level I evidence has yet appeared to support the use of Hb substitutes instead of blood.

The O_2 transport characteristics of modified Hb solutions and PFC solutions are fundamentally different (Table 4.3). The Hb solutions exhibit a sigmoid O_2 dissociation curve similar to that of blood, while PFC emulsions are characterized by a linear relationship between the partial pressure and the content of O_2. Haemoglobin solutions therefore provide O_2 transport and unloading characteristics similar to blood. This means that at a

Table 4.3 Advantages and Disadvantages of Haemoglobin-Based Solutions Compared with Hydrocarbons

Haemoglobin-Based Solutions	PFC-Based Emulsions
Advantages	**Advantages**
• Carries and unloads O_2	• Carries and unloads O_2
• Sigmoidal O_2 dissociation curve	• Few and mild side effects
• 100% FiO_2 not mandatory for maximum potency	• No known organ toxicity
• Easy to measure	
Disadvantages	**Disadvantages**
• Side effects	• 100% FiO_2 is mandatory for maximal efficacy
○ Vasoconstriction	• Additional colloid is often necessary, with potential side effects
○ Interference with laboratory methods (colorimetric)	

relatively low arterial O_2 pressure, substantial amounts of O_2 are being transported. In contrast, relatively high arterial O_2 partial pressures are necessary to maximize the O_2 transport of PFC emulsions (Figure 4.2).

Note that 5 per cent O_2 can be offloaded by both blood and PFCs, PFC O_2 being more completely offloaded than blood-transported O_2.

Figure 4.3 Oxygen transport characteristics of haemoglobin and perfluorocarbons.

4.7 MASSIVE HAEMORRHAGE/ MASSIVE TRANSFUSION

4.7.1 Definition

Blood volume is approximately 70 mL/kg. Massive transfusion[19] is defined as:

- The replacement of 100 per cent of the patient's blood volume in less than 24 hours.
- The administration of 50 per cent of the patient's blood volume in 1 hour.

There is a danger of death when blood loss is more than 150 mL per minute or 50 per cent of blood volume in 20 minutes. Each trauma unit should have a policy for massive transfusion, which should be activated as soon as a potential candidate is admitted.

Also germane to the initial period of massive blood transfusion are the potential complications of acidosis,

hypothermia and hypocalcaemia. Hypothermia (<34°C) causes platelet sequestration and inhibits the release of platelet factors that are important in the intrinsic clotting pathway. In addition, it has consistently been associated with a poor outcome in trauma patients. Core temperature often falls insidiously because of exposure at the scene and in the emergency department, and because of the administration of resuscitation fluids stored at ambient temperature.

The use of bicarbonate in the treatment of systemic acidosis remains controversial. Moderate acidosis (pH <7.20) impairs coagulation, myocardial contractility and oxidative metabolism. Acidosis in the trauma patient is caused primarily by a rise in lactic acid production secondary to tissue hypoxia and hypothermia, and usually resolves when the volume deficit has been corrected and the efficiency of the circulation restored. Administration of sodium bicarbonate may cause a leftward shift of the oxyhaemoglobin dissociation curve, reducing tissue O_2 extraction, and may worsen intracellular acidosis caused by carbon dioxide production. On the other hand, adrenergic receptors may become desensitized with protracted acidosis. Bicarbonate infusion, therefore, should be limited to persons with protracted shock.

Hypocalcaemia caused by citrate binding of ionized calcium does not occur until the blood transfusion rate exceeds 100 mL per minute (equivalent to one unit every 5 minutes). Decreased serum levels of ionized calcium depress myocardial function before impairing coagulation. Calcium gluconate or calcium chloride should be reserved for cases in which there is ECG evidence of QT interval prolongation or, in rare instances, for cases of unexplained hypotension during massive transfusion.

4.7.2 Protocol

An algorithm of coordinated action incorporating many hospital departments (surgery, blood bank, ICU, anaesthesiology) is activated upon the arrival of a trauma patient with massive haemorrhage. The protocol provides roles for the personnel, actions to be taken, medications and blood products to be transfused. The target is the increase of survival of these patients. The basis of these protocols has been the knowledge recently acquired from modern battlefields, which has dramatically changed the way we manage these patients (Tables 4.4 and 4.5).

Table 4.4 Guidelines for Massive Transfusion

Definition

Replacement of the whole blood volume within 24 hours, or 50% of the blood volume in 3 h.

Activation

The protocol will be activated **automatically by the blood bank** after two units of packed red blood cells (pRBCs) have been issued to a patient, *and* a request for a further four units of blood or more is subsequently requested within any 24-h period. A prospective tool utilizing PR >120 bpm and BP <90 + free blood in the abdomen can be used[17]. Activation can also be done at the discretion of the treating physician.

Blood Specimens

Group and cross-match

- Leukodepleted blood should be used wherever it is available.
- Cross-matched blood if available.
- Un-cross-matched group O blood.

The following **baseline blood specimens** are required:

- Full blood count including platelets.
- Prothrombin time (PT), activated partial thromboplastin time (aPTT), thrombin time, international normalized ratio (INR), fibrinogen, D-dimer, thromboelastography (TEG) or rotational thromboelastometry (ROTEM).

The following are required **after every six units of transfused blood**:

- Repeat baseline blood samples.
- Full TEG or ROTEM.

Avoid hypothermia (patient and transfused fluid)

- Use an appropriate blood warmer.
- Keep the patient warm using an appropriate patient-warming device.
- Maintain a warm environment.

Blood and Blood Products

The blood bank will issue the following products (as part of a two- or six-unit 'massive transfusion pack'):

(*Note*: Multiple **two-unit packs** are preferable as they can be returned if the 'cold chain' is intact.)

- Two units or six units of pRBC s using the *freshest blood available*.
- Two units or six units of **thawed** fresh frozen plasma (FFP).
- Two units or six units of platelets *or*
- For every six units of blood issued, one apheresis unit of platelets ('platelet mega-unit') (*Note*: This may be five or six units of pooled platelets.)

Administration

Microaggregate filters are **not** advised.

Once administration of the 'massive transfusion pack' blood is begun, administer all the above in a **1:1:1 ratio** (blood:FFP:platelets) or **6:6:1/5:5:1/4.4.1** (blood:FFP:apheresis mega-platelet unit – depends on local interpretation of a 'megaplatelet unit'). After every six units of red cells, if ongoing bleeding or need for transfusion is present:

- Give a further four units of FFP if PT or APTT is >1.5 times mid-normal or according to TEG/ROTEM.
- Give 10 units of cryoprecipitate if fibrinogen <1 g/L or according to TEG/ROTEM.
- Give 10 mL 10% calcium chloride **only** if the above additional doses are given.
- Give at least one megaunit of pooled platelets if the platelet count is <75 000 /mm^3.

   Return all unused 'massive transfusion packs' to the blood bank as soon as possible.

Endpoints of Transfusion

- Any active surgical bleeding has been controlled.
- No further need for red cells.
- Temperature >35°C.
- pH >7.3.
- Fibrinogen >1.5 g/L.
- INR better than 1.5, PT less than 16 sec., aPTT less than 42 sec.
- Haemoglobin 8–10 g/dL (4–6 mmol/L).

Table 4.5 Guidelines for Use of Recombinant Activated Factor VII (rFVIIa) in Trauma

Definition

This guideline describes the use of rFVIIa as an *adjunct* in the management of coagulopathy following trauma with massive bleeding or the need to enter the massive transfusion protocol.

Issue

The blood bank will issue the required rFVIIa for administration immediately **after completion** of the 6th and 12th units of transfused blood.

Limitation

rFVIIa should **only** be used:

- **If all <u>surgical</u> bleeding has been controlled**
- **In the presence of active bleeding**
- **Where possible, its use should be backed up with a thromboelastogram (TEG)**
  Increased R (reaction) time despite fresh frozen plasma
- After transfusion of >6 units of blood
- If the platelet count is >50 000/mm^3
- If the pH is >7.2
- If the temperature is >34° C

Blood specimens

Disseminated intravascular coagulopathy screen:

- Full blood count and platelets
- Prothrombin time, activated partial thromboplastin time, thrombin time, International Normalized Ratio, D-dimer
- Fibrinogen
- TEG or rotary thromboelastomer

Dose

The dose of rFVIIa should be 90 µg/kg

- Round UP to the nearest 1.2 mg
  (Example: a 75-kg male receives 75 × 90 µg/kg = 6.75 mg rFVIIa. Round UP to 7.2 mg.)

If the patient continues to bleed:

- Repeat the dose after 1 h and after 3 h from first dose
- Repeat the dose after completion of the **12th** unit of transfused blood

End points of administration

The first of:

- Cessation of bleeding
  or
- Three doses

REFERENCES AND RECOMMENDED READING

References

1. Huraux C, Ankri AA, Eyraud D, et al. Hemostatic changes in patients receiving hydroxyethyl starch: the influence of ABO blood group. *Anesth Analg.* 2001;92(6):1396–1401.
2. Allen CJ, Valle EJ, Jouria JM, et al. Differences between blunt and penetrating trauma after resuscitation with hydroxyethyl starch. *J Trauma.* 2014;77(6):859–864.
3. Kauvar DS, Holcomb JB, Norris GC, Hess JR. Fresh whole blood transfusion: a controversial military practice. *J Trauma.* 2006;61:181–184.
4. Spinella PC, Holcomb JB. Resuscitation and transfusion principles for traumatic hemorrhagic shock. *Blood Rev.* 2009;23:231–240.
5. Hess JR, Brohi K, Dutton RP, et al. The coagulopathy of trauma: a review of mechanisms. *J Trauma.* 2008;65:748–754.
6. British Committee for Standards in Haematology, Blood Transfusion Task Force. Guidelines for the use of fresh frozen plasma, cryoprecipitate, and cryosupernatant. *Brit J Haemat.* 2004;126:11–28.

7. Pandit TN, Sarode R. Blood component support in acquired coagulopathic conditions: is there a method to the madness? *Am J Hematol.* 2012;Suppl 1:S56–S62. doi:10.1002/ajh.23179.

8. Dutton RP, Carson JL. Indications for early red blood cell transfusion. *J Trauma.* 2006;60(6):Suppl. S35–S40.

9. Napolitano LM, Kurek S, Luchette FA, et al. Clinical practice guideline: red blood cell transfusion in adult trauma and critical care. *Crit Care Med.* 2009;37:3124–3157.

10. Holcomb JB, del Junco DJ, Fox EE, et al. The Prospective, Observational, Multicenter, Major Trauma Transfusion (PROMMTT) study: comparative effectiveness of a time-varying treatment with competing risks. *Arch Surg.* 2012;15:1–10.

11. Boffard KD, Riou B, Warren B, et al. NovoSeven Trauma Study Group. Recombinant factor VIIa as adjunctive therapy for bleeding control in severely injured trauma patients: two parallel randomized, placebo-controlled, double-blind clinical trials. *J Trauma.* 2005;59(1):8–15; discussion 15–18.

12. Hauser CJ, Boffard KD, Dutton R, et al., for the CONTROL Study Group. Results of the CONTROL Trial: efficacy and safety of recombinant activated factor VII in the management of refractory traumatic hemorrhage. *J Trauma.* 2010;69:489–500.

13. CRASH-2 Trial Collaborators. Effects of tranexamic acid on death, vascular occlusive events, and blood transfusion in trauma patients with significant haemorrhage (CRASH-2): a randomised, placebo-controlled trial. *Lancet.* 2010;376:27–32.

14. Moore HB, Moore EE, Gonzales E, et al. Hyprinofibrinolysis, physiologic fibrinolysis, and fibrinolysis shutdown: the spectrum of post injury fibrinolysis and relevance to antifibrinolytic therapy. *J Trauma Acute Care Surg.* 2014;77(6);811–817.

15. Stensballe J, Ostrowski SR, Johansson PI. Viscoelastic guidance of resuscitation. *Curr Opin Anaesthesiol.* 2014;27(2):212–218.

16. TEG/ROTEM. www.surgicalcriticalcare.net/Guidelines. Accessed January 2015.

17. Hughes LG, Thomas DW, Wareham K, Jones JE, John A, Rees M. Intra-operative blood salvage in abdominal trauma: a review of 5 years' experience. *Anaesthesia.* 2001;56:217–220.

18. Bowley DM, Barker P, Boffard KD. Intraoperative blood salvage in penetrating abdominal trauma: a randomised controlled trial. *World J Surg.* 2006;30:1074–1080.

19. Nunez TC, Young PP, Holcomb JB, Cotton BA. Creation, implementation, and maturation of a massive transfusion protocol for the exsanguinating trauma patient. *J Trauma.* 2010;68:1498–1505.

Recommended Reading

Johansson PI, Ostrowsky SR, Secher NH. Management of major blood loss: an update. *Acta Anaesthesiol Scand.* 2010;54:1039–1049.

Journal of Trauma-Injury Infection and Critical Care. Early massive trauma transfusion: current state of the art. *J Trauma* 2006;60(6, Suppl.).

Malone DL, Hess JR, Fingerhut A. Massive transfusion practices around the globe and a suggestion for a common massive transfusion protocol. *J Trauma.* 2006;60(6, Suppl.):S91–S96.

Marino PC. Transfusion practices in critical care. In: *The ICU Book.* 3rd ed. Baltimore, MD: Lippincott Williams & Wilkins; 2007:659–686.

Pierocci FM, Kashuk JL, Moore EE. Postinjury hemotherapy and hemostasis. In: Mattok KL, Moore EE, Feliciano DV, eds. *Trauma,* 7th ed. New York: NY: McGraw-Hill; 2013:216–235.

West MA, Shapiro MB, Nathens AB, et al. Inflammation and the host response to injury. Large Scale Collaborative Research Program Investigators. IV: Guidelines for transfusion in the trauma patient. *J Trauma.* 2006;61:436–439.

Damage Control Surgery 5

5.1 INTRODUCTION

The concept of 'damage control' (also known as 'staged laparotomy' or 'abbreviated laparotomy') has as its objective the delay in imposition of additional surgical stress at a moment of physiological frailty[1].

Damage control resuscitation (DCR) and damage control surgery (DCS) are a deliberate and pre-emptive set of nontraditional resuscitative and surgical manoeuvers used to reverse the pre-terminal effect of exsanguination, massive injury and shock. The primary goal is to temporize injuries with abbreviated surgery to allow for resuscitation and restoration of normal physiology, prior to the definitive surgery. Classically described for catastrophic abdominal injury, the DCS concept has been applied to all types of injury. Currently DCS techniques are described for thoracic, orthopaedic, vascular and massive cerebral trauma.

Briefly stated, this is a technique whereby the surgeon minimizes operative time and intervention in the grossly unstable patient. The primary reason for this is to minimize hypothermia, metabolic acidosis and coagulopathy ('the lethal triad'), which are often apparent after the patient rapidly loses significant blood volume and has sustained massive tissue destruction. After a post-operative intensive care resuscitation and stabilization period, the patient is returned to the operating room for definitive surgical care. Although the principles are sound, extreme care has to be exercised to avoid over-utilization of the concept, thereby causing secondary insults to viscera. Furthermore, enough appropriate surgery has to be carried out in order to minimize activation of the inflammatory cascade and the consequences of systemic inflammatory response syndrome (SIRS) and organ dysfunction.

The concept is not new, and livers were packed as long as 100 years ago by Pringle. However, with the failure to understand the underlying physiological rationale, the results were disastrous. Over time, the concept has evolved into the modern technique of an abbreviated laparotomy, establishment of intra-abdominal pack tamponade, control of contamination and delayed definitive management after the restoration of normal physiological parameters and coagulation. The use of angiography and embolization has been beneficial where packing of the viscera has failed, such as in uncontrolled pelvic bleeding or soft tissue destruction. Most recently, the combination of DCS with a blood component resuscitation scheme allowing permissive hypotension, limiting crystalloid volume and expedited administration of plasma and platelets – damage control resuscitation (DCR) – appears to increase survival.

Damage control surgery may be performed in smaller hospitals before transfer to a larger centre. Damage control surgery procedures, on properly selected patients, can be life-saving measures, and may have to be performed in any hospital admitting trauma cases.

Damage control concepts are not restricted to the abdomen, but extend to every cavity on the body as well as vascular damage control. In military conflicts, thoracic damage control has proven to be of great value. The need for damage control in children is much less common than in adults, but it is well described. Children are much more prone to hypothermia given their large surface area and small blood volume. Although the physiological parameters are very different in children, the principles of damage control are the same. At the other end of the spectrum, the application of damage control to the elderly has also been successful. The elderly (often defined as over 55 years) have decreased physiological reserve, and high morbidity and mortality is demonstrated in this population. That said, a study published by Newell et al.[2] demonstrates a survival of greater than 50 per cent when damage control is applied to this group. This has been supported even in the octogenarian population and clearly demonstrates that damage control is not futile in the elderly.

Damage control is becoming more common in the general surgery population in patients with intra-abdominal catastrophes such as perforated viscous, pancreatitis, ischemia or gastrointestinal haemorrhage. One difference between this group and the trauma group is that the initial resuscitation phase is often longer in duration. In trauma, the initial resuscitation is generally minutes before proceeding to stage 1. In the general surgery patient, it is often hours as compared to minutes, allowing for reasonable restoration of normal physiology. The DCS allows for rapid source control with the ability to re-evaluate the source easily. It also allows for frequent re-evaluation of bowel viability in the setting of ischaemia. Finally, and possibly most importantly, it decreases (but does not eliminate) the incidence of abdominal compartment syndrome (Critical Care – Chapter 14). This patient population often receives a massive amount of intravenous volume during the initial resuscitation that leads to bowel oedema and increases in intra-abdominal pressure. A temporary abdominal closure lowers the risk of this potentially devastating process.

The application of damage control principles has influenced military care and disaster planning. The need to triage mass casualty scenarios makes an abbreviated surgical and damage control approach advantageous in maximizing the use of limited resources to many patients in a restricted time span or space. A recent prospective observational military study reported that damage control was utilized in 77 per cent of abdominal operations performed in Afghanistan. Damage control was safe. The study concluded that damage control was the optimal approach to abdominal war injury and should be considered in logistical planning for future military operations[3]. Recent events, such as the Boston Marathon bombing, showed that the critical patient surge placed on hospitals within minutes of an incident was well handled with good outcomes when the abbreviated DCS strategy was used to manage all patients[4].

5.2 **DAMAGE CONTROL RESUSCITATION (DCR)**

Damage control resuscitation (DCR) is a critical adjunct to the abbreviated laparotomy of damage control surgery (DCS) and must occur in parallel[5]. The DCR is the proactive, anticipatory treatment of coagulopathy, hypothermia and acidosis that present with critical injury and shock. The DCR priorities include the following[6,7]:

- Permissive hypotension with resuscitation to a pressure which allows organ *perfusion* rather than *normotension.*

- Early use of blood products over crystalloid products, often facilitated by use of a massive transfusion protocol (see Chapter 4).
- Blood product administration with liberal use of fresh frozen plasma (FFP) and platelets.

  The optimal ratio of blood component therapy has yet to be determined, but a ratio approaching 1:1:1 has been suggested. In certain environments properly crossed and matched whole blood may also be used.

- Reversal of coagulopathy – TEG or ROTEM, if available, may be used to guide product therapy.
- Restoration of normothermia.

5.3 **DAMAGE CONTROL SURGERY (DCS)**

Damage control can be divided into five distinct stages: This begins with patient selection (stage 1) and continues through potential late abdominal wall reconstruction (stage 5).

5.3.1 **Stage 1: Patient Selection**

Proper patient selection is crucial to optimize outcomes following DCS. All patients should undergo a very rapid trauma evaluation. The establishment of large-bore intravenous access, initial neurologic evaluation and appropriate blood transfusion are important early steps as one diagnoses the source of bleeding. The duration of this stage is dictated by the patient's physiologic stability as well as the underlying pathology. During this stage, initiation of a massive transfusion protocol (see Chapter 4) and commencement of a haemostatic resuscitation are critical. Delays to the operating room must be avoided. Rapid manoeuvers to control external bleeding (tourniquets, digital control of non-compressible bleeding, etc.) are indicated as transition to the operating room occurs.

In any hospital managing trauma or a high number of emergency surgical cases protocols for massive transfusion supporting haemostatic resuscitation should be in place and supported by anaesthesia, blood bank and intensive care staff. The surgeon is well advised to call for an additional surgeon to assist, if available.

The indications to select a patient for damage control generally can be divided into the following:

- Haemodynamic instability.
  - Systolic blood pressure <90 mm Hg for more than 60 minutes.
  - Temperature <35°C.
- Metabolic instability.
  - pH <7.2.
  - Base excess ≥5 and worsening.
  - Serum lactate >5 mmol/L.
- Coagulopathy.
  - Prothrombin time (PT) >16 seconds.
  - Partial thromboplastin time (PTT) >60 seconds.
  - Viscoelastic haemostatic assays (VHAs): TEG or ROTEM.
- Surgical anatomy.
  - Inaccessible major venous injury (e.g. retrohepatic vena cava, pelvis, etc.).
  - Anticipated need for a time-consuming surgical procedure in a patient with a suboptimal response to resuscitation.
  - Inability to perform the definitive repair in a timely fashion.
  - Demand for non-operative control of other injuries, for example a fractured pelvis.
  - Inability to approximate the abdominal incision.
- Environment.
  - Blood requirement >10 units of blood.
  - Operating time >60 minutes.
- Logistics.
  - Multiple patients/mass casualty situation.
- Minimal resources (e.g. personnel, medical equipment, safety concerns).

If resources allow, the use of a hybrid operating room expedites definitive haemorrhage control and can complement damage control therapy in the exsanguinating patient.

Irrespective of the setting, a coagulopathy is the single most common reason for abortion of a planned procedure or curtailment of definitive surgery. It is important to abort the surgery *before* the coagulopathy becomes obvious.

The technical aspects of the surgery are dictated by the injury pattern.

5.3.2 Stage 2: Operative Haemorrhage and Contamination Control

The primary objectives are as follows (see also Chapter 8.1).

5.3.2.1 INITIAL INCISION

A very large incision is necessary to allow for wide retraction of the abdominal wall and rapid visualization of the liver, abdominal great vessels and all other retroperitoneal structures. Two experienced surgeons are recommended. Rapid control of the largest source of blood loss is critical and in those cases with several sources of bleeding and manual pressure, packing and temporary ligation may be necessary. Each case is unique in presentation; however, the principle is to control active large blood loss first.

5.3.2.2 HAEMORRHAGE CONTROL

The operative process works through the following (see also Chapter 8.1):

- Arrest arterial and major venous bleeding:

  Major arterial bleeding must be controlled at the index procedure. A temporary intravascular shunt is preferred for named vessels; however, ligation may be required to save an exsanguinating patient. Failure to control ongoing bleeding will lead to the patient's demise.

  Trans-arterial catheterization is effective in controlling arterial haemorrhage in areas that are difficult to access such as the pelvis, the retroperitoneum, the kidney, the liver, intercostals or soft tissue injuries.

- Tamponade using wraps or packs.
- Occlusion of inflow into the bleeding organ (e.g. Pringle manoeuvre for bleeding liver).
- Repair or ligation of accessible blood vessels.
- Temporary intravascular shunting (Figure 5.1).
- Intra-operative or post-operative catheter-directed embolization.

Figure 5.1 Diagram of an intravascular shunt.

5.3.2.3 CONTROL OF CONTAMINATION (HOLLOW VISCOUS ORGANS)

- Defects in the bowel or hollow viscous organs can be controlled with simple suturing or stapler applications.
- Damaged segments can be resected with clamps or staples.
- Biliary and genitourinary injuries can be temporized with external drainage (T-tube, ureterostomy, etc.).
- Pancreatic injuries should be widely drained and packed.

Avoid definitive repair, restoration of intestinal continuity, stoma formation and creation of feeding access at this stage.

5.3.2.4 COPIOUS WASHOUT

At the end of the procedure, before closure, the abdominal cavity must be washed out with copious amounts (several litres) of normal saline, especially if there has been contamination by, for example, faeces. After washing out, suck out all fluid. Leave the cavity as dry as possible.

5.3.2.5 TEMPORARY ABDOMINAL CLOSURE (TAC)

The abdominal cavity should be closed to prevent heat and moisture loss, and to protect the viscera.

Delayed closure is required when any combination of the factors listed above under damage control, or re-look surgery, exists. In particular, patients with multiple injuries who have undergone protracted surgery with massive volume resuscitation to maintain haemodynamic stability will develop tissue interstitial oedema. This may predispose to the development of abdominal compartment syndrome (ACS) or may simply make primary closure of the sheath impracticable. In addition, significant enteric or other contamination will raise the risk of intra-abdominal sepsis, or the extent of tissue damage may raise doubt over the viability of any repair; these conditions usually mandate planned re-laparotomy and thus a temporary closure.

In these circumstances, a temporary abdominal closure is required. The needs of such a closure can be summarised as

- Quick to do
- Cheap
- Keeps the abdominal contents inside the abdominal cavity
- Allows drainage of fluid

- Minimizes sepsis
- Facilitates delayed primary fascial closure

Vacuum-based closure is recommended for the management of the open abdomen. A review of the literature available suggests that negative-pressure wound vacuum therapy may have improved fascial closure rates, and may be associated with improved outcomes over alternative abdominal closure techniques (mesh, Velcro, bag-type dressings).

Many temporary closure systems are available, of which the most cost-effective is the 'sandwich technique' as first described by Schein in 1986[8] and popularized by Rotundo and Schwab[1].

A sheet of self-adhesive incise drape (Opsite, Smith & Nephew, London, UK; Steri-Drape or Ioban, 3M Corporation, St. Paul, MN) is placed flat, sticky side up, and an abdominal swab is placed upon it. The objective is to create a non-stick membrane on one side of the abdominal swab to place against the visceral organs. The size should be large enough that, when inserted, the sheet will extend laterally to the paracolic gutters, and 10 cm cranial and caudal to the incision. The edges are folded over to produce a composite sheet with a membrane (i.e. the drape) on one side and an abdominal swab on the other. The membrane is utilized as an onlay with the margins 'tucked in' under the edges of the open sheath as far as the paracolic gutters, with only the membrane in contact with the bowel.

5.3.2.5.1 Pitfalls

- Cover only *one* side of the swab. Covering both sides impedes drainage by preventing capillary wicking through the weave of the swab.
- Do not make any holes (slits) in the membrane. Holes would allow the suction to be transmitted directly to the serosa of the bowel, with possible risk of fistula formation.
- Keep the vacuum to between 5 and 10 mm Hg. Higher suction pressures, especially in cold hypotensive patients, transmitted directly onto the bowel may exceed capillary pressure.
- Preferably avoid the commercial equivalents (e.g. VAC Kinetic Concepts Incorporated (KCI), San Antonio, TX, or Renasys, Smith & Nephew at this time. These should be reserved for the *definitive* closure of a wound, both for cost reasons and the higher vacuum suction pressure often present.

The appreciable drainage of serosanguineous fluid that occurs is best dealt with by placing a pair of drainage tubes (e.g. sump-type nasogastric tubes or closed-system suction drains) through separate stab incisions, with the tips placed in the caudal end of the incision. The tubes lie on either side of the incision, under the edge of the anterior abdominal peritoneum and the gauze of the swab, and utilize continuous low-vacuum suction.

This arrangement is covered by an occlusive incise drape applied to the skin, thus providing a closed system (the 'sandwich'; Figures 5.2 and 5.3).The 'Bogota bag' and towel clips, etc. are no longer used, and for temporary abdominal closure, no sutures should be placed in the sheath.

The timing of transfer of the patient from the operating theatre to the intensive care unit (ICU) is critical. Prompt transfer is cost effective; premature transfer is counterproductive. Control of bleeding and contamination must be achieved. On the other hand, once haemostasis has been properly achieved, it may not be necessary to abort the procedure in the same fashion.

In the operating room, efforts must be started to reverse all the associated adjuncts, such as acidosis, hypothermia and hypoxia, and it may be possible to improve the coagulation status through these methods alone. Adequate time should still be allowed for this, following which reassessment of the abdominal injuries should take place, as it is not infrequent to discover further injuries or ongoing bleeding.

Conversely, there are some patients with severe head injuries in whom the coagulopathy is induced secondary to severe irreversible cerebral damage, and further surgical energy is futile.

5.3.3 Stage 3: Physiological Restoration in the Intensive Care Unit

Priorities in the ICU are as follows.

5.3.3.1 RESTORATION OF BODY TEMPERATURE

- Passive re-warming using warming blankets, convection blankets, warmed fluids, heat lamps, elevation of the ambient room temperature, etc.
- Active re-warming with lavage of the chest or abdomen.

5.3.3.2 OPTIMIZATION OF OXYGEN DELIVERY

- Volume loading to restore circulating blood volume.
- Haemoglobin optimization to a haemoglobin level of 8–10 g/dL (4–6 mmol/L).
- Monitoring of cardiac output.
  - Ultrasonic cardiac output devices.
  - Cardiac arterial output monitors.
  - Swan-Ganz pulmonary pressure monitoring.
- Correction of acidosis to a pH >7.3.
- Measurement and correction of lactic acidosis to <2.5 mmol/L.
- Inotropic support as required.

5.3.3.3 CORRECTION OF CLOTTING PROFILES

- Blood component repletion.
- Assessment and normalization of any coagulopathy
  - Coagulation studies.
- Thromboelastography (TEG) or rotational thromboelastometry (ROTEM).

5.3.3.4 IMPROVEMENT OF PHYSIOLOGICAL ENDPOINTS

Evidence of improvement of physiological endpoints is shown by:

- Lactate clearance.
- SvO_2.
- Urine output.
- Haemodynamics.
- Resolution of acidaemia.

Figure 5.2 Diagrammatic representation of the sandwich technique ('VacPac').

Figure 5.3 Technique of insertion of the membrane sandwich.

- Inotropic support once intravascular volume has been repleted.

5.3.3.5 MONITORING FOR AND MINIMIZING THE INCIDENCE OF INTRA-ABDOMINAL HYPERTENSION (AH) AND ABDOMINAL COMPARTMENT SYNDROME (ACS) (SEE SECTION 14.9)

- Measurement of intra-abdominal pressure (IAP).
  - Foley (bladder) catheter.
- Intragastric catheter.

5.3.3.6 RECOGNITION OF ADDITIONAL INJURIES

Review injury mechanism, presentation and those steps in the standard trauma resuscitation, along with diagnostics and therapies that were not completed, to facilitate damage control:

- Tertiary survey.
- Additional imaging as needed.
- Review of history, co-morbid conditions, and medications.
- Tetanus immunization.

5.3.4 **Stage 4: Definitive Surgery**

The patient is returned to the operating theatre as soon as physiological stability has been achieved.

Ideally this would be within 24–48 hours, as delaying beyond 48 hours can be detrimental; however, the timing for this is determined by:

- The indication for damage control in the first place.
- The pattern of injury.
- The physiological response to resuscitation, warming and evaluation as above.
- Patients with ongoing bleeding despite correction of the other parameters require immediate return to the operating theatre or angiography suite.
- Patients who develop major ACS must undergo re-look surgery early, and any further underlying causes must be corrected. Every effort must be made to return *all* patients to the operating theatre within 24 hours of their initial surgery. By leaving matters longer, other problems such as acute respiratory distress syndrome, SIRS and sepsis may intervene (cause or effect) and may preclude further surgery.

5.3.4.1 THE 'RE-LOOK LAPAROTOMY'

The re-look laparotomy may be:

- *Planned*, that is decided upon at the time of the initial procedure and usually for reasons of contamination, doubtful tissue viability, for retrieval of intra-abdominal packs or for further definitive surgery after a damage control exercise.
- *On demand*, that is, when evidence of intra-abdominal complication develops. In these cases, the principle applies of re-operation 'when the patient fails to progress according to expectation'. Failure to act in these circumstances may have dire consequences in terms of morbidity and mortality.

Re-exploration should be thorough, with careful evaluation for previously undiagnosed injuries. If the patient's physiological parameters deteriorate again, then the damage control philosophy should be reapplied with aggressive resuscitation, abbreviated laparotomy and possible adjunctive procedures such as angiography, pelvic stabilization or evaluation of extra-abdominal injury. In many cases, repacking combined with aggressive correction of physiologic endpoints including coagulopathy, along with further warming and coagulopathy, are necessary.

If a stoma (colostomy or ileostomy) is needed, consideration of a lateral ostomy is pragmatic. The stoma is positioned between the musculature of the anterior and mid-axillary lines. The rectus fascia and musculature is thereby spared for future reconstruction, and the stoma is positioned well away from the midline wound, thus minimizing contamination. As the abdominal wall is re-approximated the stoma will move toward the anterior midline.

5.3.5 **Stage 5: Abdominal Wall Closure**

Once the patient has completed definitive surgery and no further operations are contemplated, the abdominal wall can be closed. In most series the majority of patients can have the fascia closed after the first re-look, or within 7–8 days from injury. This varies greatly depending on patient size and body habitus, time to achieve physiologic stabilization, volume of fluid used to resuscitate and injuries sustained.

5.3.5.1 DELAYED PRIMARY ABDOMINAL CLOSURE

Delayed closure will be required once the reasons for the temporary surgery have been removed or treated. This is usually possible after an interval of 24–48 hours (or longer). Usually, the abdominal wall can be closed in layers using normal closure techniques. However, this should only be performed when no further surgery is contemplated, and should be accomplished without any fascial tension.

If abdominal viscera are protruding above the fascia in the supine anaesthetized patient, further management with temporary closure (vacuum assisted) is recommended. Return to the operating room after another 24–48 hours of intensive care and fluid mobilization in most cases will then allow primary fascial closure. Both surgeon and anaesthetist must be aware of the danger of causing ACS as a result of the closure, and intra-abdominal or respiratory pressures must be closely monitored.

5.3.5.2 SECONDARY ABDOMINAL CLOSURE

If for various reasons a delayed primary closure is not possible, then it will be necessary to accept (but minimize) the defect that results. The skin of the abdominal wall and the underlying fascia retract, and thus prevent a primary closure from being achieved. During the period of the open abdomen, in this situation, several techniques are usually combined to get to a point where the fascia can be closed without tension and safely. The goal is to achieve fascial closure and subsequent skin closure.

Methods involved which will minimize or reduce the eventual defect include

- Vacuum-assisted closure: Commercial closures have been shown to reduce the defect and assist in closure of the sheath. These include V.A.C. (Kinetic Concepts Inc., San Antonio, TX) and Renasys (Smith & Nephew, London, UK)[9,10].
- Skin-only closure.
- Grafts using Vicryl mesh (Johnson & Johnson, New Brunswick, NJ) or Gore-Tex sheets (W. L. Gore & Associates, Flagstaff, AZ) or other synthetic sheets.
- Biologic meshes – human dermal matrix (AlloDerm, LifeCell, Bridgewater, NJ) or porcine dermal matrix (Permacol, Covidien, Mansfield, MA).
- Split-thickness skin grafts directly on granulated bowel or mesh.

5.3.5.3 SECONDARY CLOSURE

If delayed primary closure is not possible after several days or a week, there are several options

- Closure of skin only, allowing the formation of a hernia.
- Biologic material such as human (AlloDerm) or porcine (Permacol) dermal matrix used as mesh early to prevent hernia formation, providing skin coverage.
- Continued vacuum-assisted temporary abdominal closure (VAC) until granulation over bowel occurs, for subsequent split-thickness skin grafting.
- If a synthetic mesh is left *in situ*, skin coverage of the resulting defect by split-grafting or flap transfer.
- For large hernias, often the need for later reconstruction using different techniques such as component separation and flap construction.
- Mesh-assisted closure[10,11] such as V.A.C. (Kinetic Concepts Inc., KCI) and Renasys (Smith & Nephew).
- A Wittmann patch.

An absorbable mesh of polyglycolic acid such as Vicryl elicits minimal tissue reaction and ingrowth. Thus, it has a low risk of infection or fistula formation.

Membranes such as polytetrafluoroethylene (PTFE; Gore-Tex), which elicit minimal tissue reaction and ingrowth, and thus minimize risk of infection or fistula formation, can be used, but this is considerably more

costly. Recently, composite meshes have shown promise. The mesh can then have a skin graft placed upon it (or even directly on the bowel), and definitive abdominal wall reconstruction can take place at a later stage.

Should any mesh be used and left *in situ*, however, the resulting defect will require skin coverage by split-grafting or flap transfer.

5.3.5.4 PLANNED HERNIA

A planned hernia approach aims at skin coverage with subsequent delayed abdominal wall reconstruction. Conditions favouring a planned hernia strategy include the inability to reapproximate the retracted abdominal wall edges, sizeable tissue deficit, risk of tertiary abdominal compartment syndrome, inadequate infection source control, anterior enteric fistula and poor nutritional status of the patient. Various techniques have been applied. Autologous split-thickness skin grafting over the visceral content of the abdomen allows coverage of the exposed bowel. Maturation of the skin graft requires about 6–12 months, after which the grafted skin can be easily removed from the bowel surface for reconstruction.

Bridging mesh is often employed and absorbable mesh is preferred. Non-absorbable mesh (polypropylene mesh, etc.) has been abandoned because of infection and high rates of fistula formation.

More commonly a component separation is performed. A large relaxing incision is placed in the exterior oblique muscle component of the anterior rectus muscle bilaterally. This can be combined with mobilization of the rectus muscle from the posterior fascial sheath to provide local advancement across the hernia defect. Modification of this technique has been described with division of the internal oblique to the arcuate line. Large abdominal wall defects can be reconstructed with pedicular or microvascular flaps. The most commonly used is the tensor fascia lata (TFL) flap.

5.3.6 Outcomes

In a recent study of 88 damage control patients with a mean injury severity score of 34, Brenner et al. reported of the 63 survivors, 81 per cent had gone back to work and resumed normal daily activities[11].

REFERENCES AND RECOMMENDED READING

References

1. Rotondo MF, Schwab CW, McGonigal MD, et al. Damage control: an approach for improved survival in exsanguinating penetrating abdominal injury. *J Trauma.* 1993;35:375–383.

2. Newell MA, Schlitzkus LL, Waibel BH, White MA, Schenarts PJ, Rotondo MF. "Damage control" in the elderly: futile endeavour or fruitful enterprise? *J Trauma.* 2010;69(5):1049–1053.

3. Smith IM, Beech ZKM, Lundy JB, Bowley DM. A prospective observational study of abdominal injury management in the contemporary military operations: damage control laparotomy is associated with high survivability and low rates of fecal diversion. *Ann Surg.* 2014. doi: 10.1097/SLA 0000000000000657.

4. Gates J, Arabian S, Biddinger P, et al. The initial response to the Boston Marathon bombing: lessons learned to prepare for the next disaster. *Ann Surg.* 2014;260(6):960-6.

5. Holcomb JB, Jenkins D, Rhee P, et al. Damage control resuscitation: directly addressing the early coagulopathy of trauma. *J Trauma.* 2007;62(2):307–310.

6. Hess JR, Holcomb JB, Hoyt DB. Damage control resuscitation: the need for specific blood products to treat the coagulopathy of trauma. *Transfusion.* 2006;46(5):685–6.

7. Lamb CM, MacGoey P, Navarro AP, Brooks AJ. Damage control surgery in the era of damage control resuscitation. *Br J Anaes.* 2014;113:242–249.

8. Schein M, Saadia R. Jamieson JR, Decker GA. The 'sandwich technique' in the management of the open abdomen. *Br J Surg.* 1986;73:369–370.

9. Petersson U, Acosta S, Björck M. Vacuum-assisted wound closure and mesh-mediated fascial traction – a novel technique for late closure of the open abdomen. *World J Surg.* 2007;31:2133–2137.

10. Roberts DJ, Zygun DA, Grendar J, et al. Negative-pressure wound therapy for critically ill adults with open abdominal wounds: a systematic review. *J Trauma.* 2012;73:629–639.

11. Brenner M, Bochicchio G, Bocchicchio K, et al. Long term impact of damage control laparotomy: a prospective study. *Arch Surg.* 2010;146(4):395–399.

Recommended Reading

Chovanes J, Cannon JW, Nunez TC. The evolution of damage control surgery. *Surg Clin North Am.* Aug 2012;92(4):859–875, vii–vi.

Cirocchi R, Abraha I, Montedori A, et al. Damage control surgery for abdominal trauma. *Cochrane Database Syst Rev.* 2010;(1):CD007438.

Godat L, Kobayashi L, Costantini T, Coimbra R. Abdominal damage control surgery and reconstruction: World Society of Emergency Surgery position paper. *World J Emerg Surg.* 2013;8:53.

Lamb CM, MacGoey P, Navarro AP, Brooks AJ. Damage control surgery in the era of damage control resuscitation. *Br J Anaesth.* 2014;113(2):242–249. doi: 10.1093/bja/aeu233.

Hoey BA, Schwab CW. Damage control surgery. *Scand J Surg.* 2002;91:92–103.

Lee JC, Peitzman AB. Damage-control laparotomy. *Curr Opin Crit Care.* 2006;12:346–350.

Loveland JA, Boffard KD. Damage control in the abdomen and beyond. *Br J Surg.* 2004;91;1095–1101.

Moore EE, Burch JM, Franciose RJ, et al. Staged physiologic restoration and damage control surgery. *World J Surg.* 1998;22:1184–1191.

O'Connor JV, DuBose J, Scalea TM.Damage-control thoracic surgery: management and outcomes. *J Trauma Acute Care Surg.* 2014;77:660–665.

Waibel BH, Rotondo MF. Damage control for intra-abdominal sepsis. *Surg Clin North Am.* 2012;92(2):243–257, viii.

6.1 **OVERVIEW**

The high density of critical vascular, aerodigestive and neurological structures within the neck makes the management of penetrating injuries difficult and contributes to the morbidity and mortality seen in these patients.

Before World War II, non-operative management of penetrating neck trauma resulted in mortality rates of up to 15 per cent. Therefore, the exploration of all neck wounds penetrating the platysma muscle became mandatory. However, in recent years, numerous centres have challenged this principle of mandatory exploration, since up to 50 per cent of neck explorations may be negative for significant injury.

6.2 **MANAGEMENT PRINCIPLES**

The current management of penetrating cervical injuries depends on several factors.

6.2.1 **Initial Assessment**

Patients with signs of significant neck injury with active bleeding or an expanding haematoma will require prompt exploration. However, initial assessment and management of the patient should be carried out according to Advanced Trauma Life Support principles.

The major initial concern in any patient with a penetrating neck wound is early control of the airway. Supplemental oxygen is critical. Intubation in these patients is complicated by the possibility of associated cervical spine injury, laryngeal trauma and large haematomas in the neck. Appropriate protective measures for possible cervical spine injury must be implemented. The route of intubation must be carefully considered in these patients since it may be complicated by distortion of anatomy, haematoma, dislodging of clots, laryngeal trauma and a significant number of cervical spinal injuries.

The following points should be noted:

- Cervical spine injury. While it is important to protect the unstable/potentially unstable cervical spine with immobilization a rapid risk/benefit assessment must be done in the presence of a deteriorating airway. Cervical spine immobilization techniques make endotracheal intubation more difficult.
- Oxygenate the patient with simple measures first (i.e. basic airway opening techniques). Note that laryngeal mask airways (LMAs) do *not* provide a definitive airway in the presence of complex neck injuries but can be used to attempt oxygenation prior to establishing an endotracheal tube or surgical airway.
- Recent UK military experience in Afghanistan is that the majority of patients can be managed with a rapid sequence induction of anaesthesia followed by endotracheal intubation with a relatively small tube (e.g. size 6.5 mm or 7 mm ID in an adult male) aided by a gum-elastic bougie or stylet.
- The caveat is that a surgeon is scrubbed and ready to perform a cricothyroidotomy or emergency tracheostomy if it becomes immediately obvious that the trachea cannot be intubated following rapid sequence induction (RSI).
- Patients have also been managed by a gas induction of anaesthesia (supplemented with small boluses of ketamine – 10 mg IV), laryngoscopy while still breathing then endotracheal intubation.
- Cricothyroidotomy or tracheostomy under local anaesthesia in the awake, spontaneously breathing patient is another option.
- Fibre-optic techniques may have a role in neck injury – but be aware that bleeding into the airway will rapidly obscure the view through the scope.

- Laryngeal masks do not provide a definitive airway and may be hazardous in the presence of penetrating neck injury.

Endotracheal intubation should be considered at the very early stage in the presence of large haematoma as subsequent cricothyroidotomy or emergency percutaneous tracheostomy (only to be considered if the enabling environment and extensive experience in the technique are available) can be technically difficult by entering the haematoma planes, resulting in torrential bleeding via the skin incision.

Fibre-optic bronchoscopy may be useful, and it is possible to pass the bronchoscope through an endotracheal tube, enter the trachea under direct vision and then slide the endotracheal tube into place. Video-assisted laryngoscopy further facilitates introduction of the endotracheal tube under direct vision.

Managing complicated airway injuries should be rehearsed along with backup plans for alternate techniques to secure the airway if the initial one fails. The decision as to what technique is the most appropriate should be made rapidly and jointly by the surgeon, anaesthetist and trauma team leader.

> NB: The use of paralysing agents in these patients is contraindicated, since the airway may be held open only by the patient's use of muscles.

Abolishing the use of muscles in such patients may result in the immediate and total obstruction of the airway and, with no visibility due to the presence of blood, may result in catastrophe. Ideally, local anaesthetic spray should be used with sedation, and a cricothyroidotomy below the injury should be considered when necessary.

Control of haemorrhage should be done by direct pressure where possible. If the neck wound is not bleeding, do not probe or finger the wound as a clot may be dislodged.

If the wound is actively bleeding, the bleeding should be controlled by digital pressure or, if ineffective, a Foley catheter may be inserted into the wound and the balloon inflated. This is often useful for stopping haemorrhage deep in the neck. Occasionally, the wound may need to be swiftly sutured around the catheter to produce the required tamponade. However, this may result in converting external haemorrhage into continued bleeding deep within the neck and further compromise an already compressed airway, and hence the importance of securing an early definitive airway. More than one Foley catheter is sometimes needed.

There should be no hesitation in performing an emergency cricothyroidotomy should circumstances warrant it.

Patients with signs of significant neck injury, and those whose condition is unstable, should be explored urgently in the operating room, with good light, good instruments and good assistance, once rapid initial assessment has been completed and the airway has been secured. There should be no hesitation in performing an emergency cricothyroidotomy should circumstances warrant it. Tracheostomy has no place in the emergency department. Cricothyroidotomies should be converted to formal tracheostomies within about 48 hours.

Figure 6.1 (a) Anterior view showing zones of the neck. (b) Lateral view showing triangles of the neck.

6.2.1.1 INJURY LOCATION

Division of the neck into anatomical zones (Figure 6.1) helps the categorization and management of neck wounds:

- *Zone I* extends from the level of the sternal notch to the lower border of the cricoid cartilage. Within zone 1 lie the great vessels, the trachea, the oesophagus, the thoracic duct and the upper mediastinum and lung apices.
- *Zone II* includes the area between the cricoid cartilage and the angle of the mandible. Enclosed within its region are the carotid and vertebral arteries, jugular veins, pharynx, larynx, oesophagus and trachea.
- *Zone III* includes the area above the angle of the mandible to the base of the skull, the pharynx, and the distal extracranial carotid and vertebral arteries, as well as segments of the jugular veins.

Injuries in zone II are readily evaluated and exposed operatively. Therefore in trauma centres with a high volume of penetrating trauma, a decision on immediate surgery can be reached on clinical grounds without any pre-operative investigations. Zones I and III are difficult to assess clinically and also difficult to access operatively. Therefore, in those two zones it is important in the physiologically stable patient to proceed with diagnostic work-up so that the presence or absence of injury is established, the possibility of dealing with it without an operative procedure is decided (e.g. embolization of bleeding artery) and if operation is necessary as a last resort, this will be facilitated by knowing the type of injury and its topography.

One pitfall is assuming that a wound in one zone means an injury in that zone. Not infrequently, a wound in one zone is associated with the injury in quite another area. For example, a long knife may penetrate the skin in zone I or II, but the injury may lie in the superior mediastinum. Similarly, bullets and missile fragments often transgress zone boundaries. Either may cross the midline, giving rise to contralateral injured structures.

6.2.1.2 MECHANISM

Gunshot wounds carry a higher risk of major injury than stab wounds because of their tendency to penetrate more deeply and their ability to damage tissue outside the tract of the missile due to cavitation or a percussion wave injury.

6.2.1.3 FREQUENCY OF INJURY

The carotid artery and internal jugular vein are the most frequently injured vessels. Due to its relatively protected position, the vertebral artery is involved less frequently. The larynx and trachea, and pharynx and oesophagus are frequently injured. The spinal cord is damaged less often, but injury should not be ruled out until examination has confirmed its integrity.

6.2.2 Use of Diagnostic Studies

In the stable patient without indications for immediate neck exploration, additional studies are often obtained, including angiography, endoscopy, contrast radiography and bronchoscopy. (A few recent studies have even suggested that asymptomatic patients can be observed safely by serial examination, but this is a highly selective approach.)

6.2.2.1 COMPUTED TOMOGRAPHY SCANNING WITH CONTRAST/COMPUTED TOMOGRAPHY ANGIOGRAPHY

Modern computed tomography (CT) scanners have provided a means of creating a three-dimensional (3D) image of high quality, and CT scanning is now the investigation of choice for penetrating injury in the stable patient. Angiography has been largely replaced by CT angiography that should include both internal and external carotid arteries as well as vertebral arteries on both sides (four-vessel CT angiography). Angiography is only practiced as part of arterial embolization following a diagnostic CT angiography.

6.2.2.2 ANGIOGRAPHY

Especially in zone I or zone III injuries, where surgical exposure can be difficult, angiography is invaluable to plan the conduct of operation. Angiography should visualize both the internal and external carotid arteries on both sides ('four-vessel angiography'), as well as the vertebral arteries on both sides.

Using a selective approach to the management of zone II wounds, angiography is useful in excluding carotid injuries, especially with soft signs of injury, including stable haematoma and history of significant bleeding, or when the wound is in close proximity to the major vessels.

6.2.2.3 OTHER DIAGNOSTIC STUDIES

The selective management of penetrating neck wounds involves evaluation of the oesophagus, larynx and trachea. Either contrast oesophagography or oesophagoscopy alone will detect 60 per cent of oesophageal injuries. The two tests used together increase the diagnostic accuracy to nearly 90 per cent. Laryngoscopy and bronchoscopy are useful adjuncts in localizing or excluding injury to the hypopharynx or trachea. A recent development is 3D CT reconstruction of the trachea and bronchi which can replace endoscopy in suspected injuries of these anatomical structures.

6.3 TREATMENT

6.3.1 Mandatory versus Selective Neck Exploration

Recommendations for the management of patients with penetrating cervical trauma depend on the zone of injury and the patient's clinical status. If the platysma is not penetrated, the patient may be observed. Mandatory exploration for penetrating neck injury in patients with hard signs of vascular or aerodigestive tract injury is still appropriate.

The mandatory exploration of all stable patients is controversial. Missed injuries associated with a high morbidity and mortality due to missed visceral injuries, as well as the negligible morbidity caused by negative exploration, are reasons to operate on all patients with penetrating wounds. However, exploration of all stab wounds of the neck may yield a high rate of non-therapeutic procedures. Thus, the selective management of penetrating neck wounds with thorough non-operative evaluation has been recommended.

In the stable patient with a wound that penetrates the platysma, either mandatory exploration or non-operative evaluation (angiography, oesophagography, bronchoscopy and thorough endoscopy) is appropriate.

6.3.2 Treatment Based on Anatomical Zones

6.3.2.1 VASCULAR INJURIES

If associated injuries allow, a 5000–10000 unit bolus of heparin should be given before any of the arteries in the neck are occluded. Because they have no branches, the common and internal carotid arteries can be safely

mobilized for some distance from the injury to ensure a tension-free repair.

All patients with zones I and III neck injuries should undergo angiography as soon as their vital signs are stable. Zone I injuries require angiography because of the increased association of vascular injuries with penetrating trauma to the thoracic outlet. Angiography helps the surgeon plan the surgical approach. Zone III injuries require angiography because of the relationship of the blood vessels to the base of the skull. Often these injuries can be best managed by either non-operative techniques or manoeuvres remote from the injury site such as balloon tamponade or embolization. Injuries in zone II may require angiography if the vertebral vessels are thought to be injured. Venous phasing should be requested. However, CT angiography will *not* rule out significant injury to the trachea or oesophagus.

The patient is placed in the supine position on the operating table with the arms tucked at the sides. Active bleeding from a penetrating wound should be controlled digitally. However, penetrating wounds to the neck should not be probed, cannulated or locally explored because these procedures may dislodge a clot and cause uncontrollable bleeding or air embolism. Skin preparation should include the entire chest and shoulder, extending above the angle of the mandible. If possible, the head should be extended and rotated to the contralateral side. A sandbag may be placed between the shoulder blades. A vascular set should be open, and a sternotomy set should be available in the operating room.

Zone III injuries, at the very base of the skull, are complex and should be explored with great care. Access is often extremely difficult. On rare occasions, it may not be possible to control the distal stump of a high internal carotid artery injury. While techniques for mandibular dislocation or division of the sternomastoid muscle off the mastoid process may be helpful, bleeding from this injury can be controlled either temporarily or permanently by inserting a Fogarty catheter into the distal segment and inflating the balloon. The catheter is secured, transected and left in place. It may be necessary to control the internal carotid artery from within the cranial cavity (usually the realm of the neurosurgeon).

Zone II injuries are explored by an incision made along the anterior border of the sternocleidomastoid muscle, as for carotid endarterectomy. An extended collar incision or bilateral incisions along the anterior edge of the sternocleidomastoid muscles may be used for wounds that traverse both sides of the neck. Proximal and distal control of the blood vessel is obtained. If the vessel is actively bleeding, direct pressure is applied to the bleeding site while control is obtained. Use of anticoagulation is optional. If there are no injuries that preclude its use, heparin may be given in the management of carotid injuries. Vascular shunts are rarely needed in patients with carotid injuries, especially if the distal clamp is applied proximal to the bifurcation of the internal and external carotid arteries. Repair techniques for cervical trauma do not differ significantly from those used for other vascular injuries.

- The intraoperative decisions are influenced by the patient's preoperative neurological status. If the patient has no neurological deficit preoperatively, the injured vessel should be repaired. (The one exception may be if a complete obstruction of blood flow is found at the time of surgery, because restoration of flow may cause distal remobilization or haemorrhagic infarction.)
- Operative management of the patient with a carotid injury and a preoperative neurological deficit is controversial. Vascular reconstruction should be performed in patients with mild-to-moderate deficits in whom retrograde flow is present. Ligation is recommended for patients with severe preoperative neurological deficits greater than 48 hours old, and without evidence of retrograde flow at the time of operation.

Zone I vascular injuries at the base of the neck require aggressive management. Frequently, uncontrollable haemorrhage will require immediate thoracotomy for initial proximal control. In an unstable patient, quick exposure often may be achieved via a median sternotomy and a supraclavicular extension.

The location of the vascular injury will dictate the definitive exposure. For right-sided great vessel injuries, a median sternotomy with a supraclavicular extension allows optimal access. On the left side, a left anterolateral thoracotomy may provide initial proximal control. Further operation for definitive repair may require a sternotomy, or extension into the right side of the chest or up into the neck. Trapdoor incisions are *not* recommended as they are often difficult to perform and do not significantly improve the exposure, but significantly increase the postoperative disability. Care must be taken to avoid injury to the phrenic and vagus nerves as they enter into the thorax. In the stable patient in whom the vascular injury has been confirmed by CT, the right subclavian artery or the distal two-thirds of the left subclavian artery can be exposed through an incision immediately superior to the medial third of the clavicle. Injuries to the vessels behind the clavicle can be controlled by combining supra- and infra-clavicular incisions. The clavicle does not need to be divided or resected. Grafts can easily be tunnelled underneath the bone, avoiding risk to the subclavian vein.

- Injuries to the internal jugular vein should be repaired if possible. In severe injuries that require extensive debridement, ligation is preferred. Venous interposition grafts should not be performed.
- Vertebral artery injuries are generally found only on angiographic study. These rarely require surgical repair, as they are best dealt with by angioembolization. Operative exposure may be difficult and it may be easier to ligate it at its origin off the subclavian artery, or pass a size-3 or size-4 Fogarty catheter into the lumen and inflate the balloon to provide tamponade. This may be left permanently if required, with very small incidence of neurological damage. Venous bleeding can be stopped by packing around the area of injury.

There is increasing support for the treatment of carotid artery injuries with intraluminal stenting. This approach is now common and is most frequently used in situations where arterial lesions are not surgically accessible or when anticoagulation is contraindicated.

6.3.2.2 TRACHEAL INJURIES

Injuries to the trachea should be closed in a single layer with absorbable sutures. Larger defects may require a fascia flap. These injuries should be drained.

6.3.2.3 PHARYNGEAL AND OESOPHAGEAL INJURIES

Oesophageal injuries are often missed at neck exploration. Injuries to the hypopharynx and cervical oesophagus may also be difficult to diagnose preoperatively. Perforations of the hypopharynx or oesophagus should be closed in two layers if possible, though the mucosal layer is the key to leak-proof repair. The site should be widely drained. Identification may be aided by the passage of a nasogastric tube. For devastating oesophageal injuries requiring extensive resection and debridement, a cutaneous oesophagostomy for feeding, and pharyngostomy for diversion, may be necessary.

6.3.3 **Rules**

- The first concern in the patient with a penetrating injury of the neck is early control of the airway.
- The next concern is to stop bleeding, either by digital pressure or by the use of a Foley catheter.
- The stability of the patient decides the appropriate diagnostic and treatment priorities. Never make the operation more difficult than necessary by inadequate exposure. Adequate exposure of the area involved is critical.

6.4 **ACCESS TO THE NECK**

The operative approach selected to explore neck injuries is determined by the structures known or suspected to be injured. Surgical exploration should be done formally and systematically in a fully equipped operating room under general anaesthesia with endotracheal intubation. Blind probing of wounds or mini-explorations in the emergency department should never be attempted.

6.4.1 **Incision**

Always expect the worst, and plan the incision to provide optimal access for early proximal vascular control or immediate access to the airway. The most universally applicable approach is via an incision along the anterior border of sternomastoid, which can be lengthened proximally and distally, extended to a median sternotomy or augmented with lateral extensions. The patient is positioned supine with a bolster between the shoulders, and the neck extended and rotated away from the side of injury – provided that the cervical spine has been cleared pre-operatively. The face, neck and anterior chest should be prepped and widely draped.

Having made the sternocleidomastoid muscle incision, platysma is divided, and the sternomastoid is retracted laterally to expose the fascial sheath covering the internal jugular vein. The vein cannot be mobilized until the common facial vein is divided. Omohyoid muscle is the only strap muscle that crosses the carotid sheath obliquely and acts as a landmark for the common carotid artery. Lateral retraction of the jugular vein and underlying carotid artery allows access to the trachea, oesophagus and thyroid, and medial retraction of the carotid sheath and its contents will allow the dissection to proceed posteriorly to the prevertebral fascia and vertebral arteries. Posterior to the carotid sheath, the sympathetic chain lies on the longus colli, which separates it from the transverse processes of the cervical vertebrae.

6.4.2 **Carotid Artery**

Exposure of the carotid artery is obtained by ligating the middle thyroid and common facial veins and retracting the internal jugular laterally together with the sternocleidomastoid. The vagus nerve lying posteriorly within the carotid sheath must be preserved. The occipital artery and inferior branches of the ansa cervicalis may be divided. To expose the carotid bifurcation, the dissection is carried upward to the posterior belly of the digastric muscle, which is divided behind the angle of the jaw. Care must be taken to find and preserve the hypoglossal nerve, which runs forward across both internal and external carotid artery to enter the floor of the mouth. It usually is found either at the lower border of the posterior belly of digastric, or just deep to that muscle.

Access to the internal carotid can be improved by dividing the sternocleidomastoid muscle near its origin at the mastoid. Care must be taken not to injure the accessory nerve where it enters the sternomastoid muscle 3 cm below the mastoid, or the glossopharyngeus nerve crossing anteriorly over the internal carotid artery. More distal exploration of the internal carotid artery may require unilateral mandibular subluxation or division of the ascending ramus. The styloid process may be excised after division of the stylohyoid ligament and styloglossus and stylopharyngeus muscles. The facial nerve lies superficial to these muscles and must be preserved. To reach the internal carotid artery where it enters the carotid canal, part of the mastoid bone can be removed. Fortunately, this is rarely required. Figures 6.2 and 6.3 show the surgical approach to the neck.

The proximal carotid artery is exposed by division of the omohyoid muscle between the superior and inferior bellies. More proximal control may require a midline sternotomy.

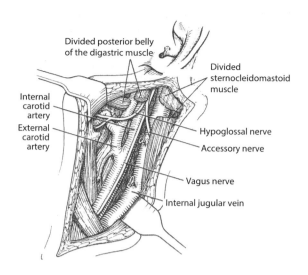

Figure 6.2 Approach to the left side of the neck with divided sterno-mastoid and digastric muscles.

6.4.3 **Midline Visceral Structures**

The trachea, oesophagus and thyroid are approached by retracting the carotid sheath laterally. The inferior thyroid artery should be divided laterally near the carotid artery, and the thyroid lobe is lifted anteriorly to expose the trachea and oesophagus posteriorly. Oesophageal identification is aided by passing a large dilator or nasogastric tube. The recurrent laryngeal nerves should be carefully preserved: the left nerve runs vertically in the tracheo-oesophageal groove, but the right nerve runs obliquely across the oesophagus and trachea from infero-lateral to superomedial. Both nerves are at risk of injury with circumferential mobilization of the oesophagus. Bilateral exposure of the midline structures may require transverse extension of the standard incision.

6.4.4 **Root of the Neck**

The structures at the root of the neck can be approached by extending the incision laterally above the clavicle. The clavicular head of the sternocleidomastoid is divided, and the supraclavicular fat pad is cleared by blunt dissection. This fat pad is a constant feature, even in the thinnest of individuals. Its removal is complicated because it contains many small blood vessels, lymph nodes and the thoracic duct. Removal reveals the scalenus anterior muscle, with the phrenic nerve crossing it from the lateral side. Division of the scalenus anterior, with preservation of the phrenic nerve, allows access to the second part of the subclavian artery. The distal subclavian artery can be exposed by a further infra-clavicular incision and obtaining control of the proximal axillary artery, or dividing the clavicle at its mid-point, and dissecting away the subclavius muscle and fascia. The clavicle should not be re-sected as this leads to considerable morbidity. To fix the divided bone, the periosteum should be approximated with strong polyfilament absorbable sutures, or a mini-plate can be inserted.

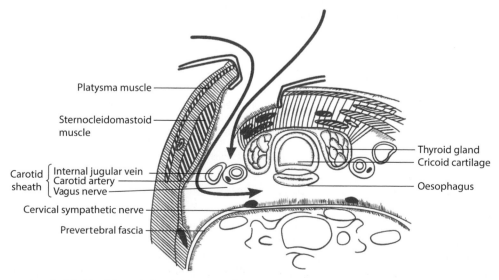

Figure 6.3 Approach to the left side of the neck showing retraction of the platysma and sternomastoid muscles.

6.4.5 **Collar Incisions**

These are rarely used unless there is absolute certainty that the injury is limited to the area about to be exposed. In trauma in general, it is wiser to make incisions that can be extended both proximally and distally, therefore utilizing bilateral sternomastoid incisions that can be joined for bilateral injuries in the form of a 'U'.

However, some surgeons adopt the collar incisions. Horizontal or 'collar' incisions placed either over the thyroid or higher up over the thyroid cartilage can sometimes be useful to expose bilateral injuries or injuries limited to the larynx or trachea. The transverse incision is carried through the platysma, and subplatysmal flaps are then developed: superiorly up to the thyroid cartilage notch, and inferiorly to the sternal notch. The strap muscles are divided vertically in the midline and retracted laterally to expose the fascia covering the thyroid. The thyroid isthmus can be divided to expose the trachea. A high collar incision, placed over the larynx, is useful for repairing isolated laryngeal injuries.

6.4.6 **Vertebral Arteries**

The proximal part of the vertebral artery is approached via the anterior sternomastoid incision, with division of the clavicular head of the sternomastoid. The internal jugular vein and common carotid artery are mobilized, the vein is retracted medially, and the artery and nerve are retracted laterally. The proximal vertebral artery lies deeply between these structures. The vertebral artery is crossed by branches of the cervical sympathetic chain and on the left side by the thoracic duct. The inferior thyroid artery crosses in a more superficial plane just before the vertebral artery enters its bony canal.

Access to the distal vertebral artery is challenging and rarely needed. The contents of the carotid sheath are retracted anteromedially, and the prevertebral muscles are longitudinally split over a transverse process above the level of the injury. The anterior surface of the transverse process can be removed with a small rongeur, or a J-shaped needle may be used to snare the artery in the space between the transverse processes.

The most distal portion of the vertebral artery can be approached between the atlas and the axis after division of the sternocleidomastoid near its origin at the mastoid process. The pre-vertebral fascia is divided over the transverse process of the atlas. With preservation of the C2 nerve root, the levator scapulae and splenius cervicis muscles are divided close to the transverse process of the atlas. The vertebral artery can now be visualized between the two vertebrae and may be ligated with a J-shaped needle. This area of dissection more commonly requires expertise of a neurosurgeon if available.

Neck exploration wounds are closed in layers after acquiring homeostasis. Drainage is usually indicated, mainly to prevent haematomas and sepsis.

RECOMMENDED READING

Demetriades D, Asensio JA, Velmahos G, Thal E. Complex problems in penetrating neck trauma. *Surg Clin North Am.* 1996;76:661–683.

Fabian TC, George SM Jr, Croce MA, Mangiante EC, Voeller GR, Kusdk KA. Carotid artery trauma: management based on mechanism of injury. *J Trauma.* 1990;30:953–961.

Osborn TM, Bell RB, Qaisi W, et al. Computed angiography as an aid to clinical decision making in the selective management of penetrating injuries of the neck: a reduction in the need for operative exploration. *J Trauma.* 2008;64:146–171.

Part 3

Physiology and the body's response to trauma

7.1 OVERVIEW

7.1.1 Introduction: Scope of the Problem

Thoracic injury constitutes a significant problem in terms of mortality and morbidity. In the United States during the early 1990s, there were approximately 180 000 deaths per annum from injury. Several investigators have shown that 50 per cent of fatal injuries are due to primary brain injury, 25 per cent of fatal accidents are due to chest trauma, and in another 25 per cent (including brain injury) thoracic injury contributes to the primary cause of mortality[1]. Approximately 15 per cent of thoracic injuries will require definitive surgery.

Somewhat less clearly defined is the extent of appreciable morbidity following chest injury, most usually the long-term consequences of hypoxic brain damage. There are a number of important points to be taken in this regard.

A significant proportion of these deaths occur virtually immediately (i.e. at the time of injury), for example, rapid exsanguination following traumatic rupture of the aorta in blunt injury or major vascular disruption after penetrating injury.

Of survivors with thoracic injury who reach hospital, a significant proportion dies in hospital as the result of mis-assessment or delay in the institution of treatment. These deaths occur *early* as a consequence of shock, or *late* as the result of adult respiratory distress syndrome, multiple organ failure and sepsis. Most life-threatening thoracic injuries can be simply and promptly treated after identification by tube placement for drainage. These are simple and effective techniques that can be performed by any trained physician.

Emergency department thoracotomy (EDT) has specific indications; these virtually always relate to patients in extremis with penetrating injury. Indiscriminate use of EDT, however, especially in blunt trauma, will not alter patient outcome, but will increase the risk of communicable disease transmission to health workers.

Injuries to the chest wall and thoracic viscera can directly impair oxygen transport mechanisms. Hypoxia and hypovolaemia resulting as a consequence of thoracic injuries may cause secondary injury to patients with brain injury or may directly cause cerebral oedema.

Conversely, shock and/or brain injury can secondarily aggravate thoracic injuries and hypoxaemia by disrupting normal ventilatory patterns or by causing loss of protective airway reflexes and aspiration.

The lung is a target organ for secondary injury following shock and remote tissue injury. Microemboli formed in the peripheral microcirculation embolize to the lung, causing ventilation–perfusion mismatch and right heart failure. Tissue injury and shock can activate the inflammatory cascade, which can contribute to pulmonary injury (reperfusion).

7.1.2 Spectrum of Thoracic Injury

Thoracic injuries are grouped into two types, as described below.

7.1.2.1 IMMEDIATELY LIFE-THREATENING INJURIES

- Airway obstruction due to any cause, including laryngeal or tracheal disruption with obstruction or extensive facial bony and soft tissue injuries.
- Impaired ventilation due to tension pneumothorax, major bronchial disruptions, open pneumothorax or flail chest.
- Impaired circulation due to massive haemothorax or pericardial tamponade.
- Air embolism.

7.1.2.2 POTENTIALLY LIFE-THREATENING INJURIES

- Blunt cardiac injury.
- Pulmonary contusion.

- Flail chest (multiple fractured ribs with paradoxical chest wall movement).
- Traumatic rupture of the aorta.
- Traumatic diaphragmatic herniation.
- Tracheobronchial tree disruption.
- Oesophageal disruption.
- Haemothorax.
- Pneumothorax.

Penetrating wounds traversing the mediastinum warrant specific mention. Injuries of this type frequently damage a number of mediastinal structures, and are thus more complex in their evaluation and management.

7.1.3 **Pathophysiology of Thoracic Injuries**

The well-recognized pathophysiological changes occurring in patients with thoracic injuries are essentially the result of

- Impairment of ventilation.
- Impairment of gas exchange at the alveolar level.
- Impairment of circulation due to haemodynamic changes.
- Impairment of cardiac function due to tamponade or air embolus.

The approach to the patient with thoracic injury must therefore take all these elements into account.

Specifically, hypoxia at a cellular or tissue level results from inadequate delivery of oxygen to the tissues, with the development of acidosis and associated hypercapnia. The late complications resulting from mis-assessment of thoracic injuries are directly attributable to these processes.

Penetrating chest injuries should be obvious. Exceptions include small puncture wounds such as those caused by ice picks, or ballistic fragments. Bleeding is generally minimal secondary to the low pressure within the pulmonary system. Exceptions to these management principles include wounds to the great vessels as they exit over the apex of the chest wall to the upper extremities, or injury to any systemic vessel that may be injured in the chest wall, such as the internal mammary or intercostal vessels.

Penetrating injuries to the mid-torso generate more controversy. These will require a fairly aggressive approach, particularly with anterior wounds. If the wound is between one posterior axillary line and the other and obviously penetrates the abdominal wall, laparotomy is indicated. If the wound does not obviously penetrate, an option is to explore the wound under local anaesthesia to determine whether or not it has penetrated the peritoneal lining or the diaphragm. If peritoneal penetration has occurred, laparotomy is indicated. Other options include laparoscopy or thoracoscopy to determine whether the diaphragm has been injured and for evacuation of clots (see Section 15)[2].

Patients arrive in one of two general physiological states:

- Haemodynamically stable.
- Haemodynamically unstable.

In the patient with penetrating injury to the upper torso who is haemodynamically unstable, and whose bleeding is occurring into the chest cavity, it is important to insert a chest tube as soon as possible during the initial assessment and resuscitation. In the patient in extremis who has chest injuries or in whom there may be suspicion of a transmediastinal injury, bilateral chest tubes may be indicated. X-ray is *not* required to insert a chest tube, but it *is* useful after the chest tubes have been inserted to confirm proper placement.

In patients who are haemodynamically stable, X-ray remains the gold standard for diagnosis of a pneumothorax or haemothorax. In these patients, it is preferable to have the X-ray completed before placement of a chest tube. The decrease in air entry may not be due to a pneumothorax, and especially following blunt injury may be due to a ruptured diaphragm with bowel or stomach occupying the thoracic cavity, or simply pulmonary contusion.

The widespread use, free availability and training in performing the extended focussed assessment with sonography for trauma (eFAST) and other clinician-performed modalities has further reduced the need for plain X-rays in thoracic trauma

When it comes to the removal of chest tubes, bedside thoracic ultrasonography of the fourth intercostal space can reliably determine safe removal of tube thoracostomy after traumatic injury, by excluding the presence of an ongoing pneumothorax, and ensuring a new pneumothorax has not redeveloped by repeating the examination in 4–6 hours[3].

7.1.4 **Paediatric Considerations**

There are a number of important considerations in the assessment and management of paediatric and adolescent chest trauma[4]:

In children, the ribs are more flexible, so the presence of rib fractures implies a high-energy injury, and a higher incidence of associated head, thoracic and abdominal solid organ injuries[5].

Penetrating cardiac wounds in the paediatric age have a poorer prognosis than in adults, and are associated with a low in-hospital survival (<30%)[6].

- In children, the thymus may be very large, and care should be taken to avoid damage to it.
- The sternum is relatively soft and can be divided using a pair of heavy scissors.
- Intercostal drains should be tunnelled subcutaneously over at least one rib space to facilitate later removal without air leaks. The child may not cooperate with a Valsalva manoeuvre, and pressure on the extended tract may prevent iatrogenic pneumothorax on removal.

Paediatric patients with blunt torso trauma and pneumothoraces are uncommon, and most are not identified on the ED chest X-ray. Nearly half of pneumothoraces, and most occult pneumothoraces, can be managed without tube thoracostomy[7]. An important issue in dealing with severe paediatric chest trauma is the unavailability and unsuitability of adult-sized aortic stent grafts for the very rare occasions of traumatic aortic injuries in this age group.

7.1.5 **Applied Surgical Anatomy of the Chest**

It is useful to broadly view the thorax as a container with an inlet, walls, a floor and contents.

7.1.5.1 **CHEST WALL**

This is the bony 'cage' constituted by the ribs, thoracic vertebral column and sternum with the clavicles anteriorly and the scapula posteriorly. The associated muscle groups and vascular structures (specifically the intercostals vessels and the internal thoracic vessels) are further components.

Remember the 'safe area' of the chest. This triangular area is the thinnest region of the chest wall in terms of musculature. This is the area of choice for tube thoracostomy insertion. In this area, there are no significant structures within the walls that may be damaged; however, note that there is a need to avoid the intercostal vascular and nerve bundle on the undersurface of the rib (Figure 7.1).

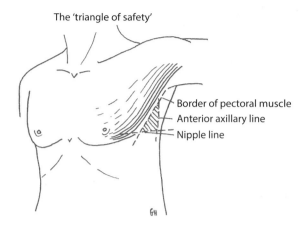

Figure 7.1 Anatomy of the chest wall.

7.1.5.2 **CHEST FLOOR**

This is formed by the diaphragm with its various openings. This broad sheet of muscle with its large, trefoil-shaped central tendon has hiatuses through which pass the aorta, the oesophagus and the inferior vena cava, and is it innervated by the phrenic nerves. The oesophageal hiatus also contains both vagus nerves. The aortic hiatus contains the azygos vein and the thoracic duct.

During normal breathing, the diaphragm moves about 2 cm, but it can move up to 10 cm in deep breathing. During maximum expiration, the diaphragm may rise as high as the fifth intercostal space. Thus, any injury below the fifth intercostal space may involve the abdominal cavity.

7.1.5.3 **CHEST CONTENTS**

The chest contents are as follows:

- The left and right pleural spaces containing the lungs, lined by the parietal and visceral pleurae, respectively.
- The mediastinum and its viscera, located in the centre of the chest. The mediastinum has anterior, middle, posterior and superior divisions. The superior mediastinum is contiguous with the thoracic inlet and zone I of the neck (Figure 7.2).

7.1.5.3.1 Tracheobronchial Tree

The trachea extends from the cricoid cartilage at the level of the fifth cervical vertebra, to the carina at the level of the upper border of the sixth thoracic vertebra,

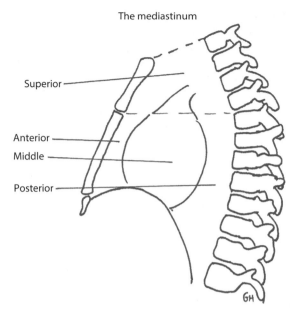

The mediastinum

Superior

Anterior

Middle

Posterior

Figure 7.2 Chest contents.

where it bifurcates. The right main bronchus is shorter, straighter and at less of an angle compared with that on the left side. It lies just below the junction between the azygos vein and the superior vena cava, and behind the right pulmonary artery.

7.1.5.3.2 Lungs and Pleurae

The right lung constitutes about 55 per cent of the total lung mass and has oblique and transverse fissures that divide it into three lobes. The left lung is divided into upper and lower lobes by the oblique fissure. Both lungs are divided into bronchopulmonary segments corresponding to the branches of the lesser bronchi, and are supplied by branches of the pulmonary arteries. The right and left pulmonary arteries pass superiorly in the hilum, anterior to each respective bronchus. There are superior and inferior pulmonary veins on each side, the middle lobe usually being drained by the superior vein.

The pleural cavities are lined by parietal and visceral pleura. The parietal pleura lines the inner wall of the thoracic cage. The visceral pleura is intimately applied to the surface of the lungs, and is reflected onto the mediastinum to join the parietal pleura at the hilum.

7.1.5.3.3 Heart and Pericardium

The heart lies in the middle mediastinum, extending from the level of the third costal cartilage to the xiphisternal junction. The majority of the anterior surface

of the heart is represented by the right atrium and its auricular appendage superiorly and the right ventricle inferiorly. The aorta emerges from the cranial aspect and crosses to the left as the arch. The pulmonary artery extends cranially and bifurcates in the concavity of the aortic arch. The left pulmonary artery is attached to the concavity of the arch of the aorta, just distal to the origin of the left subclavian artery, by the ligamentum arteriosum. The pericardium is a strong fibrous sac that completely invests the heart and is attached to the diaphragm inferiorly. Pericardial tamponade can be created by less than 50 mL or up to more than 200 mL of blood.

7.1.5.3.4 Aorta and Great Vessels

The thoracic aorta is divided into three parts: the ascending aorta, arch and descending aorta. The innominate artery is the first branch from the arch, passing upward and to the right, posterior to the innominate vein. The left common carotid artery and left subclavian artery arise from the left side of the arch.

7.1.5.3.5 Oesophagus

The oesophagus, approximately 25cm long, extends from the pharynx to the stomach. It starts at the level of the sixth cervical vertebra, and passes through the diaphragm about 2.5 cm to the left of the midline at the level of the 11th thoracic vertebra. The entire intrathoracic oesophagus is surrounded by loose areolar tissue, which allows for rapid spread of infection if the oesophagus is breached.

7.1.5.3.6 Thoracic Duct

The duct arises from the cysterna chyli overlying the first and second lumbar vertebrae. It lies posteriorly and to the right of the aorta. It ascends through the oesophageal hiatus of the diaphragm between the aorta and the azygos vein, anterior to the right intercostal branches from the aorta. It overlies the right side of the vertebral bodies, and injury can result in a right-sided chylothorax. It drains into the venous system at the junction of the left subclavian and internal jugular veins.

From a functional and practical point of view, it is useful to regard the chest in terms of a 'hemithorax and its content', both in evaluation of the injury and in choosing the option for access. Figures 7.3 and 7.4 illustrate the hemithoraces and their respective contents.

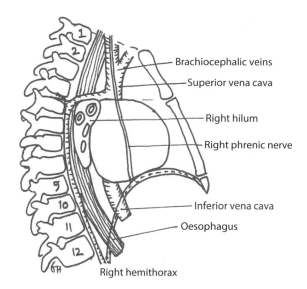

Figure 7.3 Right hemithorax and mediastinum.

Labels (Figure 7.3):
- Brachiocephalic veins
- Superior vena cava
- Right hilum
- Right phrenic nerve
- Inferior vena cava
- Oesophagus
- Right hemithorax

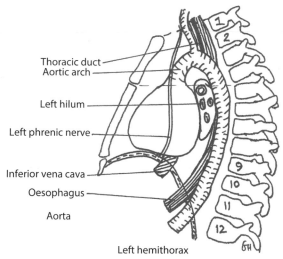

Figure 7.4 Left hemithorax and mediastinum.

Labels (Figure 7.4):
- Thoracic duct
- Aortic arch
- Left hilum
- Left phrenic nerve
- Inferior vena cava
- Oesophagus
- Aorta
- Left hemithorax

7.1.6 **Diagnosis**

Penetrating injuries to the chest may be clinically obvious. It is, however, important to log-roll the patient to make sure that the entire back has been examined. Log-rolling is just as important in patients with penetrating trauma as it is in blunt trauma, until injuries to the thoracic or lumbar spine have been ruled out.

The surgeon should auscultate each hemithorax, noting whether there are diminished or absent breath sounds. A chest X-ray should be obtained early in the patient with penetrating injuries. This is the key diagnostic study, and in most instances it will reveal the presence of a pneumothorax and haemothorax. Furthermore, missiles often leave metallic fragments outlining the path of the bullet, and areas of pulmonary contusion are additional indicators of the missile tract. It is good practice to place metallic objects such as paper clips on the skin over any wounds on the chest wall. This also can be useful for stab wounds. Tracking the missile helps the surgeon to determine which visceral organs may be injured and, in particular, whether or not there is potential transgression of the diaphragm and/or mediastinum.

Ultrasound has a role primarily in determining whether or not a patient has pericardial blood, assessing for the presence of pneumothoraces, with greater accuracy than with a supine plain chest X-ray. It is also superior to plain radiology in differentiating between fluid and lung contusion[8].

Using the E-FAST technique, pericardial blood can be detected. Similarly, transoesophageal echocardiography is a useful adjunct in determining whether tamponade is present in the haemodynamically stable patient. Computed tomography is not routinely used in patients with penetrating chest injury, except in *stable* patients with transmediastinal wounds. It may have some utility in determining the extent of pulmonary contusion caused by higher-velocity injuries or shotgun blasts, but is not generally indicated in the initial resuscitation or treatment. Arteriography can be quite useful in the haemodynamically stable patient with penetrating injuries to the thoracic outlet or upper chest. This can detect arteriovenous fistulas and false aneurysms.

7.1.7 **Management**

7.1.7.1 CHEST DRAINAGE

Chest tubes are placed according to the technique described in the Advanced Trauma Life Support (ATLS) programme. The placement is in the triangle between the mid-axillary line, anterior axillary line, via the fifth intercostal space – the triangle of safety. Care must be taken to avoid placement of the drain through breast tissue or the pectoralis major muscle.

In the conscious patient, a wheal of 1 per cent lignocaine (lidocaine) is placed in the skin, followed by a further 20 mL subcutaneously and down to the pleura.

Adequate local anaesthesia is critical. The aim is to block the relevant intercostal nerves.

Remember that local anaesthetic may take 5–10 minutes to work adequately. The chest is prepped and draped in the usual way, and after topical analgesia, an incision is made over about 2 cm in length, onto the underlying rib (Figure 7.5).

Using blunt dissection, the tissue is lifted upwards off the rib, and penetration is made over the top of the rib towards the pleura (Figure 7.6). In this manner, damage to the intercostal neurovascular bundle is avoided.

Once the incision has been made, the wound is explored with the index finger for adults and the fifth finger for children. This ensures that the chest cavity has been entered, and also allows limited exploration of the pleural cavity (Figure 7.7). In patients with minor adhesions (e.g. following tuberculosis) it allows the lung tissue to be cleared from the path of the drain.

Once the tract has been dilated with the finger, a large (34 or 36 FG) chest tube is inserted. The incision should be of sufficient size to allow the introduction of a finger *and* the tube together, allowing the tube to be directed cranially *behind* the lung towards the posterior gutter. This provides optimal drainage of both blood and air. When the chest tube is in place, it is secured to the chest wall with a size 0 monofilament suture as follows:

- A vertical mattress suture is inserted into the centre of the wound (Figure 7.8). A *single* throw is placed in the suture at skin level, and then the suture is knotted halfway up its length.
- The suture is then wound around the chest tube until 1 cm before the 'halfway knot' mark is reached. The suture with knot is then threaded *under* the vertical mattress loop (Figure 7.9).

Rib IV–V
Rib V–VI

Figure 7.5 Anatomical placement of the incision for a chest drain.

Figure 7.7 Use of a finger to clear adhesions.

Figure 7.6 Blunt dissection over the top of the rib.

Figure 7.8 Insertion of a vertical mattress suture in the centre of the wound.

Figure 7.9 Securing the tube: first stage.

- The suture is then tied around the chest tube at the level of the knot, about 1 cm from the skin (Figure 7.10).

An additional simple suture may be required to close the wound in a linear fashion.

7.1.7.1.1 Pitfalls

- Do not use a 'purse-string' closure as this is both painful in the long term and less effective.
- Do not 'weave' the drain tie as, if it becomes loose, the entire securing suture will be loose. The securing suture should be wound around the drain in one plane, as shown (Figure 7.10).

All connectors are taped to prevent inadvertent disconnection or removal of the chest tube.

After the chest tube has been placed, it is prudent to obtain an immediate chest film or further ultrasound, to assess the adequate removal of air and blood and the position of the tube. If, for any reason, blood accumulates and cannot be removed, another chest tube is inserted. Persistent air leak or bleeding should alert the surgeon that there is significant visceral injury that may require operative intervention.

7.1.7.1.2 Pitfall

- The surgeon should be aware that the blood may be entering the chest via a hole in the diaphragm.

The tube is removed once the lung has expanded. The suture is cut at the 'halfway knot'. The remaining suture is unwound, and the skin can then be pinched, or sealed with petroleum gauze, as the tube is withdrawn (Figure 7.11); the preplaced suture, now unwound, is then pulled tight and secured. The wound should thus be closed as a linear incision (Figure 7.12).

Complications of tube thoracostomy include wound tract infection and empyema. With meticulous aseptic techniques, the incidence of both of these should be well under 1 per cent.

There is sufficient (class I and II) data to recommend prophylactic antibiotic use in patients receiving tube

Figure 7.10 Securing the tube: second stage.

Figure 7.11 Removal of drain showing pinching of the skin.

Figure 7.12 End result after drain removal.

thoracostomy following chest trauma. The data suggest there may be a reduction in the incidence of pneumonia but *not* empyema in trauma patients receiving prophylactic antibiotics when a tube thoracostomy is placed[9].

Routine antibiotics are not a substitute for good surgical technique.

On the frequently discussed issue of negative suction, a recent prospective study concluded that negative suction confers no advantage in patients with uncomplicated traumatic pneumothorax, haemothorax or haemopneumothorax[10].

7.1.7.2 NON-OPERATIVE MANAGEMENT

As noted above, non-operative management can be used in the majority of penetrating injuries. These patients should be observed in a monitored setting to ensure haemodynamic stability, monitoring of ventilatory status and output of blood from the pleural cavity.

Non-operative management of mid-torso injuries is problematic until injury to the diaphragm or abdominal viscera has been ruled out. Various modalities have been described to try to identify the trajectory of penetrating injuries in these regions, including triple-contrast CT scan and, recently, CT tractography with radiopaque contrast[11]. Thoracoscopy and laparoscopy have been successful in diagnosing diaphragm penetration. Laparoscopy may have a small advantage in that if the diaphragm has been penetrated, it also allows some assessment of the intraperitoneal viscera; however, in many ways, thoracoscopy is better for assessment of the diaphragm, particularly in the right hemithorax. The disadvantage is that once an injury has been detected, this does not rule out associated intraperitoneal injuries.

Failures of non-operative management include patients who continue to bleed from the pleural cavity and those patients who go on to develop a clotted haemothorax.

If placement of additional chest tubes does not remove the thoracic clots, video-assisted thoracoscopic surgery (VATS) is indicated, optimally within 72 hours of the injury, to aid in the removal of these clots[12].

7.1.7.3 OPERATIVE MANAGEMENT

In general, patients who have penetrating injuries to the torso should be left in the supine position in the operating room. The importance of this cannot be over-emphasized. The surgeon must be prepared to extend incisions up into the neck or along the supraclavicular area if there are thoracic outlet injuries. Similarly, once it has been determined that the diaphragm has been penetrated or there are associated injuries to the lower torso, it is important the patient *not* be in a lateral decubitus position that would compromise exploration of the peritoneal cavity or pelvis. Similarly, the posterolateral approach is not appropriate in this situation. The surgeon must be comfortable in dealing with injuries on both sides of the diaphragm.

The trauma patient must be prepared and the drapes positioned over a large area so that the surgeon can expeditiously gain access to any body cavity and can properly place drains and chest tubes. The entire anterior portion and both lateral aspects of the torso should be prepared with antiseptic solution and draped so that the surgeon can work in a sterile field from the neck and clavicle above to the groin below, and from tabletop to tabletop laterally. Prepping should not involve more than a few minutes, and is preferably carried out before induction of anaesthesia so that if deterioration should occur, immediate laparotomy or thoracotomy can be carried out.

For an emergency thoracotomy, performed either in the emergency department or in the operating room, an anterior lateral thoracotomy in the fifth intercostal space is preferred. Most often, this is done on the left chest, particularly if it is a resuscitative thoracotomy. The rationale for this left thoracotomy is that posterior myocardial wounds will necessitate traction of the heart. If this is done through a median sternotomy and the heart is lifted, decreased venous return and fatal dysrhythmia may occur. In patients who are in extremis, and a left thoracotomy has been performed that turns out to be inadequate for the extensive injuries, there should be no hesitation in extending this into the right chest in a 'clamshell' fashion, which gives excellent exposure to all the intrathoracic viscera. Occasionally, a right anterolateral thoracotomy is indicated in emergencies if air embolism is suspected (see Section 7.3.1).

In patients who are haemodynamically stable, a median sternotomy is often the best incision when the visceral injury is undetermined or if there may be multiple injuries. An alternative is the butterfly or clamshell incision, which gives superb exposure to the entire thoracic viscera, but may carry increased morbidity. Sternotomy is generally preferred for upper mediastinal injuries or injuries to the great vessels as they exit the thoracic outlet. The sternotomy can be extended up the sternocleidomastoid muscle or laterally along the top of the clavicle. Re-section of the medial half of the clavicle exposes most of the vessels, except possibly the proximal left subclavian vein. When this diagnosis is known, it is best approached by a left posterior lateral thoracotomy. In an emergency, it may be necessary to go through a fourth or fifth intercostal space for a left anterolateral thoracotomy. Care should be taken in female patients not to transect the breast.

An adjunctive measure to exploratory thoracotomy, after injuries have been dealt with, is the pleural toilet. It is extremely important to evacuate all clots and foreign objects. Foreign objects can include clothing, wadding from shotgun blasts and any spillage from hollow viscous injury. In general, it is best to place a chest tube to drain the diaphragmatic sulcus and a further tube to drain the posterior gutter up towards the apex. These chest tubes should be placed so that they do exit the chest wall in the anterior axillary line. All chest tubes are sutured to the skin with a size 0 monofilament suture. Another useful adjunct is to inject 0.25 per cent bupivacaine (Marcaine) into the intercostal nerve posteriorly in the inner space of the thoracotomy and intercostal nerves just above and below the thoracotomy; this provides excellent analgesia in the immediate postoperative period. This can then be supplemented with a thoracic epidural if necessary after the initial 12 hours of the postoperative period.

Emergency department thoracotomy (see Section 7.2) is indicated in the agonal or dying patient with thoracic injuries. The intent of the emergency thoracotomy is to either aid in resuscitation or to control bleeding and bronchopulmonary vein fistulas (air embolism). The best results have been obtained with penetrating injuries to the torso, but some authors report up to 5 per cent salvage in patients with blunt injuries. Specific indications include resuscitative thoracotomy from hypovolaemic shock, suspected pericardial tamponade and air embolism. Patients who have signs of life in the pre-hospital setting and arrive with an electrical complex are also candidates. Ultrasound is very helpful in looking for signs of cardiac activity. Good results can also be obtained in centres with limited exposure but with well-established protocols for emergency thoracotomies if required.

7.1.7.4 MANAGEMENT OF SPECIFIC INJURIES

7.1.7.4.1 Damage Control in the Chest

Damage control surgery can be applied to the chest, through packing and temporary vacuum closure[13]. Reconstruction can be carried out after physiological stabilization. This often takes the form of myocutaneous flaps such as latissimus dorsi or pectoralis major particularly when cartilage or ribs must be debrided.

7.1.7.4.2 Open Pneumothorax

The incidence of open pneumothorax or significant chest wall injuries following civilian trauma is low, less than 1 per cent of all major thoracic injuries. Although all penetrating wounds are technically open pneumothoraces, the tissue of the chest wall serves as an effective seal. True open pneumothorax is most often associated with close-range shotgun blasts and high-velocity missiles. There is usually a large gaping wound commonly associated with frothy blood at its entrance. Respiratory sounds can be heard with to-and-fro movement of air. The patient often has air hunger and may be in shock from associated visceral injuries.

The wound should be immediately sealed with an occlusive clean or sterile dressing such as petroleum-soaked gauze, thin plastic sheets, sealed on three sides to create a valve, or even aluminium foil as a temporary dressing. Once the chest wound has been sealed, it is important to realize that a tube thoracostomy may be immediately necessary because of the risk of converting the open pneumothorax into a tension pneumothorax, if there is associated parenchymal injury to the lung. Large gaping wounds will invariably require debridement, including resection of devitalized tissue back to bleeding tissue and removal of all foreign bodies including clothing, wadding from shotgun shells or debris from the object that penetrated the chest. The majority of these patients will require thoracotomy to treat visceral injuries and to control bleeding from the lung or chest wall.

After the wounds have been thoroughly debrided and irrigated, the size of the defect may necessitate reconstruction. The use of synthetic material such as Marlex to repair large defects in the chest wall has mostly been abandoned. Instead, myocutaneous flaps such as latissimus dorsi or pectoralis major have proven efficacy, particularly when cartilage or ribs must be debrided. The flap provides prompt healing and minimizes infection to the ribs or costal cartilages. If potential muscle flaps have been destroyed by the injury, a temporary dressing can be placed, and the patient stabilized in the intensive care unit and then returned to the operating room in 24–48 hours for a free myocutaneous graft or alternative reconstruction. Complications include wound infection and respiratory insufficiency, the latter usually due to associated parenchymal injury. Ventilatory embarrassment can persist secondary to the large defect. If the chest wall becomes infected, debridement, wound care and myocutaneous flaps should be considered.

7.1.7.4.3 Tension Pneumothorax
(Pneumo/Haemothorax)

Tension pneumothorax is a common threat to life. The importance of making the diagnosis is that it is the most easily treatable life-threatening surgical emergency in the emergency department. 'Simple' closed pneumothorax, which is not quite as dramatic, occurs in approximately 20 per cent of all penetrating chest injuries. Haemothorax, in contrast, is present in about 30 per cent of penetrating injuries, and haemopneumothorax is found in 40–50 per cent of penetrating injuries.

The diagnosis of tension pneumothorax can be difficult in a noisy emergency department. The classic signs are decreased breath sounds and percussion tympany on the ipsilateral side, and tracheal shift to the contralateral side. The diagnosis is clinical. In the patient who is dying, there should be no hesitation in performing a tube thoracostomy. Massive haemothorax is equally life-threatening.

7.1.7.4.4 Massive Haemothorax

The diagnosis of massive haemothorax is invariably made by the presence of shock, ventilatory embarrassment and a shift in the mediastinum.

Chest X-ray will confirm the extent of blood loss, but most of the time tube thoracostomy is done immediately to relieve the threat of ventilatory embarrassment. If a gush of blood is obtained when the chest tube is placed, autotransfusion should be considered. There are simple devices for this that should be available in all major trauma resuscitation centres. The only contraindication to autotransfusion is a high suspicion of hollow viscus injury. Lesser forms of haemothorax are usually diagnosed by routine chest X-ray.

The treatment of massive haemothorax is to restore blood volume. Essentially, all such patients will require thoracotomy. In approximately 85 per cent of patients with massive haemothorax, a systemic vessel has been injured such as the intercostal artery or internal mammary artery. In a few patients, there may be injury to the hilum of the lung or the myocardium. In about 15 per cent of instances, the bleeding is from deep pulmonary lacerations. These injuries are treated by oversewing the lesion, making sure that bleeding is controlled to the depth of the lesion, or, in some instances, performing tractotomy or resection of a segment or lobe.

Complications of haemothorax or massive haemothorax are almost invariably related to the visceral injuries. Occasionally, there is a persistence of undrained blood that may lead to a cortical peel necessitating thoracoscopy or thoracotomy and removal of this peel. The aggressive use of two chest tubes should minimize the incidence of this complication. If that is not sufficient, early VATS evacuation of retained clots and fibrin is likely to be successful if performed within 72 hours.

7.1.7.4.5 Tracheobronchial Injuries

Penetrating injuries to the tracheobronchial tree[14] are uncommon and constitute less than 2 per cent of all major thoracic injuries. Disruption of the tracheobronchial tree is suggested by massive haemoptysis, airway obstruction, progressive mediastinal air, subcutaneous emphysema, tension pneumothorax and significant persistent air leak after placement of a chest tube. Fibreoptic bronchoscopy in the relatively stable patient is a useful diagnostic adjunct in diagnosis, tube placement, postoperative tracheobronchial toilet and post-operative follow-up of tracheobronchial repairs.

Treatment for tracheobronchial injuries is straightforward. If it is a distal bronchus, there may be persistent air leak for a few days, but it will usually close with chest tube drainage alone. If, however, there is persistent air leak or the patient has significant loss of minute volume through the chest tube, bronchoscopy is used to detect whether or not this is a proximal bronchus injury, and the involved haemothorax is explored usually through a posterolateral thoracotomy. If possible, the bronchus is repaired with monofilament suture. In some instances, a segmentectomy or lobectomy may be required.

7.1.7.4.6 Oesophageal Injuries

Penetrating injuries to the thoracic oesophagus are quite uncommon. Injuries to the cervical oesophagus are somewhat more frequent and are usually detected at the time of exploration of zone I and zone II injuries of the neck. In those centres where selective management of neck injuries is practised, the symptoms found are usually related to pain on swallowing and dysphagia. Occasionally, patients may present late with signs of posterior mediastinitis – a grave situation with a high mortality rate, even with aggressive and comprehensive treatment. Injuries to the thoracic oesophagus may present with pain, fever, pneumomediastinum, persistent pneumothorax in spite of tube thoracostomy and pleural effusion with extravasation of contrast on a Gastrografin swallow.

Treatment of cervical oesophageal injuries is relatively straightforward. As noted above, the injury is usually found during routine exploration of penetrating wounds beneath the platysma. Once found, a routine closure is performed. In more devitalizing injuries, it may be necessary to debride and close using drainage to protect the anastomosis. Injuries to the thoracic oesophagus should be repaired if the injury is less than 6 hours old and there is minimal inflammation and devitalized tissue present. A two-layer closure is all that is necessary. Post-operatively, the patient is kept on intravenous support and supplemental nutrition. Antibiotics may be indicated during the 24-hour peri-operative period.

If the wound is between 6 and 24 hours old, a decision will be necessary to determine whether primary closure can be attempted or whether drainage and nutritional support is the optimal management. Almost all injuries older than 24 hours will not heal primarily when repaired. Optimal management consists of open drainage, antibiotics, nutritional support and consideration of diversion. Complications following oesophageal injuries include wound infection, mediastinitis and empyema.

The more recent technique of non-operative endoscopic expanding silicon-coated stent placement in selected cases is gaining acceptance in practice, although further experience is required to establish its correct application. Injuries of up to 30–40 mm in extent, with localized mural damage and located in the middle and lower third of the oesophagus, are suited to this technique. Cervical (upper third) and gastro-oesophageal junction injuries are not suitable, due to incomplete sealing by the stent. Some authorities advise a concomitant thoracotomy to place mediastinal drains when the stenting method is used. Accurate localization and assessment of the extent of the injury by contrast radiography and endoscopy is mandatory in selecting cases for stenting.

7.1.7.4.7 Diaphragmatic Injuries

See Chapter 8.2 (Bowel and Diaphragm).

7.1.7.4.8 Complications

As noted in the preface, the lung is a target organ for reperfusion injury, and any injury to the viscera within the thorax can result in impaired oxygen transport. Conversely, severe chest trauma is a potent initiator for the release of multiple inflammatory mediators, which allow bacterial translocation and apoptotic processes to occur, which explains the high incidence of pulmonary sepsis following major injuries of any kind. The lungs are at high risk from aspiration, which can accompany shock or substance abuse, and is often associated with penetrating injuries. Finally, pulmonary sepsis is one of the more common sequelae following major injuries of any kind.

7.1.7.4.9 Pulmonary Contusion (PC)

Pulmonary contusions represent bruising of the lung and are usually associated with direct chest trauma, high-velocity missiles and shotgun blasts. The pathophysiology is the result of ventilation–perfusion defects and shunts. Its anatomical composition makes the extent of lung damage easily quantifiable on CT scanning.

The treatment of significant pulmonary contusion consists primarily of cardiovascular and tailored ventilatory support; adjunctive measures such as steroids and diuretics are used *selectively* as required to modulate the development of significant systemic inflammatory response syndrome (SIRS).

Antibiotics are not generally used, as this will simply select out nosocomial, opportunistic and resistant organisms. It is preferable to obtain a daily Gram stain of the sputum and chest X-rays when necessary. If the Gram stain shows the presence of a predominant organism with an associated increase in polymorphonuclear cells, antibiotics are indicated.

7.1.7.4.10 Flail Chest (FC)

Traditionally, flail chest has been managed by internal splinting ('internal pneumatic stabilization') utilizing positive pressure ventilation. This modality remains the gold standard method of management, as it treats both the flail segment by splinting and the associated (often severe) pulmonary contusion.

While this is undoubtedly the method of choice in most instances, there has been increasing interest in the open reduction and fixation of multiple rib fractures[15]. In uncontrolled trials, there have been considerable benefits shown, with a shortening of ventilation time and thus a reduction of risk for ventilator-associated pneumonia (VAP), and improved earlier mobilization resulting from reduced analgesic requirements.

A flail chest may be stabilized using pins, plates, wires, rods or, more recently, absorbable plates. Exposure for the insertion of these can be via a conventional posterolateral thoracotomy or via incisions made over the ribs.

Table 7.1 presents the Eastern Association for the Surgery of Trauma (EAST) guidelines for the management of pulmonary contusion and flail chest (PC-FC)[15,16].

7.1.7.4.11 Pulmonary Laceration

Lung preservation wherever possible is critically important, with conservative resections if required, using a combination of techniques such as tractotomy, wedge resection and segmentectomy, reserving lobectomy or pneumonectomy for only the most critical patients. Currently available stapling devices are invaluable.

7.1.7.4.12 Air Embolism

Air embolism is an infrequent event following penetrating trauma[16]. It occurs in 4 per cent of all major thoracic trauma. Sixty-five per cent of the cases are due to penetrating injuries. The key to diagnosis is to be aware of the possibility. The pathophysiology is a fistula between

Table 7.1 Evidence-Based Guidelines for Selective Non-operative Management of Pulmonary Contusion-Flail Chest (PC-FC)[15]

Level of Evidence	Recommendation
I	There are no recommendations for the management of PC-FC.
II	**1.** A pulmonary artery may be useful to avoid fluid overload during resuscitation.
	2. Obligatory mechanical ventilation in the absence of respiratory failure solely for the purpose of overcoming chest wall instability should be avoided.
	3. Patients with PC-FC requiring mechanical ventilation should be supported in a manner based on institutional and physician preference and separated from the ventilator at the earliest possible time. Positive end expiratory pressure (PEEP) and continuous positive airway pressure (CPAP) should be included in the ventilatory regimen.
	4. The use of optimal analgesia and aggressive chest physiotherapy should be applied to minimize the likelihood of respiratory failure and ensuing ventilatory support. Epidural catheter is the preferred mode of analgesia delivery in severe injury.
	5. Steroids should not be used in therapy of pulmonary contusion.
III	**1.** A trial of mask CPAP should be considered in alert compliant patients with marginal respiratory status in combination with optimal regional anaesthesia.
	2. There is insufficient evidence to prove the effectiveness of paravertebral analgesia in the trauma population. However, this modality may be equivalent to epidural analgesia and may be considered in certain situations when epidural is contraindicated.
	3. Independent lung ventilation may be considered in severe unilateral PC when shunt cannot otherwise be corrected owing to maldistribution of ventilation, or when crossover bleeding is problematic.
	4. High-frequency oscillatory ventilation (HFOV) has not been shown to improve survival in blunt chest trauma patients with PC, but has been shown to improve oxygenation in certain cases where other modalities have failed.
	5. Diuretics may be used in the setting of hydrostatic fluid overload, as evidenced by elevated pulmonary capillary wedge pressures in haemodynamically stable patients, or in the setting of known concurrent congestive cardiac failure.
	6. Although improvement has not been definitively shown in any outcome parameters after surgical fixation of FC, this modality may be considered in cases of severe FC failing to wean from the ventilator, when thoracotomy is required for other reasons. Patient subgroups that would benefit from early fracture fixation have not been identified.
	7. There is insufficient clinical evidence to recommend any type of proprietary implant for surgical fixation of rib fractures. However, trend studies indicate that replacing or wrapping devices are likely superior to intramedullary wires.
	8. Self-activating multidisciplinary protocols for the treatment of chest wall injuries may improve outcome.

Source: Simon B, Ebert J, Bokhari F, et al., *J Trauma Acute Care Surg.*, 73, S351–S361, 2012. With permission.

a bronchus and the pulmonary vein. Those patients who are breathing spontaneously will have a pressure differential from the pulmonary vein to the bronchus that will cause approximately 22 per cent of these patients to have haemoptysis on presentation. If, however, the patient has a Valsalva-type respiration or grunts, or is intubated with positive pressure in the bronchus, the pressure differential is from the bronchus to the pulmonary vein, causing systemic air embolism.

These patients present in one of three ways: focal or lateralizing neurological signs, sudden cardiovascular collapse and froth when the initial arterial blood specimen is obtained. Any patient who has obvious chest injury or, does not have obvious head injury and yet has focal or lateralizing neurological findings should be assumed to have air embolism. Confirmation can occasionally be obtained by funduscopic examination, which shows air in the retinal vessels. Patients who are intubated and have a sudden unexplained cardiovascular collapse with an absence of vital signs should be immediately assumed to have an air embolism to the coronary vessels. Finally, those patients who have a frothy blood sample drawn for initial blood gas determination will have air embolism.

When a patient comes in to the emergency department in extremis and an EDT is carried out, air should always be looked for in the coronary vessels. If air is found, the hilum of the offending lung should be clamped immediately to reduce the ingress of air into the vessels.

The treatment of air embolism is immediate thoracotomy, preferably in the operating room. In the majority of patients, the left or right chest is opened depending on the side of penetration. If a resuscitative thoracotomy has been carried out, it may be necessary to extend this across the sternum into the opposite chest if there is no parenchymal injury to the lung on the left. Definitive treatment is to oversew the lacerations to the lung, in some instances perform a lobectomy and only rarely a pneumonectomy.

Other resuscitative measures in patients who have asystolic arrest due to air embolism include internal cardiac massage and reaching up and holding the ascending aorta with the thumb and index finger for one or two beats – this will tend to push air out of the coronary vessels and thus establish perfusion. Adrenaline (epinephrine) 1:1000 can be injected intravenously or down the endotracheal tube to provide an alpha effect, driving air out of the systemic microcirculation. It is prudent to vent the left atrium and ventricle as well as the ascending aorta to remove all residual air once the lung hilum has been clamped. This prevents further air embolism when the patient is moved.

Using aggressive diagnosis and treatment, it is possible to achieve up to a 55 per cent salvage rate in patients with air embolism secondary to penetrating trauma.

7.1.7.4.13 Cardiac Injuries

In urban trauma centres, cardiac injuries are most common after penetrating trauma, and constitute about 5 per cent of all thoracic injuries. The diagnosis of cardiac injury is usually fairly obvious. The patient presents with exsanguination, cardiac tamponade and, rarely, acute heart failure. In addition to the well-described globular heart shape on X-rays, a straight left heart border has been associated with the presence of a haemopericardium. Patients with tamponade due to penetrating injuries usually have a wound in proximity, decreased cardiac output, increased central venous pressure, decreased blood pressure, decreased heart sounds, narrow pulse pressure and occasionally paradoxical pulse. Immediate clinician-performed E-FAST will usually demonstrate the presence of pericardial fluid, but in cases where the diagnosis of pericardial tamponade cannot be confirmed on clinical signs and on E-FAST, formal echocardiogram is useful.

The treatment of all cardiac injuries is immediate thoracotomy, ideally in the operating room. In the patient who is in extremis, thoracotomy in the emergency department can be life-saving. The great majority of wounds can be closed with simple sutures or horizontal mattress sutures of a 3/0 or 4/0 monofilament. Bolstering the suture with Teflon pledgets is *not* essential, but may occasionally be required, particularly if there is surrounding contusion, or there is proximity of the wound to a coronary artery. If the stab wound or gunshot wound is in proximity to the coronary artery, care must be taken not to suture the vessels. This can be achieved by passing horizontal mattress sutures beneath the coronary vessels, avoiding ligation of the vessel.

If the coronary arteries have been transected, two options exist. Closure can be accomplished in the beating heart using a fine 6-0 or 7-0 polypropylene suture, under magnification if necessary. The second option is to temporarily initiate inflow occlusion and fibrillation. However, both of these measures have a high risk associated with them. Heparinization is optimally avoided in the trauma patient, and fibrillation in the presence of shock and acidosis may be difficult to reverse. Bypass is usually reserved for patients who have injury to the valves, chordae tendineae or septum. In most instances, these injuries are not immediately life-threatening, but become evident over a few hours or days following the injury.

Complications from myocardial injuries include recurrent tamponade, mediastinitis and post-cardiotomy syndrome. The former can be avoided by placing a mediastinal chest tube or leaving the pericardium partially open following repair. Most cardiac injuries are treated through a left anterolateral thoracotomy and only occasionally via a median sternotomy. If mediastinitis does develop, the wound should be opened (including the sternum), and debridement carried out with secondary closure in 4–5 days.

Another complication is herniation of the heart through the pericardium, which may occlude venous return and cause sudden death. This is avoided by loosely approximating the pericardium after the cardiac injury has been repaired.

7.1.7.4.14 Injuries to the Great Vessels

Injuries to the great vessels from penetrating forces are infrequently reported. The reason for this is that extensive injury to the great vessels results in immediate exsanguination into the chest, and most of these patients die at the scene of injury.

The diagnosis of penetrating great vessel injury is usually obvious. The patient is in shock, and there is an injury in proximity to the thoracic outlet or posterior mediastinum. If the patient stabilizes with resuscitation, an arteriogram should be performed to localize the injury. Approximately 8 per cent of patients with major vascular injuries do not have clinical signs, stressing the need for arteriograms when there is a wound in proximity. These patients usually have a false aneurysm or arteriovenous fistula. Treatment of penetrating injuries to the great vessels can almost always be accomplished using lateral repair, since larger injuries that might necessitate grafts are usually incompatible with survival long enough to permit the patient to reach the emergency department alive[17].

Complications of injuries to the great vessels include rebleeding, false aneurysm formation and thrombosis. A devastating complication is paraplegia, which usually occurs following blunt injuries but rarely after penetrating injuries, either because of associated injury to the spinal cord or because at the time of surgery important intercostal arteries are ligated. The spinal cord has a segmental blood supply to the anterior spinal artery (artery of Adamkiewicz), and every effort should be made to preserve the intercostal vessels, particularly those that appear to be larger than normal, as these may constitute an important collateral feeder system.

7.2 EMERGENCY DEPARTMENT THORACOTOMY

7.2.1 History

Rapid emergency medical response times and advances in prehospital care have led to increasing numbers of patients arriving in resuscitation in extremis. Salvage of these patients often demands immediate control of haemorrhage and desperate measures to resuscitate them. This has often been attempted in hopeless situations, following both blunt and penetrating injury, and failure to understand the indications and sequelae will almost inevitably result in the death of the patient. With the increasing financial demands on medical care, and the increasing risk of transmission of communicable diseases, a differentiation must be made between the true EDT and futile care.

In 1874, Schiff described open cardiac massage, and in 1901, Rehn sutured a right ventricle in a patient presenting with cardiac tamponade. The limited success of EDT in most circumstances, however, prohibited the use of the technique for the next six or seven decades. A revival of interest occurred in the 1970s, when the procedure was initially revived by Ben Taub General Hospital in Houston for the treatment of cardiac injuries. It has subsequently been applied as a means of temporary aortic occlusion in exsanguinating abdominal trauma. More recently, there has been decreased enthusiasm and a more selective approach, particularly with respect to blunt trauma.

It must be noted that there is an extremely high mortality rate associated with all thoracotomies performed anywhere outside the operating theatre, especially when performed by non-surgeons.

It is important early on to differentiate between the definitions of thoracotomy:

- Thoracotomy performed in the emergency department (EDT) for patients in extremis.
- To control haemorrhage.
- To control the aortic outflow (aortic 'cross-clamping').
- To perform internal cardiac massage.
- *Planned* resuscitative thoracotomy (i.e. in operating theatre or intensive care unit minutes to hours after

injury in acutely deteriorating patients for control of haemorrhage).

It is also important to differentiate between:

- Patients with 'no signs of life'.
- Patients with 'no vital signs' in whom cardiac electrical activity, pupillary activity and/or respiratory effort is still evident. (This is where cardiac ultrasound can be very helpful.)

Obviously, the results of EDT in these two circumstances will differ. This section concentrates on the thoracotomies performed by the surgeon in those patients who present in extremis in the resuscitation area.

7.2.2 **Objectives**

The primary objectives of EDT in this set of circumstances are to:

- Release cardiac tamponade.
- Control intrathoracic bleeding.
- Control air embolism or bronchopleural fistula.
- Permit open cardiac massage.
- Allow for temporary occlusion of the descending aorta to redistribute blood to the upper body and possibly limit subdiaphragmatic haemorrhage.

Emergency department thoracotomy has been shown to be most productive in life-threatening penetrating cardiac wounds, especially when cardiac tamponade is present. Patients requiring EDT for anything other than isolated penetrating cardiac injury rarely survive, even in established trauma centres. The outcome in the field is even worse. Indications for the procedure in military practice are essentially the same as in civilian practice.

The EDT and the necessary rapid use of sharp surgical instruments, as well as exposure to the patient's blood, pose certain risks to the resuscitating surgeon. Contact rates of patient's blood to the surgeon's skin approximate to 20 per cent. 'Invisible pathogens' such as human immunodeficiency virus (HIV), hepatitis C and others must be considered. The use of universal precautions and the selective use of EDT may minimize this risk.

7.2.3 **Indications and Contraindications**

There are instances where EDT has been shown to have clear benefit. These indications include:

- Those patients in whom there is a witnessed arrest and a high likelihood of isolated intrathoracic injury, especially penetrating cardiac injury ('salvageable' post-injury cardiac arrest).
- Those with severe post-injury hypotension (blood pressure <60 mm Hg) due to cardiac tamponade, air embolism or thoracic haemorrhage.

Less clear benefit occurs for:

- Patients presenting with moderate post-injury hypotension (blood pressure <80 mm Hg) potentially due to intra-abdominal aortic injury (e.g. an epigastric gunshot wound).
- Major pelvic fractures.
- Active intra-abdominal haemorrhage.

The first group of patients constitutes those in whom EDT is relatively indicated. One must consider the patient's age, pre-existing disease, signs of life and injury mechanism, as well as the proximity of the emergency department to the operating theatre and the personnel available, when applying the principles related to EDT. Although optimal benefit from the procedure will be obtained with an experienced surgeon, in cases where a moribund patient presents with a penetrating chest wound, the emergency physician should not hesitate to perform the procedure.

The EDT is contraindicated in the following situations:

- When there has been cardiopulmonary resuscitation (CPR) in the absence of endotracheal tube intubation in excess of 5 minutes.
- When there has been CPR for more than 10 minutes with or without endotracheal tube intubation.
- In cases of blunt trauma, when there have been no signs of life at the scene or only pulseless electrical activity is present in the emergency department.

Consider the use of cardiac ultrasound to aid the diagnosis.

7.2.4 **Results**

The results of EDT vary according to the injury mechanism and location and the presence of vital and life signs.

Emergency department thoracotomy has been shown to be beneficial in around 50 per cent of patients presenting with signs of life after isolated penetrating cardiac injury, and only rarely in those patients presenting without signs of life (<2 per cent). With non-cardiac penetrating wounds, 25 per cent of patients benefit when signs of life and detectable vital signs are present, compared with 8 per cent of those with signs of life only and 3 per cent of those without signs of life.

Only 1–2 per cent of patients requiring EDT are salvaged after blunt trauma regardless of their clinical status on admission. A decision-making algorithm has been formulated based on these findings, and the four factors found to be most predictive of outcome following EDT are reported to be

- Absence of signs of life at the scene.
- Absence of signs of life in the emergency department.
- Absence of cardiac activity at EDT.
- Systolic blood pressure less than 70 mm Hg after aortic occlusion.

At the scene, patients in extremis and without cardiac electrical activity are declared dead. Those with electrical activity are intubated, supported with CPR and transferred to the emergency department. If blunt injury is present, EDT is embarked on only if pulsatile electrical activity is present. (In penetrating trauma, all patients undergo EDT.) If no blood is present in the pericardial cavity and there is no cardiac activity, the patient is declared dead. All others are treated according to the type of injury, as above. Those with intra-abdominal injury who respond to aortic occlusion with a systolic blood pressure of more than 70 mm Hg and all other surviving patients are rapidly transported to the operating theatre for definitive treatment.

7.2.5 **When to Stop Emergency Department Thoracotomy**

Emergency department thoracotomy is a 'team event'. It should not be prolonged unduly but should have specific endpoints. If an injury is repaired and the patient responds, he or she should be moved to the operating room for definitive repair or closure.

Emergency department thoracotomy should be terminated if:

- Irreparable cardiac damage has occurred.
- The patient is identified as having massive head injuries.
- Pulseless electrical activity is established.
- Systolic blood pressure is less than 70 mm Hg after 20 minutes.
- Asystolic arrest has occurred.

7.2.6 **Conclusion**

Success in the management of thoracic injury in those cases requiring operation lies in rapid access to the thoracic cavity with good exposure. Thus, good lighting, appropriate instrumentation, functioning suctioning apparatus and a 'controlled, aggressive but calm frame of mind' on the part of the surgeon will result in acceptable, uncomplicated survival figures.

7.3 **SURGICAL APPROACHES TO THE THORAX**

The choice of approach to the injured thorax should be determined by three factors:

- The hemithorax and its contents.
- The stability of the patient.
- Whether the indication for surgery is acute or chronic (non-acute).

A useful distinction can be made with respect to indications (Table 7.2). It will be noted that the acute indications include all acutely life-threatening situations, while the chronic or non-acute indications are essentially late presentations.

The surgical approaches in current use include:

- Anterolateral thoracotomy.
- Median sternotomy.
- Bilateral thoracotomy ('clamshell' incision).

Table 7.2 Indications for Surgery in the Thorax

Acute Indications	Chronic Indications
Cardiac tamponade	Unevacuated clotted haemothorax
Acute deterioration	Chronic traumatic diaphragmatic hernia
Vascular injury at the thoracic outlet	
	Traumatic atrioventricular fistula
Loss of chest wall substance	Traumatic cardiac septal or valvular lesions
Endoscopic or radiological evidence of tracheal, oesophagus or great vessel injury	
	Missed tracheobronchial injury or tracheo-oesophageal fistula
Massive or continuing haemothorax	Infected intrapulmonary haematoma
Bullet embolism to the heart/ pulmonary artery	
Penetrating mediastinal injury	

- Posterolateral thoracotomy.
- The 'trapdoor' incision.

In the *unstable* patient, the choice of approach usually will be an anterolateral thoracotomy or median sternotomy, depending upon the suspected injury. In the case of the *stable* patient, the choice of approach must be planned after proper evaluation and work-up has clearly identified the nature of the injury.

If time permits, intubation (or reintubation) with a double-lumen endotracheal tube, to allow selective deflation or ventilation of each lung, can be very helpful and occasionally life-saving; however, advice should be sought from an experienced anaesthetist.

It is seldom necessary to resort to the remaining three approaches in the acute situation. Of these, the bilateral trans-sternal thoracotomy (the 'clamshell' incision) and the 'trapdoor' incision are complex and somewhat mutilating, with significant postoperative morbidity and difficulty in terms of access and closure.

7.3.1 **Anterolateral Thoracotomy**

This is the approach of choice in most unstable patients and is utilized for EDT (Figure 7.13):

- This approach allows rapid access to the injured hemithorax and its contents.
- It is made with the patient in the supine position with no special positioning requirements or instruments.

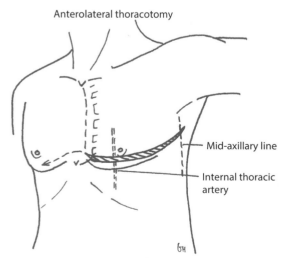

Figure 7.13 Anterolateral thoracotomy.

- It has the advantages that it
  - May be extended across the sternum into the contralateral hemithorax (the 'clamshell' incision or bilateral thoracotomy).
  - May be extended downward to create a thoracoabdominal incision.

7.3.1.1 TECHNIQUE

A slight tilt of the patient to the right is advisable; this is achieved by use of either a sandbag or other support, or by tilting the table.

The incision is made through the fourth or fifth intercostal space from the costochondral junction anteriorly to the mid-axillary line posteriorly, following the upper border of the lower rib in order to avoid damage to the intercostal neurovascular bundle.

The muscle groups are divided down to the periosteum of the lower rib. The muscle groups of the serratus anterior posteriorly and the intercostals medially and anteriorly are divided. The trapezius and the pectoralis major are avoided. Care should be taken at the anterior end of the incision, where the internal mammary artery runs and may be transected.

The periosteum is opened, leaving a cuff of approximately 5 mm for later closure. The parietal pleura is then opened, taking care to avoid the internal mammary artery adjacent to the sternal border. These vessels are ligated if necessary.

A Finochietto retractor is placed with the handle away from the sternum (i.e. laterally placed), the ribs are spread and intrathoracic inspection for identification of injuries is carried out after suctioning. In cases of ongoing bleeding, an autotransfusion suction device is advisable.

Note that it is important to identify the phrenic nerve in its course across the pericardium if this structure is to be opened – the pericardiotomy is made 1 cm anterior and vertical to the nerve trunk in order to avoid damage and subsequent morbidity.

7.3.1.2 CLOSURE

Following definitive manoeuvres, the anterolateral thoracotomy is closed in layers over one or two large-bore intercostal tube drains and after careful haemostasis and copious lavage.

- The ribs and intercostal muscles should be closed with synthetic absorbable sutures.

- Closure of discrete muscle layers reduces both pain and long-term disability.
- The skin is routinely closed.

7.3.2 **Median Sternotomy**

This incision is the approach of choice in patients with a penetrating injury at the base of the neck (zone 1) and the thoracic outlet, as well as to the heart itself. It allows access to the pericardium and heart, the arch of the aorta and the origins of the great vessels. It has the attraction of allowing upwards extension into the neck (as a Henry incision), extension downwards into a midline laparotomy or lateral extension into a supraclavicular approach (Figure 7.14). It has the relative disadvantage of requiring a sternal saw or chisel (of the Lebsche type). In addition, the infrequent but significant complication of sternal sepsis may occur post-operatively, especially in the emergency setting.

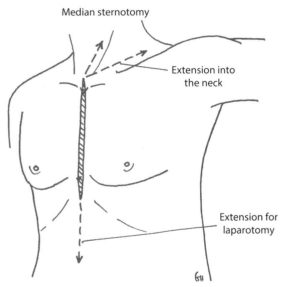

Figure 7.14 Median sternotomy.

7.3.2.1 TECHNIQUE

The incision is made with the patient fully supine, in the midline from the suprasternal notch to below the xiphoid cartilage. A finger-sweep is used to open spaces behind the sternum, above and below. Excision of the xiphoid cartilage may be necessary if this is large and intrusive, and can be done with heavy scissors.

Split section (bisection) of the sternum is carried out with a saw (either oscillating or a braided-wire Gigli saw)

or a Lebsche knife, commencing from above and moving downwards. This is an important point to avoid inadvertent damage to vascular structures in the mediastinum. In addition, be aware of the possible presence of the large transverse communicating vein, which may be found in the areolar tissue of the suprasternal space of Burns, and must be controlled.

7.3.2.2 CLOSURE

- The pericardium is usually left open or only partially closed. It is advisable to close the pericardium with an absorbable suture to avoid adhesion formation.
- Two mediastinal tube drains are brought out through epigastric incisions.
- Closure of the sternotomy is made with horizontal sternal wires or encircling heavy non-absorbable suture (braided, non-absorbable).
- Closure of the linea alba should be by non-absorbable suture.

7.3.3 **'Clamshell' Thoracotomy**

The 'clamshell' is essentially a bilateral fourth or fifth interspace thoracotomy, linked by division of the sternum, which allows the chest to be opened very widely anteriorly. Care should be taken to ligate the internal mammary arteries and to ensure haemostasis prior to closure.

The incision is particularly effective in those situations where it is important to achieve rapid access to the opposite side of the chest, especially posteriorly, such as for

- Transmediastinal injury.
- Lung injury.
- Injury on the right, where aortic control may be necessary.

As mentioned earlier, the incision allows access to the most thoracic structures. It has been recently demonstrated through cadaveric studies that the clamshell incision gives access to most intrathoracic organs[26], but it is considered to be inferior to median sternotomy in accessing upper mediastinal vascular structures[27].

7.3.4 **Posterolateral Thoracotomy**

This approach requires appropriate positioning of the patient and is usually used in the elective setting for definitive lung and oesophageal surgery. It is not usually employed in the acute setting. It is more time-consuming in approach and closure, since the bulkier muscle groups of the posterolateral thorax are traversed, and scapular retraction is necessary.

7.3.5 'Trapdoor' Thoracotomy

This is a combination of an anterolateral thoracotomy, a partial sternotomy and an infra- or supraclavicular incision with resection or dislocation of the clavicle (Figure 7.15). The incision is considered *obsolete*.

It has the disadvantages of being relatively more time-consuming, retraction of the bony 'trapdoor' created is often difficult, resulting in multiple fractures of the ribs laterally or posteriorly, and closure is difficult. A median sternotomy with extension of the incision into the neck will provide more rapid and efficient exposure of injury in this region.

Post-operative morbidity is very high.

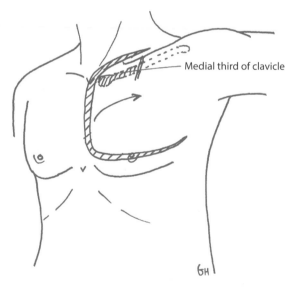

Figure 7.15 'Trapdoor' incision.

Medial third of clavicle

7.4 EMERGENCY DEPARTMENT THORACOTOMY TECHNIQUE

7.4.1 Requirements

The numbers of instruments and types of equipment necessary to perform EDT do not even begin to approach those used for formal thoracotomy in the operating theatre and really include only the following:

- A scalpel, with a #20 or #21 blade.
- Forceps.
- A suitable retractor such as a Finochietto chest retractor or a Balfour abdominal retractor.
- A Lebsche knife and mallet or Gigli saw for the sternum.
- Large vascular clamps such as Satinsky vascular clamps (large and small).
- Mayo scissors.
- Metzenbaum scissors.
- Long needle-holders.
- Internal defibrillator paddles.
- Sutures, swabs and Teflon pledgets.
- Sterile skin preparation and drapes.
- Good light.

7.4.2 Approach

Two basic incisions are used in EDT. These are applied according to the best incision for the particular injury suspected (based on the entrance and exit wounds, the trajectory and the most likely diagnosis from clinical examination) and may be extended in various ways according to need.

Routine immediate resuscitation protocols as per the ATLS are instituted, and once indications for EDT have been fulfilled, EDT should follow without delay.

> Pitfall
> - If the conditions are not fulfilled, you are embarking upon futile care.

The left anterolateral thoracotomy is the most common site for urgent access. The incision is placed in the fifth intercostal space through muscle, periosteum and parietal pleura from the costochondral junction anteriorly to the mid-axillary line laterally following the upper border of rib, and care is taken to avoid the internal mammary artery. This incision can be extended as a bilateral incision requiring horizontal division of the sternum and ligation of the internal mammary vessels bilaterally. It affords excellent access to both pleural cavities, the pericardial cavity and even the abdominal cavity if required. The incision also may be extended cranially in the midline by dividing the sternum for penetrating wounds involving mediastinal structures. The same incision may be employed on the right side in hypotensive patients with penetrating right chest trauma in whom massive blood loss or air embolism is suspected. This, too, may be extended trans-sternally if a cardiac wound is discovered.

The median sternotomy affords the best exposure to the anterior and middle mediastinum, including the heart and great vessels, and is typically advocated for penetrating wounds, particularly of the upper chest between the nipples. This can be extended supraclavicularly for access to control subclavian and brachiocephalic vascular injuries.

7.4.3 Emergency Procedures

7.4.3.1 SUSPECTED CARDIAC INJURY AND CARDIAC TAMPONADE

Access is achieved via lateral or midline sternotomy, the former allowing more rapid access, and the latter approach ensuring better exposure. It is important to identify the phrenic nerve prior to opening the pericardium at least 1 cm anterior to this structure. The pericardial incision is initiated using either a knife or the sharp point of a pair of scissors, and blood and clots are evacuated.

Cardiac bleeding points on the ventricle are initially managed with digital pressure, and those on the atria and great vessels by partially occluding vascular clamps. If the heart is beating, repair should be delayed until initial resuscitation measures have been completed. If it is not beating, suturing precedes resuscitation.

Foley catheters may be used to temporarily control haemorrhage prior to definitive repair in the emergency department or operating theatre. A Foley catheter with a large balloon is preferable.

Once it has been placed, great care should be taken not to exert too much traction on the catheter as it will easily tear out, making the hole dramatically bigger.

Suturing of the right ventricle requires the placement of Teflon pledgets, which are utilized selectively on the left ventricle using a horizontal mattress suture under the coronary vessels to avoid trauma to or occlusion of the coronary vessels. Low-pressure venous and atrial wounds can be repaired with simple continuous sutures. Posterior wounds are more difficult as they necessitate elevation of the heart before their closure, which can lead to further haemodynamic compromise. With large wounds of the ventricle or inaccessible posterior wounds, temporary digital inflow occlusion might be necessary to facilitate repair[18-20].

Most patients with blunt injuries to the heart who survive the initial resuscitation and require operative intervention can likewise be treated with simple off-pump methods although more complex injuries may require immediate cardiopulmonary bypass and advanced techniques.

After initial repair, fluids are best slowed down to limit further bleeding (the concept of hypotensive resuscitation), aiming for critical organ perfusion while minimizing additional haemorrhage (i.e. a blood pressure of about 85 mm Hg). The patient is best transferred to the operating theatre, where repair of the injury and closure of the access procedure are carried out under controlled circumstances with adequate resources.

7.4.3.2 PULMONARY HAEMORRHAGE

Access is best achieved by anterolateral thoracotomy on the appropriate side. With localized bleeding sites, control can be achieved with vascular clamps placed across the affected segment. The affected segment is then dealt with, preferably in controlled circumstances in the operating theatre by local oversewing, segmental resection or pulmonary tractotomy.

Pulmonary tractotomy is a means of controlling tracts that pass through multiple lung segments where the extent of injury precludes pulmonary resection. It is a means of non-anatomical lung preservation in which linear staplers are passed along both sides of the tract formed, and the lung is divided to allow blood vessels and airways in the bases to be repaired; the divided edges are then oversewn.

With massive haemorrhage from multiple or indeterminate sites, or widespread destruction of lung parenchyma leaving large areas of non-viable tissue, hilar clamping with a large soft vascular clamp or a large doubled vessel loop, or a soft catheter across the hilar structures occluding the pulmonary artery, pulmonary vein and main-stem bronchus is employed until a definitive surgical procedure can be performed.

Air embolism is controlled by placing a clamp across the hilar structures, and air is evacuated by needle aspiration of the elevated left ventricular apex.

7.4.3.3 THORACOTOMY WITH AORTIC CROSS-CLAMPING

This technique is employed to optimize oxygen transport to vital proximal structures (the heart and brain), maximize coronary perfusion and possibly limit infradiaphragmatic haemorrhage in both blunt and penetrating trauma.

The thoracic aorta is cross-clamped inferior to the left pulmonary hilum, and the area is exposed by elevating the left lung anteriorly and superiorly. The mediastinal pleura is dissected under direct vision, the aorta being separated by blunt dissection from the oesophagus anteriorly and the prevertebral fascia posteriorly. When properly exposed, the aorta is occluded using a large vascular clamp. It is important that the aortic cross-clamp time be kept to the absolute minimum (i.e. that the clamp is removed once effective cardiac function and systemic arterial pressure have been achieved), as the metabolic penalty rapidly becomes exponential once beyond 30 minutes.

7.4.3.4 BILATERAL TRANS-STERNAL THORACOTOMY ('CLAMSHELL' THORACOTOMY)

This is the thoracic equivalent of the chevron or 'bucket handle' upper abdominal incision, providing wide exposure to both hemithoraces. It is relatively time-consuming in terms of both access and closure. It may be argued that median sternotomy will provide the same degree of exposure with greater ease of access and closure. It is usually necessary to use this incision only when it becomes necessary to gain access to both hemithoraces.

The incision usually extends as a fifth intercostal space anterolateral thoracotomy, across the sternum. The sternum is divided using a Gigli saw, chisel or bone-cutting forceps. Care is taken to ligate the internal mammary arteries.

7.5 DEFINITIVE PROCEDURES

7.5.1 Pericardial Tamponade

- Open the pericardium in a cranial to caudal direction, anterior to the phrenic nerve.
- It is important to examine the whole heart to localize the source of bleeding.
- Deal with the source of bleeding.
- It is not essential to close the pericardium after the procedure.
- If the pericardium is closed, it should be drained to avoid a recurrent tamponade.

7.5.2 Myocardial Laceration

- Wherever possible, initial control of a myocardial laceration should be digital, while the damage is assessed.
- A Foley catheter can also be used.

> Pitfall
> - There is a real danger of extending the damage if the balloon pulls through the laceration. Use a 30-mL balloon, and avoid other than gentle traction.

- Use 3-0 or 4-0 non-absorbable braided sutures tied gently to effect the repair. Pledgets may be helpful.
- Care should be exercised near coronary arteries. Whereas a vertical mattress suture is normally acceptable, it may be necessary to use a horizontal mattress suture under the vessel to avoid occluding it.
- In inexperienced hands, and as a temporizing measure, a skin stapler will allow control of the bleeding, with minimal manipulation of the heart.

> Pitfall
> - Staples often eventually tear out, so the repair should not be regarded as definitive.

7.5.3 Hilar Clamping

- Wide anterolateral thoracotomy is the exposure of choice.
- A vascular clamp can be placed across the hilum, occluding the pulmonary artery, vein and main-stem bronchus.

7.5.4 Lobectomy or Pneumonectomy

- Lobectomy or pneumonectomy[21] is rarely performed. It is usually done to control massive haemorrhage from the pulmonary hilum.
- Lung preservation should be attempted wherever possible.
- A double-lumen endotracheal tube should be used whenever possible.
- For segmental pneumonectomy, use of the GIA stapler is helpful. The staple line can then be oversewn.

7.5.5 Pulmonary Tractotomy

- This is used where the injury crosses more than one segment, commonly caused by a penetrating injury. Anatomical re-section may not be possible.
- Linear staplers can be introduced along both sides of the tract, the tract being divided and then oversewn.
- This procedure is also helpful in 'damage control' of the chest.

7.5.6 **Aortic Injury**

- Most patients with these injuries do not survive to reach hospital.
- Cardiopulmonary bypass is preferable in order to avoid paraplegia.

7.5.7 **Oesophageal Injury**

- Surgical repair is mandatory.
- Two-layer repair (mucosal and muscular) is preferable.
- If possible, the repair should be wrapped in autogenous tissue.
- A feeding gastrostomy is preferable to a nasogastric tube through the area of repair, and the stomach should be drained.
- A cervical oesophagostomy may be required.

7.5.8 **Tracheobronchial Injury**

- Flexible bronchoscopy is very helpful in assessment.
- Formal repair should be undertaken under ideal conditions, with removal of devitalized tissue.

7.6 SUMMARY

The success in the management of thoracic injury in those cases requiring operation lies in the 'team approach', with good anaesthesia and rapid access to the thoracic cavity with good exposure. Thus, good lighting, appropriate instrumentation, functioning suction apparatus and a 'controlled, aggressive but calm frame of mind' on the part of the team will result in acceptable, uncomplicated survival figures.

REFERENCES AND RECOMMENDED READING

References

1. Baker CC, Oppenheimer L, Stephens B, et al. Epidemiology of trauma deaths. *Am J Surg.* 1980;140:144–150.
2. Mancini M, Smith LM, Nein A, Buechler KJ. Early evacuation of clotted blood and haemothorax using thoracoscopy: case reports. *J Trauma.* 1993;34:144–149.
3. Kwan RO, Miraflor E, Yeung L, Strumwasser A, Victorino G. Bedside thoracic ultrasonography of the fourth intercostal space reliably determines safe removal of tube thoracostomy after traumatic injury. *J Trauma Acute Care Surg.* 2012;73:1570–1575.
4. Van As AB, Manganyi R, Brooks A. Treatment of thoracic trauma in children: literature review, Red Cross War Memorial Children's Hospital data analysis, and guidelines for management. *Eur J Pediatr Surg.* 2013;23(6):434–443.
5. Kessel B, Dagan J, Swaid F, et al. Rib fractures: comparison of associated injuries between pediatric and adult population. *Am J Surg.* 2014;208(5):831–834.
6. Lustenberger T, Talving P, Lam L, et al. Penetrating cardiac trauma in adolescents: a rare injury with excessive mortality. *J Pediatr Surg.* 2013;48(4):745–796.
7. Lee LK, Rogers AJ, Ehrlich PF, et al. Occult pneumothoraces in children with blunt torso trauma. *Acad Emerg Med.* 2014;21(4):440–486.
8. Bouhemad B, Zhang M, Lu Q, Rouby JJ. Clinical review: bedside lung ultrasound in critical care practice. *Crit Care.* 2007;11:205. Review.
9. Luchette FA, Barie PS, Oswanski MF, et al. Practice management guidelines for prophylactic antibiotic use in tube thoracostomy for traumatic hemopneumothorax: EAST Practice Management Guidelines Work Group. *J Trauma.* 2000;48(4):753–757.
10. Morales CH, Mejía C, Roldan LA, Saldarriaga MF, Duque AF. Negative pleural suction in thoracic trauma patients: a randomized controlled trial. *J Trauma Acute Care Surg.* 2014;77(2):251–255.
11. Bansal V, Reid CM, Fortlage D, et al. Determining injuries from posterior and flank stab wounds using computed tomography tractography. *Am Surg.* 2014;80(4):403–407.
12. Goodman M, Lewis J, Guitron J, Reed M, Pritts T, Starnes S. Video-assisted thoracoscopic surgery for acute thoracic trauma. *J Emerg Trauma Shock.* 2013;6(2):106–109.
13. O'Connor JV, DuBose JJ, Scalea TM. Damage-control thoracic surgery: management and outcomes. *J Trauma Acute Care Surg.* 2014;77:660–665.
14. Welter S. Repair of tracheobronchial injuries. *Thorac Surg Clin.* 2014;24(1):41–50.
15. Simon B, Ebert J, Bokhari F, et al. Management of pulmonary contusion and flail chest: an Eastern Association for the Surgery of Trauma practice management guideline. *J Trauma Acute Care Surg.* 2012;73:S351–S361.
16. Yee ES, Verrier ED, Thomas AN. Management of air embolism in blunt and penetrating thoracic trauma. *J Thorac Cardiovasc Surg.* 1983;85:661–667.
17. Mattox KL. Approaches to trauma involving the major vessels of the thorax. *Surg Clin North Am.* 1989;69:77–87.

18. Telich-Tarriba JE, Anaya-Ayala JE, Reardon MJ. Surgical repair of right atrial wall rupture after blunt chest trauma. *Tex Heart Inst J.* 2012;39(4):579–581.

19. Lee CN, Leng SA, Sorokin V. Simple and quick repair of cardiac rupture due to blunt chest trauma. *Asian Cardiovasc Thorac Ann.* 2012;20(1):64–65.

20. Nakajima H, Uwabe K, Asakura T, Yoshida Y, Iguchi A, Niinami H. Emergent surgical repair of left ventricular rupture after blunt chest trauma. *Ann Thorac Surg.* 2014;98(2):e35–e36. doi:0.1016j.athoracsur.2014.03.057.

21. Kamiyoshihara M, Igai H, Ibe T, et al. Pulmonary lobar root clamping and stapling technique: return of the "en masse lobectomy." *Gen Thorac Cardiovasc Surg.* 2013;61(5):280–291. doi:10.1007/s11748-012-0159-3.

Recommended Reading

Mattox KL, Wall MJ, Tsai P. Trauma thoracotomy: principles and techniques. In: Mattox KL, Moore EE, Feliciano DV, eds. *Trauma*, 7th ed. New York, NY: McGraw-Hill; 2008:461–467.

Wall MJ, Tsai P, Mattox KL. Heart and thoracic vascular injuries. In: Mattox KL, Moore EE, Feliciano DV, eds. *Trauma*, 7th ed. New York, NY: McGraw-Hill; 2008:485–511.

The Abdomen 8

8.1 Trauma Laparotomy

8.1.1 OVERVIEW

Delayed diagnosis and treatment of abdominal injuries are common causes of preventable death from blunt or penetrating trauma. Approximately 20 per cent of abdominal injuries will require surgery. In the United Kingdom, Europe and Australia, abdominal trauma is predominantly blunt in origin, while in the military context, as well as civilian trauma in South Africa, South America and the larger US cities, it is predominantly penetrating.

The diagnosis of injury following blunt trauma can be difficult, and insight into the mechanism of injury can be helpful. Passenger restraints themselves may cause blunt trauma to the liver, duodenum or pancreas, and rib fractures are associated with hepatic or splenic injuries. Virtually all penetrating injury to the abdomen should be addressed promptly, especially in the presence of hypotension:

- Blood is not initially a peritoneal irritant, and therefore it may be difficult to assess the presence or quantity of blood present in the abdomen.
- Bowel sounds may remain present for several hours after abdominal injury, or may disappear soon after trivial trauma. This sign is therefore particularly unreliable.

Diagnostic modalities depend on the nature of the injury:

- Physical examination.
- Ultrasound – focussed abdominal sonography for trauma (FAST).
- Computed tomography (CT) scanning (stable patients only).
- Diagnostic peritoneal lavage.
- Diagnostic laparoscopy.

It is important to appreciate the difference between abdominal surgery as part of the resuscitation process, and the definitive surgical treatment for abdominal trauma:

- Surgical resuscitation includes the technique of 'damage control resuscitation' and 'damage control surgery' and implies only that the surgical procedure is primarily life-saving by stopping bleeding and preventing further contamination, as the patient's physiological derangement preludes definitive repair. (See Section 5.)
- Definitive surgical treatment implies that the physiological state of the patient allows the definitive surgical repair to take place.

During resuscitation, standard Advanced Trauma Life Support guidelines should be followed. These should include:

- Standard A-B-C-D-E priorities.
- Nasogastric or orogastric tube.
- Urinary catheter.

8.1.1.1 Difficult Abdominal Injury Complexes

There are at least four complex abdominal injury patterns:

- *Major liver injuries.* Management of actively bleeding hepatic injuries may be challenging. Improvement in computed tomography (CT) imaging has made it possible to treat more adult solid organ injuries non-operatively. Unstable patients with major liver injury require urgent laparotomy, which is technically demanding for the general surgeon, and the principle of appropriate mobilization and packing are the mainstay of treatment, followed by angioembolization. The presence of a contrast blush on CT in a relatively stable patient may be handled with angioembolization initially, if it is immediately available.
- *Pancreaticoduodenal injuries.* Difficulties in diagnosis and management are often encountered, as the extent of injury to the pancreas and bile ducts, as well as possible retropancreatic vascular injuries, may not be immediately apparent. Missed injuries lead to a significant morbidity and mortality.
- *Aortic and vena caval injuries.* Access to the retroperitoneal great vessels to obtain proximal and distal control is complicated in the presence of a large or enlarging retroperitoneal haematoma.
- *Complex pelvic fractures with associated open pelvic injury.* These are particularly difficult to treat and are associated with a high mortality.

Damage control approaches to these injuries may dramatically improve survival.

8.1.1.2 **Retroperitoneum**

Injuries to retroperitoneal structures are associated with a high mortality and are often underestimated or missed. Exsanguinating vascular injuries need rapid and efficient access techniques. Large retroperitoneal haematomas often obscure the exact position and extent of the injury.

The retroperitoneum should be explored in all central abdominal or expanding lateral haematomas as major abdominal vascular injury, or injury to the kidneys, ureters and renal vessels, pancreas, duodenum and colon may be present. In the trauma patient, the retroperitoneum is always approached via a transperitoneal incision, because of the high incidence of intraperitoneal and retroperitoneal injuries occurring simultaneously.

The decision to explore a retroperitoneal haematoma is based on its location and the mechanism of injury, and whether the haematoma is pulsating or rapidly enlarging.

The retroperitoneum is divided into

- A central zone (zone 1).
- Two lateral zones (zone 2).
- A pelvic zone (zone 3).

If the haematoma is not expanding, other intra-abdominal injuries take priority. An expanding haematoma mandates exploration. Before the retroperitoneum is opened, it is important to try to gain proximal and distal control of vessels supplying the area. Direct compression with abdominal swabs and digital pressure may help to 'buy time' while vascular control is being obtained.

Lateral retroperitoneal haematomas need not be routinely explored, unless perforation of the colon or a ureteric injury is thought to have occurred. The source of bleeding is usually the kidney, and unless expanding, the haematoma will probably not require surgery.

Non-expanding haematomas related to pelvic fractures should not be explored. Ongoing bleeding from pelvic fractures is best managed with a combination of external fixation on the pelvis and angiographic embolization. Attempts at ligation of internal iliac vessels are usually unsuccessful. If angioembolization is not available, expanding pelvic haematomas should be packed. Extraperitoneal packing is more effective than intraperitoneal pelvic packing, and is advocated in unstable patients with pelvic fractures who require surgery for haemodynamic instability.

Upper midline central retroperitoneal haematomas *must* be explored to rule out underlying duodenal, pancreatic or vascular injuries. It is wise to ensure that proximal and distal control of the aorta and distal control of the inferior vena cava (IVC) has been achieved, before the haematoma is explored.

8.1.1.3 **Non-operative Management of Penetrating Abdominal Injury**

There is universal agreement that patients with generalized peritonism or haemodynamic instability should undergo urgent laparotomy after penetrating injury to the abdomen. In some institutions with a high volume of penetrating trauma to the abdomen, certain haemodynamically stable patients are managed non-operatively. (See Chapter 8.3 on the liver and Chapter 8.4 on the spleen for the non-operative management of solid organ injury.)

However, it is imperative that serial examination of these patients is undertaken in a meticulous fashion, and that a laparotomy is done if any concerns arise.

The majority of patients with penetrating abdominal trauma managed non-operatively may be discharged after 24 hours of observation in the presence of a reliable abdominal examination and minimal to no tenderness. In addition, diagnostic laparoscopy may be considered as a tool to evaluate diaphragmatic lacerations and peritoneal penetration in an effort to avoid unnecessary laparotomy (see Chapter 15 on minimally invasive surgery in trauma). If the laparoscopy is positive, one should convert to a full trauma laparotomy to explore the intraabdominal cavity fully for other injuries.

The Eastern Association for the Surgery of Trauma (EAST) Practice Management Guidelines provide the following evidence-based guidelines for the management of penetrating abdominal trauma (Table 8.1.1)[1].

8.1.2 TRAUMA LAPAROTOMY

The trauma laparotomy contains several essential steps:

- Rapid entry
- Adequate (large) incision
- Control of massive haemorrhage by
  - · Identification of all injuries
  - · Packing
  - · Direct control
  - · Proximal control (i.e. source control)
- Identification of injuries
- Control of contamination
- Reconstruction (if possible)

8.1.2.1 Pre-operative Adjuncts

8.1.2.1.1 ANTIBIOTICS

Routine single-dose pre-operative intravenous antibiotic prophylaxis should be employed[2,3]. Subsequent antibiotic policy will depend on the intraoperative findings (Table 8.1.2).

The antibiotics commonly recommended include a second-generation cephalosporin, plus metronidazole, or where available, amoxicillin/clavulanate. There is some evidence that aminoglycosides should not be used in acute trauma, partly because of the shift in fluids which requires substantially higher doses of aminoglycoside to reach the appropriate minimum inhibitory concentration (MIC), and partly because they work

Table 8.1.1 Evidence-Based Guidelines for the Management of Penetrating Injury of the Abdomen

Level I	There are no level I evidence-based guidelines.
Level II	Patients who are haemodynamically unstable or who have diffuse abdominal tenderness after penetrating abdominal trauma should be taken emergently for laparotomy.
	Patients with an unreliable clinical examination (i.e. severe head injury, spinal cord injury, severe intoxication or need for sedation or intubation) should be explored or further investigation done to determine if there is intraperitoneal injury.
	Others may be selected for initial observation. In these patients:
	1. Triple-contrast (oral, intravenous and rectal contrast) abdominopelvic computed tomography should be strongly considered as a diagnostic tool to facilitate initial management decisions as this test can accurately predict the need for laparotomy.
	2. Serial examinations should be performed, as physical examination is reliable in detecting significant injuries after penetrating trauma to the abdomen. Patients requiring delayed laparotomy will develop abdominal signs.
	3. If signs of peritonitis develop, laparotomy should be performed.
	4. If there is an unexplained drop in blood pressure or hematocrit, further investigation is warranted.
Level III	The vast majority of patients with penetrating abdominal trauma managed non-operatively may be discharged after 24 hours of observation in the presence of a reliable abdominal examination and minimal to no abdominal tenderness.
	Patients with penetrating injury to the right upper quadrant of the abdomen with injury to the right lung, right diaphragm and liver may be safely observed in the presence of stable vital signs, reliable examination and minimal to no abdominal tenderness.
	Angiography and investigation for and treatment of diaphragm injury may be necessary as adjuncts to the initial non-operative management of penetrating abdominal trauma.
	Mandatory exploration for all penetrating renal trauma is not necessary.

Table 8.1.2 Antibiotic Prophylaxis and Empiric Therapy in Major Abdominal Injury after First Dose

No pathology found	No further antibiotics
Blood only	No further antibiotics
Small bowel or gastric contamination	Continuation for 24 hours only Copious peritoneal wash-out
Large bowel, minimal contamination	Continuation for 24 hours only
Large bowel, gross contamination	Copious peritoneal wash-out 24–72 hours of antibiotics

best in an alkaline environment (traumatized tissue is acidotic).

The administered dose should be increased twofold to threefold, and repeated after every 10 units of blood transfusion until there is no further blood loss. If intra-abdominal bleeding is significant, it may be necessary to give a further dose of antibiotic therapy intra-operatively, due to dilution of the pre-operative dose.

8.1.2.1.2 TEMPERATURE CONTROL

Temperature control[4] is fundamental in preventing complications in the injured patient. Minimizing patient hypothermia by raising the operating room temperature to a higher than normal level, and warming the patient with warm air blankets, warmed intravenous fluids and warmed anaesthetic gases, is very important.

Theatre preparations should where possible commence well before the arrival of the patient. These include warming of the operating theatre, warming of all intravenous fluids, warming of anaesthetic gases and activating external warming devices such as a Bair Hugger (3M Corporation, St. Paul, MN).

8.1.2.1.3 BLOOD COLLECTION AND AUTOTRANSFUSION

Preparations must be made for collection of blood in a saline and heparin primed drainage system, or a cell saving device, for autotransfusion if indicated.

8.1.2.2 **Draping**

During the trauma laparotomy, it may become necessary to extend the incision, if required. All patients should therefore be prepared and draped to allow access to the thorax, abdomen and groin if required (Figure 8.1.1).

8.1.2.3 **Incision**

All patients undergoing a laparotomy for abdominal trauma should be explored through a long midline incision. This incision is generally placed through, or to the left of, the umbilicus, to avoid the falciform ligament. The incision is made from the xiphisternum to the pubis, and if necessary, can be further extended into a sternotomy, or can be extended right or left as a thoracotomy for access to the liver, diaphragm, etc. (Figure 8.1.1). The incision should initially involve the skin and the subcutaneous tissues, the linea alba only. The peritoneum should be opened last, once the entire incision as indicated above has been performed. This is essentially for two reasons: first, a closed peritoneum maintains a tampon effect and keeps the incision visible, and second, this avoids losing time extending the incision in an abundantly bleeding situation. Usually, the peritoneum can be opened quickly with two fingers without having to resort to any instrument (which may be dangerous).

Figure 8.1.1 Exploration of the abdomen, showing extent of skin preparation and draping prior to surgery.

In patients with gross haemodynamic instability, or who have had significant previous midline surgery, a bilateral subcostal ('clamshell' or 'chevron') incision extending from the anterior axillary line on each side transversely across the midline just superior to the umbilicus may be used.

8.1.2.4 **Procedure**

A quick exploratory 'trauma laparotomy' is performed to identify any other associated injuries:

1. As soon as the abdomen has been opened, scoop out as much blood as possible into a receiver. Do not use a sucker at this time as it is too slow and will block with clots.
2. Eviscerate the small bowel. Perform a rapid exploration to any obvious site of large-volume (audible) bleeding. Assess the midline structures where packing is inefficient – the aorta, IVC and mesentery, and if necessary control with direct pressure or proximal control, e.g. on the aorta. Active bleeding *must* be controlled before proceeding further with a laparotomy.
3. Perform resuscitative technique (haemostatic packing) using large dry abdominal swabs:
   3.1. Under the left diaphragm.
   3.2. In the left paracolic gutter.
   3.3. In the pelvis.
   3.4. In the right paracolic gutter.
   3.5. Into the subhepatic pouch.
   3.6. Above and lateral to the liver.
   3.7. Directly on any other bleeding area.
   - Use dry swabs throughout. Dry swabs work better and will not cool the patient further. Pack them open and loosely into the above-mentioned anatomical areas. This type of packing is focussed on identifying the origin of bleeding by removing the excess blood from the uninjured parts of the peritoneal cavity.
   - Packing does not control arterial bleeding.
4. Remove the abdominal packs, one at a time, starting in the area *least* likely to be the site of the bleeding. Then, apply pressure, or compress the organ or area where active bleeding is identified.
5. Allow the anaesthetist to 'catch up' and achieve an adequate blood pressure, and to establish any lines required.
6. Perform definitive packing and haemorrhage control. (See also chapters on individual organs.)

- Preferably keep the dry swabs folded as it is easier to 'layer' them into a cavity.
- Use the folded dry packs 'flat' against the organ.
- Packs must exert sufficient force on the organ to tamponade venous bleeding, but arterial perfusion should be preserved.

6.1 Liver (See also Chapter 8.3.)

When the packs are removed from the right upper quadrant, injury to the liver is assessed. It is prudent at this time to dissect the gastrohepatic ligament using blunt and sharp dissection so that a vessel loop (Rumel tourniquet) or vascular clamp can be placed across the portal triad.

- The liver is mobilized *only* if necessary.
   6.1.1 Bleeding from the liver may require manual compression.
   6.1.2 If compression of the liver controls the bleeding, the bleeding is probably venous in nature, and can be arrested with definitive therapeutic liver packing. If not, a Pringle manoeuvre should be performed.
   6.1.3 If a Pringle manoeuvre controls the bleeding, the surgeon should suspect hepatic artery or portal vein injury. Hepatorrhaphy is then performed to control intrahepatic vessels, alone or in combination with packing.
   6.1.4 If a Pringle manoeuvre fails to control bleeding, the likely source is hepatic veins or IVC. Compression of the liver against the posterior abdominal wall and diaphragm can be useful, and packing should be performed.

6.2 Spleen (See Chapter 8.4.)

When the packs in the left upper quadrant are removed, and if there is associated bleeding from the spleen, a decision should be made on whether the spleen should be preserved or removed.

   6.2.1 A vascular clamp placed across the hilum will allow temporary haemorrhage control.

6.3 Pelvis (See Chapter 9.)

   6.3.1 If the pelvis seems to be a major source of bleeding, intraperitoneal packing should be converted to extraperitoneal pelvic packing, once intra-abdominal haemorrhage has been achieved.

7. Use definitive packing as required:

 7.1 Use dry packs.

 7.2 Do *not* cover them in plastic – they will slip and will be too rigid.

 7.3 Place the packs flat against the organ.

 7.4 Packs only work in venous injury (arteries must be controlled directly).

 7.5 Packs must exert sufficient force on the organ to tamponade the bleeding.

 7.6 Use the least number of packs that will achieve the desired result.

8. Deal with lesions in order of their lethality:

 8.1 Injuries to major blood vessels.

 8.2 Major haemorrhage from solid abdominal viscera.

 8.3 Haemorrhage from mesentery and hollow organs.

 8.4 Retroperitoneal haemorrhage.

 8.5 Contamination.

9. Replace the small intestine in the abdominal cavity with great care at the conclusion of the operation, and perform temporary abdominal closure as required.

 · Convert to a damage control procedure as appropriate.

8.1.2.5 Retroperitoneum

8.1.2.5.1 LESSER SAC

The stomach is grasped and pulled inferiorly, allowing the operator to identify the lesser curvature and the superior aspect of the pancreas visible through the lesser omentum. The coeliac artery and the body of the pancreas can also be accessed through this approach.

8.1.2.5.2 GREATER SAC

The omentum is then grasped and drawn upwards. A window is made in the omentum (via the gastrocolic ligament), and provides access into the lesser sac posterior to the stomach. This allows excellent exposure of the entire body and tail of the pancreas, as well as the posterior aspect of the first part of the duodenum and the medial aspect of the second part. Any injuries to the pancreas can be easily identified. If there is a possibility of an injury to the head of the pancreas, a Kocher manoeuvre should be performed. Additional exposure can be achieved using the right medial visceral rotation.

8.1.2.5.3 MOBILIZATION OF ASCENDING COLON (RIGHT HEMICOLON)

The hepatic flexure is retracted medially, dividing adhesions along its lateral border down to the caecum (Figure 8.1.2).

Figure 8.1.2 Mobilization of the right hemicolon.

8.1.2.5.4 KOCHER MANOEUVRE

The Kocher manoeuvre is performed by initially dividing the lateral peritoneal attachment of the duodenum, allowing medial rotation of the duodenum (Figure 8.1.3).

The loose areolar tissue around the duodenum is bluntly dissected, and the entire second and third portions of the duodenum are identified, and are mobilized medially with a combination of sharp and blunt dissection. This dissection is carried all the way medially to expose the IVC and a portion of the aorta.

The posterior wall of the duodenum can be inspected, together with the right kidney, porta hepatis and IVC. By reflecting the duodenum and pancreas towards the anterior midline, the posterior surface of the head of the pancreas can be completely exposed (Figure 8.1.4). Better

Figure 8.1.3 Kocher manoeuvre.

Figure 8.1.4 Reflection of the duodenum and right hemicolon to show the right kidney and IVC.

inspection of the third part, and inspection of the fourth part, of the duodenum can be achieved by mobilizing the ligament of Treitz and performing a right medial visceral rotation.

8.1.2.5.5 RIGHT MEDIAL VISCERAL ROTATION

Right medial visceral rotation[5] was previously known as the Cattel and Braasch manoeuvre (Figure 8.1.5).

After mobilizing the right hemicolon from the hepatic flexure to the caecum and performing a Kocher manoeuvre, the small bowel mesentery is mobilized by sharply incising its retroperitoneal attachments from the right lower quadrant, to the ligament of Treitz, by progressively lifting up the caecum. The entire ascending colon, and caecum are then reflected superiorly towards the left upper quadrant of the abdomen. A Kocher manoeuvre is performed as well. This will expose the right retroperitoneum (Figure 8.1.4). The small bowel mobilization is undertaken by sharply incising its retroperitoneal attachments from the right lower quadrant to the ligament of Treitz. The entire ascending colon and the caecum are then reflected superiorly towards the left upper quadrant of the abdomen.

As the dissection is carried further, the inferior border of the entire pancreas can then be identified and any injuries inspected. Severe oedema, crepitation or bile staining of the peri-duodenal tissues implies a duodenal injury until proven otherwise. Mobilization of the whole duodenum is mandatory for exclusion of duodenal injury.

These manoeuvres allow for complete exposure of the first, second, third and fourth parts of the duodenum, along with the head, neck and proximal body of the pancreas. Access to the vena cava and the renal vessels is also facilitated (Figure 8.1.5).

Exposure for repair of the aorta and the distal body and tail of pancreas can be better obtained by performing a left medial visceral rotation.

8.1.2.5.6 LEFT MEDIAL VISCERAL ROTATION

Medial rotation of the left side of the abdominal contents can be performed by mobilizing the spleen and descending colon, and then displacing the spleen, descending colon and sigmoid colon to the right (left medial visceral rotation[6]). This allows inspection of the left kidney, retroperitoneum and tail of the pancreas.

Mobilize the splenorenal ligament and incise the peritoneal reflection in the left paracolic gutter, down

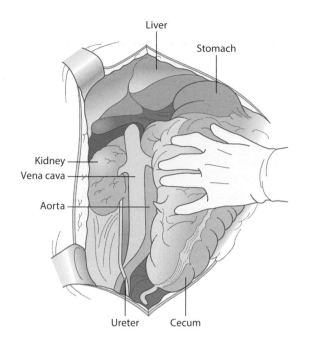

Figure 8.1.5 Right medial visceral rotation.

to the level of the sigmoid colon. The left-sided viscera are then bluntly dissected free of the retroperitoneum, and mobilized to the right. Care should be taken to

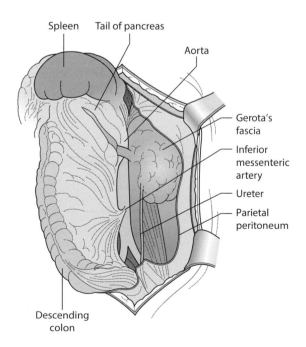

Figure 8.1.6 Left medial rotation.

remain in a plane anterior to Gerota fascia, which covers the kidney. The entire anterior surface of the abdominal aorta and the origins of its branches are exposed by this technique. This includes the coeliac axis, the origin of the superior mesenteric artery, the iliac vessels and the left renal pedicle (Figure 8.1.6). The dense and fibrous superior mesenteric and coeliac nerve plexuses overlie the proximal aorta and need to be sharply dissected in order to identify the renal and superior mesenteric arteries.

If vascular access to the kidney is required, Gerota fascia should be divided on the lateral aspect of the kidney, and the kidney rotated medially to allow access to the renal hilum, as well as the lateral side of the aorta, which can be controlled if necessary.

Pelvic haematomas should not be explored routinely. It is preferable to perform a combination of external pelvic fixation, pelvic packing and angiographic embolization. Attempts at tying the internal iliac vessels are usually unsuccessful.

8.1.3 CLOSURE OF THE ABDOMEN

8.1.3.1 Principles of Abdominal Closure

On completion of the intra-abdominal procedures, it is important to adequately prepare for closure. This preparation includes:

- Careful evaluation of the adequacy of haemostasis and/or packing.
- Copious lavage and removal of debris within the peritoneum and wound.
- Placement of adequate and appropriate drains if indicated.
- Assurance that the instrument and swab counts are completed and correct.

It is important to replace the small intestine in the abdominal cavity with great care at the conclusion of the operation.

8.1.3.2 Choosing the Optimal Method of Closure

Thal and O'Keefe[7] state that the optimal closure technique is chosen on the basis of five principal considerations and list these as follows:

- The *stability* of the patient (and therefore the need for speed of closure).
- The amount of blood loss both prior to and during operation.
- The volume of intravenous fluid administered.
- The degree of intraperitoneal and wound contamination.
- The nutritional status of the patient and possible intercurrent disease.

These factors will also dictate the decision to plan for a relaparotomy, which will naturally influence the method chosen for closure. Other factors that should be taken into consideration are hypothermia, coagulopathy and acidosis, which are indications to revert to damage control strategies.

Temporary abdominal closure is described in Chapter 5.

8.1.3.3 **Primary Closure**

Primary closure of the abdominal sheath (or fascia), the subcutaneous tissue and the skin is obviously the desired goal, and may be achieved when the conditions outlined above are optimal, that is, a stable patient with minimal blood loss and volume replacement, no or minimal contamination, no significant intercurrent problems and a patient in whom surgical procedures are deemed to be completed with no anticipated subsequent operation. Should any doubt exist regarding these conditions at the conclusion of operation, it would be prudent to consider a technique of delayed closure.

The most commonly used technique at present is that of *mass closure* of the peritoneum and sheath using a monofilament suture with a continuous (preferable, since relatively quick) or an interrupted (discontinuous) application. Either absorbable material (e.g. 1 polydioxanone loop) or non-absorbable material (e.g. nylon, polypropylene) may be used. Chromic catgut is not a suitable material.

Whichever method is used, the most important technical point is that of avoiding excessive tension on the tissues of the closure. Remember the 'one centimetre-one centimetre' rule as described by Leaper et al.[8] (the so-called 'Guildford technique'; Figure 8.1.7). This uses 4 cm of material for every 1-cm advance. This spacing seems to minimize tension in the tissues, and thus also minimize compromise of the circulation in the area, as well as using the minimum acceptable amount of suture. The use of 0 or 1 looped polydioxanone as a continuous suture is recommended.

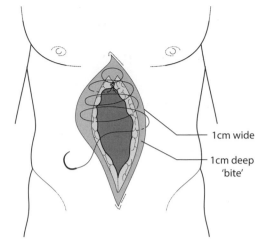

Figure 8.1.7 The Guildford technique.

Retention sutures should be avoided at all costs. A wound that seems to require these is not suitable for primary closure.

Closure of such a wound may result in abdominal compartment syndrome; such a wound should be left open, with a vacuum dressing.

Skin closure as a primary manoeuvre may be done in a case with no or minimal contamination, using monofilament sutures or staples. These latter have the advantage of speed and, while being less haemostatic, nevertheless allow for a greater degree of drainage past the skin edges and less tissue reaction.

8.1.4 **HAEMOSTATIC ADJUNCTS IN TRAUMA**

8.1.4.1 **Overview**

Haemostatic substances can be used after surgical haemostasis in trauma surgery to secure the surface of the wound. Tissue adhesives are used alone or in combination with other haemostatic measures.

The main indications for using adhesives are:

- To arrest minor oozing of blood.
- To secure the wound area to prevent subsequent bleeding.

Various forms of fibrin sealing are available and are suitable for treating injuries, especially of the parenchymatous organs. The different presentations make some suitable for superficial bleeding surfaces, and others easier to apply in deep lacerations. Some are readily available, while preparation is time-consuming in others. It is important that the surgeon knows what haemostatic agents are available and how and where they can be used.

Of the adhesives currently available, fibrin glue is the most suitable for treating injuries to the parenchymatous organs and retroperitoneum. It is also possible to make autologous fibrin from the patient's own blood (Vivostat system, Vivolution A/S, Birkeroed, Denmark); the fibrin is applied with a sprayer. The necessary volume of blood (125 mL) can already be drawn in the emergency room, and the autologous adhesive is ready within 30 minutes.

Fibrin sealing is based on the transformation of fibrinogen to fibrin. Fibrin promotes clotting, tissue adhesion and wound healing through interaction with the fibroblasts. The reaction is the same as in the last phase of blood clotting. One such heterologous fibrin is Tisseel/Tissucol (Baxter Hyland Immuno, Vienna, Austria). Heterologous fibrin is a biological two-component adhesive and has high concentrations of fibrinogen and factor XIII, which, together with thrombin and calcium, result in clotting. Resorption time and resistance to tearing depend on the size and thickness of the glue layer, and on the proportion by volume of the two components. The fibrin sealant is best applied with a sprayer or syringe injection system such as the Tissomat sprayer (Baxter Hyland Immuno).

TachoSil (Takeda Nycomed AS, Asker, Norway), is a fixed, ready-to-use combination of a collagen sponge coated with a dry layer of the human coagulation factors fibrinogen and thrombin, making it easy to employ. It is most suitable for oozing from the raw surfaces of solid organs or to seal air leaks from lung injuries. It is available in most countries in Europe and Australasia.

Similarily, HemoPatch (Baxter Hyland Immuno) has recently become available. HemoPatch is a soft, thin and flexible patch consisting of a porous collagen matrix, which facilitates clotting, coated on one side with a thin protein-binding layer (pentaerythritol polyethylene glycol ether tetra-succinimidyl glutarate [NHS-PEG]) which allows rapid adhesion (within 2 minutes) via electrophilic cross-linking. The patch consequently has a dual-method mechanism of action, in which the two components interact to achieve hemostasis by sealing off the bleeding surface and initiating the body's own clotting mechanisms. The patch is resorbed within 6–8 weeks.

Even after surgical haemostasis, deep parenchymal injuries can require a resorbable tamponade; here,

collagen fleece (e.g. TissoFleece, Baxter Hyland Immuno) is suitable. Collagen fleece is composed of heterologous collagen fibrils obtained from devitalized connective tissue and is fully resorbable. Collagen fleece promotes the aggregation of thrombocytes when in contact with blood. The platelets degenerate and liberate clotting factors, which in turn activate haemostasis. The spongy structure of the collagen stabilizes and strengthens the coagulate. Another alternative for deep parenchymal injuries is FloSeal (Baxter Hyland Immuno).

Fibrin glue and collagen fleece are used preferentially to treat slight oozing of blood. Before application, the bleeding surface should be tamponaded and compressed with a warm pad for a few minutes. Immediately after removal of the pad, air is first sprayed alone, followed by short bursts of fibrin. This creates a surface that is free from blood and nearly dry when the fibrin glue is sprayed onto it. A dry field is essential for most fibrin sprays in order to secure adequate haemostasis.

If collagen fleece is to be applied, a thin layer of fibrin is sprayed onto the fleece, which, in turn, is pressed onto the wound. After a few moments of compression, the fleece is sprayed with fibrin glue. The thickness of the fibrin layer will depend on the size and depth of the injury.

8.1.4.2 **Other Haemostatic Adjuncts**

8.1.4.2.1 CHITOSAN (CELOX, MEDITRADE LTD., CREWE, UK)/HEMCON (HEMCON MEDICAL TECHNOLOGIES, PORTLAND, OR)

Chitosan is a granular product made from a natural polysaccharide derived from chitin from shellfish. Chitosan is the deacetylated form of chitin. In the form of an acid salt, chitosan demonstrates mucoadhesive activity. Chitosan stops bleeding by bonding with red blood cells and gelling with fluids to produce a sticky pseudoclot. This reaction is not exothermic and has been used successfully within body cavities. Chitosan is broken down by enzymatic action within the body to produce glucosamine. The dressing is sold as pads or bandages.

8.1.4.2.2 MINERAL ZEOLYTE (QUIKCLOT, Z-MEDICAL CORPORATION, WALLINGFORD, CT)

Mineral zeolyte, when made moist, produces an exothermic reaction that seals blood vessels and results in haemostasis. The initial preparation was in the form of granules and was very exothermic, resulting in significant tissue damage. The current preparation is presented in bags ('tea-bags') that are packed into the wound and may cause less damage.

8.1.4.3 **Specific Applications**

8.1.4.3.1 HEPATIC INJURY

In severe liver injury, after successful surgical treatment including the removal of devascularized necrotic tissue and resectional debridement in selected cases, the liver is packed, and the injured area compressed with warm pads. After complete exploration of the abdomen and treatment of other injuries and sources of bleeding, the liver packs are removed and any slight oozing on the surface of the liver can be arrested by sealing with fibrin and collagen fleece as described above. Fibrin glue cannot, however, compensate for inadequate surgical technique.

8.1.4.3.2 SPLENIC INJURY

When possible, in the stable patient, the surgeon should try to achieve splenic repair that preserves as much of the damaged spleen as possible. For splenic preservation, the choice of procedure depends not only on the clinical findings, but also on the surgeon's experience of splenic surgery and the equipment available. In trauma cases, conservation of the spleen should not take significantly more time than would a splenectomy.

After using one of the surgical techniques described above, definitive treatment can be completed by the application of adhesives to secure the resected edge or the mesh-covered splenic tissue. Fibrin is sprayed on, and the collagen fleece is pressed on it for a few minutes. After removal of the compressing pad, a new layer of fibrin glue can help to ensure the prevention of rebleeding. When mesh is used, the collagen fleece and fibrin are placed directly on the injured splenic surface and then covered with the mesh. Additional fibrin spray may then be added.

8.1.4.3.3 PANCREATIC INJURY

When pancreatic injury is suspected, extended exploration of the whole organ is imperative. Parenchymal lacerations that do not involve the pancreatic duct can be sutured when the tissue is not too soft and vulnerable. With or without sutures, a worthwhile option in the treatment of such lacerations is fibrin sealing and collagen tamponade, for which adequate drainage is essential.

8.1.4.3.4 RETROPERITONEAL HAEMATOMA

Injuries to the retroperitoneal vessels can cause haematomas of varying size, depending on the calibre of the vessels injured and the severity of the injury. Retroperitoneal haematomas can be treated by packing after surgical control of injured vessels, and be followed by catheter embolization.

When the patient is stable, the packs may be removed after 24–48 hours. Rebleeding after removal of the packs can necessitate repacking. Slight bleeding can, however, be stopped effectively by spraying on adhesives.

8.1.5 **BRIEFING FOR OPERATING ROOM SCRUB NURSES**

A separate briefing for operating room scrub nurses forms Appendix E of this manual.

8.1.6 **SUMMARY**

The laparotomy in trauma needs to be performed in a systematic fashion. The ease with which injuries can be missed, and the potentially catastrophic consequences of a missed injury, mandate that extreme care be taken to exclude injuries, based on the injury complexes, and the way in which the laparotomy is approached. Careful examination of each organ is essential.

The trauma laparotomy is a team event, and the anaesthesiologist must be fully involved and informed of all decision making.

REFERENCES AND FURTHER READING

References

1. Como JJ, Bokhari F, Chiu WC, et al. Practice management guidelines for selective nonoperative management of penetrating abdominal trauma. *J Trauma*. 2010;68(3):721–733. doi:10.1097/TA.0b013e3181cf7d07.

2. Luchette FA, Borzotta AP, Croce MA, et al. Practice management guidelines for prophylactic antibiotics in penetrating abdominal trauma. Available from www.east.org (accessed December 2014).

3. Goldberg SR, Anand RJ, Como JJ, et al. Prophylactic antibiotic use in penetrating abdominal trauma: an Eastern Association for the Surgery of Trauma practice management guideline. *J Trauma Acute Care Surg.* 2012;Supplement 73(5):S321–S325. doi:10.1097/TA.0b013e3182701902.

4. Hardcastle TC, Stander M, Kalafatis N, Hodgson E, Gopalan D. External patient temperature control in emergency centres, trauma centres, intensive care units and operating theatres: a multi-society literature review. *S Afr Med J.* 2013;103:609–611.

5. Cattell RB, Braasch RW. A technique for the exposure of the third and fourth parts of the duodenum. *Surg Gynaecol Obstet.* 1960;111:379–385.

6. Mattox KL, McCollum WB, Jordan GL Jr, et al. Management of upper abdominal vascular trauma. *Am J Surg.* 1974;128:823–828.

7. Thal ER, O'Keefe T. Operative exposure of abdominal injuries and closure of the abdomen. In: *ACS Surgery: Principles and Practice.* New York, NY: Web MD, 2007: Section 7, Chapter 9.

8. Leaper DJ, Pollock AV, Evans M. Abdominal wound closure: a trial of nylon, polyglycolic acid and steel sutures. *Br J Surg.* 1977;64:603–606.

Recommended Reading

Hirshberg A. In: Mattox KL, Moore EE, Feliciano DV, eds. *Trauma*, 7th ed. New York, NY: McGraw-Hill; 2013:512–528.

Hoff WS, Holevar M, Nagy KK, et al. Practice management guidelines for the evaluation of blunt abdominal trauma. *J Trauma.* 2002;53:602–615. In: Eastern Association for the Surgery of Trauma, Trauma Practice Management Guidelines. Available from: www.east.org (accessed December 2014).

Ogura T1, Lefor AT, Nakano M, Izawa Y, Morita H. Nonoperative management of hemodynamically unstable abdominal trauma patients with angioembolization and resuscitative endovascular balloon occlusion of the aorta. *J Trauma Acute Care Surg.* 2015;78(1):132–135. doi:10.1097/TA.0000000000000473.

8.2 Bowel and Diaphragm

8.2.1 OVERVIEW

The surgeon must always bear in mind the three-dimensional nature of wound tracks in penetrating injury. An odd number of bowel enterotomies should prompt a second look for missed injury.

In all patients who are subjected to laparotomy after injury, the entire length of bowel, from the oesophagogastric junction, stomach, small bowel from the ligament of Treitz to the ileo-caecal valve, and large bowel from the caecum to the rectum, and their mesenteries should be inspected.

8.2.1.1 'Two hands, but four eyes'

The most common sites of missed organ injury in the abdomen are:

- Diaphragm.

> **Pitfall**
>
> - Do not fail to inspect the diaphragm, especially in the presence of penetrating injury, especially if below the fifth intercostal space.
> - Both the surgeon and the assistant independently inspect the same segment at the same time. Ideally, only one operator handles the bowel at any time, as otherwise each operator thinks that the other is doing the inspection.

- Oesophago-gastric junction.
- The posterior aspect of stomach and pancreas (in the lesser sac; a missed injury here led to the death of President McKinley in 1902[1]).
- Small bowel (a small penetrating injury to the small bowel can be easy to miss).
- Retroperitoneal colon and rectum.

8.2.2 **DIAPHRAGM**

The diaphragm divides the torso into thoracic and abdominal components. Particularly with penetrating injury, the penetration may go through the diaphragm and give misleading signs. For example, a stab wound of the lower chest with a haemothorax may be a reflection of an intra-abdominal injury to the liver, spleen or kidney, with blood draining through the diaphragm into the chest. All diaphragmatic injuries benefit from early diagnosis and repair. The presence of a defect, when the thoracic cavity is at negative pressure compared to the abdominal cavity, invariably results in a slowly enlarging defect, herniation of abdominal contents into the chest and a late presentation.

Diagnosis of small defects is notoriously difficult, and entities such as chest X-ray are unhelpful. In blunt injury, the passage of a nasogastric tube prior to the chest X-ray will show the presence of the herniated stomach in the chest if the defect is large. Likewise, computed tomography (CT) is unhelpful, though magnetic resonance imaging (MRI) in the stable patient is somewhat more accurate.

In the stable patient, laparoscopy or video-assisted thoracoscopy (VATS) is helpful. VATS is useful in those patients with a penetrating chest injury, and no indication for laparotomy. Laparoscopy, especially in the hands of a surgeon inexperienced in the techniques required for examination of the injured diaphragm, is less reliable.

> *Penetration of the diaphragm mandates exploratory laparotomy in most cases, to exclude sub-diaphragmatic visceral injuries.*

Repair of the diaphragm is relatively straightforward. It is, after all, a skeletal muscle. Most lacerations can be held at their apices by two Babcock or Allis tissue forceps. The laceration can be sutured in a continuous fashion using a 3/0 non-absorbable suture. There is no evidence that a braided suture or interrupted sutures make much difference.

> *If the laceration is close to pericardium, extra care must be taken not to inadvertently include pericardium in the suture.*

If there is major contamination of the abdominal cavity, then the thoracic cavity must be thoroughly washed out as well, using copious amounts of normal saline, and a chest drain placed. Close off the diaphragmatic defect prior to washing out the abdominal cavity to avoid further contamination.

Diaphragmatic injuries occur in approximately 6 per cent of patients with mid-torso injuries from penetrating trauma. The left diaphragm is injured more commonly than the right. The diaphragm usually rises to the fifth intercostal space during normal expiration, so that any patient with a mid-torso injury is at risk of a diaphragmatic injury.

The diagnosis of penetrating injury to the diaphragm is less problematic than injury from blunt trauma. Typically, the patient has a wound in proximity, and the surgeon's decision is how best to assess the diaphragm. Thoracoscopy is a good method because it is so easy to visualize the diaphragm from above. However, thoracoscopy does not allow the assessment or repair of intra-abdominal organs. Laparoscopy has an additional advantage in that it is possible to assess intra-peritoneal organs as well as the diaphragm for injury. However, laparoscopy has not withstood the degree of specificity and sensitivity necessary for it to be the method of choice (see Chapter 14).

Optimally, all diaphragmatic injuries should be repaired, even small penetrating puncture wounds of no apparent importance. An injury that is not repaired will present as a late complicated traumatic diaphragmatic hernia (TDH), usually with incarceration of the small bowel, colon or omentum within the hernia sac. The preferred closure of diaphragmatic injuries is with interrupted non-absorbable suture. The use of synthetic material to close large defects from high-velocity missile injuries or shotgun blasts is only rarely indicated.

The complications of injuries to the diaphragm are primarily related to late diagnosis with hernia formation and incarceration. Phrenic nerve palsy is another complication, but this is uncommon after penetrating trauma.

If the defect is very large, and the patient is haemodynamically stable, it can be closed with a patch, usually 2-mm polytetrafluoroethylene (PTFE). Ideally this is done using a trans-thoracic approach.

8.2.3 **STOMACH**

The stomach is lifted and pulled caudally, using two Babcock forceps, and the anterior surface inspected. It is helpful if there is a nasogastric tube in place – place the forceps around the tube, forming a useful gastric retractor. The lesser sac should be entered through the greater omentum, and the stomach can then be lifted to allow inspection of its posterior surface (as well as the body and tail of the pancreas)

The stomach is highly vascular, and in all injuries, life-threatening bleeding can result. All holes should be repaired using a continuous 3/0 polydioxanone suture (e.g. PDS, Johnson & Johnson, Brunswick, NJ). Simple gastric injuries can be minimally debrided and closed (usually in two layers); more complex gastric injuries should be controlled by non-anatomic resection, with reconstruction deferred to the re-look laparotomy.

8.2.3.1 Pitfall

In all penetrating injuries in which a hole is found on the anterior surface of the stomach, it is important to seek the corresponding hole on the posterior wall of the stomach. If this cannot be found, enlarge the anterior hole and inspect the stomach from within: 'penetrating holes generally go in pairs – one in, one out'.

8.2.4 THE DUODENUM

The duodenum must be carefully inspected from the pylorus to the ligament of Treitz. If there is a haematoma on the duodenum, it is mandatory to perform a Kocher manoeuvre and inspect the posterior surface of the duodenum. See section 8.6.

8.2.5 SMALL BOWEL

The fundamental decision to be made on every patient is:

Damage control laparotomy or definitive procedure?

The decision will depend on the context – the injury pattern, the physiological status of the patient and the nature and volume of other patients waiting. If decision is made to 'damage control' the patient, then management of visceral injury is usually simple. The stomach will require haemostatic sutured closure; the rest of the bowel will usually be dealt with by resecting damaged gut and leaving it stapled in discontinuity. Definitive intestinal surgery can be undertaken at re-look surgery, when the patient should be in a better physiological state.

Starting at the ligament of Treitz, each segment of small bowel is inspected and then flipped over to examine the opposite side. The mesentery is carefully inspected as well. If the bowel is dropped, start again at the ligament of Treitz!

8.2.5.1 **The Stable Patient**

Small bowel injuries should be closed, with primary repair or resection and primary anastomosis as appropriate. Consider one resection and anastomosis when several wounds are localized close to one another. Be mindful, however, that bowel should be preserved wherever possible.

Where multiple small wounds are present (e.g. following a shotgun injury), a size 35W skin stapler can be used to close individual holes safely.

8.2.5.2 **The Unstable Patient**

The first priority is haemorrhage control. If the patient is haemodynamically unstable, damage control is likely, and bowel injuries should be treated using damage control procedures. The first priority is to treat the haemorrhage and then to control contamination.

Small wounds can be closed rapidly, using a size 35W skin stapler or with mass closure. In severely injured patients, with more extensive injuries requiring damage control, simple proximal and distal closure of the injured bowel using a GIA-type stapler is the best way to prevent ongoing soiling. The bowel should be transected and closed for later repair ('clip and drop'). Umbilical tape can also be used.

Neither any anastomosis nor any stoma should be performed at this stage, as these can be time-consuming, the tissue viability is uncertain and the leak rate is much higher, especially in the presence of concomitant contamination. The non-viable or damaged areas can be removed at a later time and the need for ileostomy or colostomy assessed. Additionally, the bowel may be oedematous secondary to trauma or overenthusiastic fluid resuscitation, and suturing or stapling is then technically difficult.

In wounds caused by small penetrating missiles, for example with a shotgun, it is easy to miss multiple holes, which are often less than 2 mm in diameter. It is recommended that, in these cases, the bowel be passed through a bowl of water, so that any air leak will show itself as bubbles. All such injuries should be reinspected at 36–48 hours, and the procedure repeated.

8.2.6 **LARGE BOWEL**

World War II experience of poor outcomes following complications of repair or anastomosis after colonic injury led to a policy of mandatory colostomy for colon injury that continued into civilian practice in the post-war years. In 1979, a randomized trial of 268 patients was undertaken to challenge this doctrine. Primary repair was found to be associated with fewer complications than diversion; however, throughout the trial, approximately half of the total patients with colonic injury were excluded from randomization and had a mandatory colostomy due to the presence of factors assumed to increase risk of complications (shock, extensive faecal contamination, prolonged delay from injury to operation, destructive colonic injury or multiple associated injuries). Subsequent trials were conducted and a meta-analysis of further trials confirmed mortality is not significantly different between diversion and repair; however, morbidity is significantly less with primary repair. A further important consideration when considering optimal primary surgery is the morbidity inherent in colostomy reversal; complications following closure after colon injury have been reported to occur in up to half of patients.

In a civilian major trauma centre, primary repair appears safe even when the colonic injury is severe; however, a multicentre prospective study on destructive colon wounds confirmed that abdominal complications are more likely if the patient is critically injured: if the transfusion requirement is ≥4 units of blood or there is severe faecal contamination associated with the bowel injury. Importantly, the actual surgical method of colon wound management (colostomy or repair/anastomosis) made no difference.

Pragmatic recommendations for the management of patients with colonic injury were produced in the early years of this century; patients with non-destructive injuries should undergo minimal debridement of the colonic injury and primary repair, patients with destructive wounds of the colon but without co-existent serious injury, comorbidities or large transfusion requirement should undergo resection and anastomosis, while patients with destructive wounds, co-existing critical injury, significant medical illness or transfusion requirements of >6 units should undergo faecal diversion.

Utilizing these guidelines led to colostomy being undertaken for <10% of all colon wounds with acceptable morbidity.

8.2.6.1 **The Stable Patient**

For colonic injuries, indications for colostomy are still debated. Time from injury, haemodynamic status, co-morbid conditions and degree of contamination will influence the decision. More primary repairs/primary anastomoses are being performed, with fewer colostomies. Simple colonic injuries can be treated in much the same way as a simple small bowel injury, with local debridement and primary repair. When there are multiple small and large bowel lacerations, a protective ileostomy can be helpful.

8.2.6.2 **The Unstable Patient**

In the unstable patient (Table 8.2.1) undergoing a damage control procedure, small wounds can simply be sutured using 3/0 polydioxanone. The wounds can be re-inspected at the re-look procedure.

Larger wounds should be excluded in the same manner as small bowel. All macroscopic contamination should be washed out using copious amounts of warmed saline before (temporary) closure.

Destructive colonic injuries should be treated with resection and stapling in discontinuity. The decision to restore continuity by anastomosis or divert is made at re-look laparotomy. In a recent series, up to 75% of patients with colon injury undergoing damage control laparotomy (DCL) had anastomosis at subsequent laparotomy with acceptable rates of complications. If a damage control patient remains critically unwell at time of first re-look (typically at 48 hours) with inotropes still required, if they have a large burden of injury or if they have had a massive transfusion, it is advisable to avoid a colonic anastomosis and cover with a colostomy. If a stoma is considered to be the most appropriate management for the patient, surgeons should be aware that early colostomy closure can be achieved safely. In a trial of 49 patients undergoing colostomy for trauma in South Africa, 77% were considered fit for early closure during the same hospital stay. These patients were then randomized to early or standard closure and there was no excess morbidity associated with early closure.

Table 8.2.1 Evidence-Based Recommendations for the Management of Penetrating Injuries of the Colon[2]

Level I	There is sufficient class I and class II data to support a standard of primary repair for *non-destructive* (involvement of <50% of the bowel wall without devascularization) colon wounds in the absence of peritonitis.
Level II	Patients with penetrating intra-peritoneal colon wounds that are *destructive* (involvement of >50% of the bowel wall or devascularization of a bowel segment) can undergo resection and primary anastomosis if they:

- Are haemodynamically stable without evidence of shock (sustained pre- or intra-operative hypotension as defined by a systolic blood pressure <90 mm Hg)
- Have no significant underlying disease
- Have minimal associated injuries (penetrating abdominal trauma index <25, injury severity score <25, Flint grade <11)
- Have no peritonitis

Patients with shock, underlying disease, significant associated injuries or peritonitis should have destructive colon wounds managed by resection and colostomy.

Colostomies performed following colon and rectal trauma can be closed within 2 weeks if a contrast enema examination is performed to confirm distal colon healing. This recommendation pertains to patients who do not have non-healing bowel injury or unresolved wound sepsis, and are not unstable.

A barium enema should not be performed to rule out colon cancer or polyps prior to colostomy closure for trauma in patients who otherwise have no indications for being at risk of colon cancer and/or polyps.

Source: Cayten CG, Fabian TC, Garcia VF, Ivatury RR, Morris JA, *J Trauma*, 44(6), 941–956, 1998. With permission.

8.2.6.3 **Pitfall**

No stomas should be performed in the unstable patient as this prolongs the surgical time and may make things more complex in the presence of competing injury.

8.2.7 **RECTUM**

Surgeons consider the rectum[3] in distinct parts: the intra-peritoneal upper third and the extra-peritoneal lower two-thirds. Diagnosis of rectal injury can be difficult and, as low rectal injuries are, by definition, not within the peritoneal cavity, they can easily be missed. Any penetrating injury at the level of the lower abdomen, hips or thighs (such as penetrating injury to the buttocks) should be considered to be associated with a rectal injury.

Major pelvic fracture can also cause injury to the rectal muscle tube. Suspicion of rectal injury mandates specific investigation; luminal examination with a flexible sigmoidoscope is much more likely to identify a rectal injury than rigid sigmoidoscopy, which can have a high false-negative rate. Surgical dogma derived from wartime experience suggested that rectal injury should be treated in an aggressive surgical manner with:

- Diversion.
- Debridement.

With rectal injuries, primary repair should be considered for intraperitoneal injuries and extraperitoneal injuries that can be mobilized. A proximal diverting colostomy (often a loop sigmoidostomy) is indicated in more extensive rectal injuries and when repair is impossible.

In patients with complex abdominal injuries, peritoneal soiling is of secondary importance to haemorrhage control. Once haemorrhage has been controlled, devascularized areas accompanying deep injuries should be re-sected.

A protocol for management of rectal injury has been formulated by Weinberg and colleagues: injury to the intraperitoneal rectum should be treated as per a colon injury, with primary repair when feasible. Accessible injury to the rectum, including the extraperitoneal component is treated by direct repair (after surgical mobilization) and selective faecal diversion. Inaccessible distal extraperitoneal rectal injuries are treated with diversion and pre-sacral drainage. In an observational, non-comparative study of this protocol, infectious complications (wound infection, bacteraemia, intra-abdominal and/or retroperitoneal abscess) were reduced compared to historical controls. The optimal treatment of penetrating injury to the rectum has yet to be subjected to a satisfactory randomized controlled trial, and, as ever in trauma surgery, the nature of the extent of tissue destruction, associated injury and physiological status of the patient need to be taken into account. In a contemporary military setting, faecal diversion is still almost universally applied to patients with rectal injury.

8.2.7.1 **Pitfall**

There is no indication for routine presacral drains or distal rectal wash-out.

8.2.8 **MESENTERY**

Arterial bleeders should be tied off. Do not extend mesenteric lacerations, and if necessary oversew bleeding wounds.

8.2.9 **ADJUNCTS**

8.2.9.1 **Antibiotics**

Practice management guidelines for prophylactic antibiotic use[4] in penetrating abdominal trauma are given in Table 8.2.2.

REFERENCES

1. Pappas TN, Swanson S. Anarchy and the surgical care of President William McKinley. *J Trauma Acute Care Surg.* 2012;72(4):1106–1113.

2. Cayten CG, Fabian TC, Garcia VF, Ivatury RR, Morris JA. Patient management guidelines for penetrating intraperitoneal colon injuries. An Eastern Association for the Surgery of Trauma practice management guideline. *J Trauma.* 1998;44(6):941–956.

3. Weinberg JA, Fabian TC, Magnotti LJ, et al. Penetrating rectal trauma: management by anatomic distinction improves outcome. *J Trauma.* 2006;Mar;60(3):508–513; discussion 513–514.

4. Goldberg SR, Anand RJ, Como JJ, et al. Prophylactic antibiotic use in penetrating abdominal trauma: an Eastern Association for the Surgery of Trauma practice management guideline. *J Trauma and Acute Care Surg.* 2012;73(5 Suppl 4):S321-5 doi:10.1097/TA.0b013e3182701902.

Selected Reading

Emergency War Surgery. US Army Medical Department. 2014. http://www.cs.amedd.army.mil/borden/Portlet.aspx?ID = cb88853d-5b33-4b3f-968c-2cd95f7b7809.

Smith I, Beech Z, Lundy JB, Bowley DM. A prospective observation study of abdominal injury management in contemporary military operations: damage control laparotomy is associated with high survivability and low rates of faecal diversion. *Ann Surg.* 2015; 261(4): 765-73. do:10.1097/SLA.0000000000000657.

Table 8.2.2 Practice Management Guidelines for Prophylactic Antibiotic Use in Penetrating Abdominal Trauma[4]

Level I	There are sufficient class I and II data to recommend a single pre-operative dose of prophylactic antibiotics with broad-spectrum aerobic and anaerobic coverage as a standard of care for trauma patients sustaining penetrating abdominal wounds. Absence of a hollow viscus injury requires no further administration
Level II	There are sufficient class I and class II data to recommend continuation of prophylactic antibiotics for only 24 h in the presence of injury to any hollow viscus.
Level III	There are insufficient clinical data to provide meaningful guidelines for reducing infectious risks in trauma patients with haemorrhagic shock. Vasoconstriction alters the normal distribution of antibiotics, resulting in reduced tissue penetration. To circumvent this problem, the administered dose may be increased two- or threefold and repeated after every 10th unit of blood product transfusion until there is no further blood loss. Once haemodynamic stability has been achieved, antibiotics with excellent activity against obligate and facultative anaerobic bacteria should be continued for periods that depend on the degree of wound contamination. Aminoglycosides have been demonstrated to exhibit suboptimal activity in patients with serious injury, probably due to altered pharmacokinetics of drug distribution.

8.3 Liver and Biliary System

8.3.1 **OVERVIEW**

While most injuries to the liver do not require surgical intervention, management of severe hepatic lesions can be a devastating experience. The evolution in management of the condition has evolved since packing was first described over 100 years ago, through aggressive surgery, to refinement of techniques, and the increasing role of non-operative management of the majority of injuries[1-6].

Management of hepatic trauma demands a sound working knowledge of the anatomy of the liver including the arterial supply, portal venous supply and hepatic venous drainage.

The liver is composed of a right and a left half of the liver (hemiliver), defined by Cantlie line separating the two. The Cantlie line runs from the gallbladder fossa to the inferior vena cava (IVC). The hemilivers are divided into eight Couinaud segments. Segment I is the caudate lobe, segments II through IV make up the left hemiliver and the right hemiliver includes segments V through VIII (Figure 8.3.1).

The structures within the porta hepatis include the hepatic artery, portal vein and bile duct. The portal triad is encased in an extension of Glisson capsule and thus is relatively resistant to injury. The portal triad runs *within* the segments of the liver. The major hepatic veins (right,

left and middle) have no valves, are not protected by an extension of Glisson capsule and run *between* the segments of the liver. Difficult to control, life-threatening haemorrhage in the operating room is generally related to hepatic vein or retrohepatic inferior vena cava injury. The liver generally encases a portion of the retrohepatic cava, at times circumferentially. Full mobilization of the liver to expose the retrohepatic IVC requires division of this attachment. The major hepatic veins are 8–12 cm in length, the majority of which is intra-hepatic (Figure 8.3.2). Injury to the major hepatic veins is generally to this portion of the veins and can be controlled by compression or suture ligation. The extrahepatic segments of the major hepatic veins are <2 cm in length and are less commonly injured. Injury to the extrahepatic portion of the major hepatic veins generally presents as active haemorrhage and carries a high mortality[2]. In addition,[3-11] short hepatic veins run directly from the liver to the IVC and can also be a source of haemorrhage, and must be identified and controlled if liver re-section is necessary. Finally, the liver parenchyma will tolerate ligation or embolization of hepatic artery branches, but the bile ducts will not. The bile ducts depend on the hepatic artery for their blood supply.

Knowledge of this hepatic anatomy is important, as it explains some of the patterns of injury that follow blunt trauma. In addition, there are differences in tissue

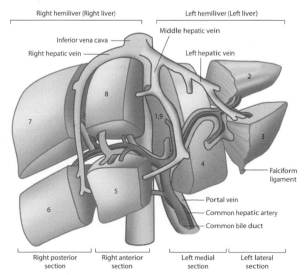

Figure 8.3.1 Hepatic anatomy, showing Couinaud segments of the liver. Image printed with permission from Peitzman A.B.

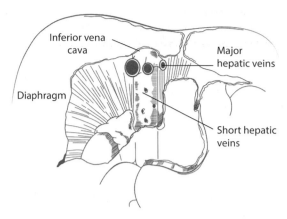

Fig 8.3.2 The liver showing the relationship of the veins.

elasticity that determine injury patterns. Segmental anatomical resection has been well documented but is usually not applicable to trauma.

The forces from blunt injury are usually direct compressive forces or shear forces. The elastic tissue within arterial blood vessels makes them less susceptible to tearing than any other structures within the liver. Venous and biliary ductal tissue is moderately resistant to shear forces, whereas the liver parenchyma is the least resistant. Thus, fractures within the liver parenchyma tend to occur along segmental fissures (remember this is where the major hepatic veins course) or directly in the parenchyma. This causes shearing of branches emanating from the major hepatic and portal veins. With severe deceleration injury and traction injury, the origin of the short retro-hepatic veins may be ripped from the cava, causing devastating haemorrhage (these veins may be as large as 1 cm in diameter). Similarly, the small branches from the caudate lobe entering directly into the cava are at high risk for shearing with linear tears on the caval surface. Direct compressive forces usually cause tearing between segmental fissures in an anterior-posterior vector. Horizontal fracture lines into the parenchyma give the characteristic burst pattern to such liver injuries. If the fracture lines are parallel, these have been dubbed 'bear claw'-type injuries and probably represent where the ribs have been compressed directly into the parenchyma. This can cause massive haemorrhage if there is direct extension or continuity with the peritoneal cavity.

Diagnosis of hepatic trauma preoperatively may be difficult (blood itself is not an irritant). The liver is at risk of damage in any penetrating trauma or blunt force injury to the upper abdomen and lower thorax, especially of the right upper quadrant.

Appropriate decision making is critical to a good outcome:

- Do not be in the operating room unless necessary with major liver injury.
- Patients actively bleeding from major liver injury must be promptly taken to the operating room with rapid haemorrhage control. Any delay in doing so increases risk of coagulopathy and mortality.
- If operation is indicated, the simplest, quickest technique that can restore haemostasis is the most appropriate.
- If simple manoeuvres fail to control haemorrhage the decision to proceed with hepatorrhaphy or re-sectional debridement must be made quickly.

8.3.2 RESUSCITATION

Haemodynamically *stable* patients without signs of peritonitis or other indication for operation are generally managed non-operatively (>80 per cent of blunt liver injuries).

Haemodynamically *unstable* patients with liver injuries require immediate surgical exploration to achieve haemostasis, and exclude other sources of bleeding. The patient in whom a surgical approach is decided upon or is mandated by haemodynamic instability should be transferred to the operating room as rapidly as possible after the following are completed:

- Establish emergency airway or ventilatory management if necessary.
- Establish adequate upper limb large-bore vascular access and initiate crystalloid resuscitation. Infuse blood products early and preferentially if the patient is profoundly hypotensive. Avoid IV access below the diaphragm as this may exacerbate bleeding from the liver or IVC.
- Initiate the massive haemorrhage (massive transfusion) protocol.

> *Consider early damage control and packing before the coagulopathy is established!*
>
> *Once the patient is cold, coagulopathic and in irreversible shock, the battle usually is lost. Call for senior help early in the operation.*

8.3.3 DIAGNOSIS

Any delay to control of bleeding will increase mortality. Surgery should not be delayed by multiple emergency department procedures such as limb X-rays, unnecessary ultrasonography, and vascular access procedures. Computed tomography (CT) scanning of the brain should be delayed until the patient is stable. Control of bleeding takes priority over any diagnostic procedure (including CT). The anaesthesiologist can continue resuscitation in the operating room.

In patients with blunt trauma there may be an absence of clear clinical signs such as rigidity, distension or unstable vital signs. Up to 40 per cent of patients with significant haemoperitoneum have no obvious signs. Focussed abdominal sonography for trauma (FAST) may be particularly useful in the setting of blunt injury and haemodynamic instability, since the presence of free fluid in the abdominal cavity will direct you quickly to the operating room in a hypotensive patient. With a haemodynamically stable patient, CT is an invaluable diagnostic aid and allows the surgeon to make decisions on the need for embolization or operative management. Diagnostic peritoneal lavage in the blunt trauma setting is also useful, particularly when CT support services are inadequate or unavailable.

The purpose of diagnostic investigation in the stable patient is to help identify those patients who can be safely managed non-operatively, to assist decision making in non-operative management and to act as a baseline for comparison in future imaging studies. Accurate, good-quality contrast-enhanced CT has enhanced our ability to make an accurate diagnosis of liver injuries.

Penetrating wounds of the liver usually do not present a diagnostic problem, as most surgeons would advocate exploration of any wound in the unstable patient.

Peritoneal lavage as a diagnostic tool in penetrating trauma has been misleading. The CT scan using contrast for penetrating liver injury can be useful in very select circumstances – in the haemodynamically stable patient who is suspected to have an injury of the right upper quadrant, isolated to the liver only. In this setting trajectory of the injury can be confirmed, delineation of vascular viability and assistance with the decision of whether to treat the injury non-operatively versus operatively, with or without embolization.

8.3.4 LIVER INJURY SCALE

The American Association for the Surgery of Trauma's Committee on Organ Injury Scaling has developed a grading system for classifying injuries to the liver (Table 8.3.1).

Hepatic injuries are graded on a scale of I to VI, with grade I representing superficial lacerations and small subcapsular haematomas and grade VI representing avulsion of the liver from the vena cava. Isolated injuries that are not extensive (grades I to III) are usually managed non-operatively; however, extensive parenchymal injuries and those involving the juxtahepatic veins (grades IV and V) may require complex manoeuvres for successful treatment. Hepatic avulsion (grade VI) is generally lethal.

Eighty per cent of blunt liver injuries are grades I to III. Grades IV and V comprise 15 to 20 per cent of blunt liver injuries and these are the patients who are unstable and require laparotomy for control of haemorrhage. In

Table 8.3.1 Liver Injury Scale (See also Appendix B: Trauma Scores and Scoring Systems)

Grade[a]	Type of Injury	Description of Injury
I	Haematoma	Subcapsular, <10% surface area
	Laceration	Capsular tear, <1 cm parenchymal depth
II	Haematoma	Subcapsular, 10% to 50% surface area: intraparenchymal <10 cm in diameter
	Laceration	Capsular tear 1–3 parenchymal depth, <10 cm in length
III	Haematoma	Subcapsular, >50% surface area of ruptured subcapsular or parenchymal haematoma; intraparenchymal haematoma >10 cm or expanding 3-cm parenchymal depth
	Laceration	Parenchymal disruption involving 25% to 75% hepatic lobe or 1–3 Couinaud segments
IV	Laceration	Parenchymal disruption involving >75% of hepatic lobe or >3 Couinaud segments within a single lobe
V	Vascular	Juxtahepatic venous injuries; i.e. retrohepatic vena cava/central major hepatic veins
VI	Vascular	Hepatic avulsion

[a]Advance one grade for multiple injuries up to grade IV.

Source: Moore EE, Cogbill TH, Jurkovich GJ, et al., *J Trauma,* 38, 323–324, 1995.

general, if the patient with blunt liver injury is stable enough for CT, the patient can be managed non-operatively. In the patient who is truly stable, without active bleeding, this generally applies irrespective of the grade of liver injury or amount of haemoperitoneum.

8.3.5 MANAGEMENT

Traditionally, discussion of liver injuries differentiates between those arising from blunt and those arising from penetrating trauma. In general blunt hepatic injury carries higher mortality than penetrating liver injury due to the magnitude of parenchymal injury. Most stab wounds cause relatively minor liver injury unless a critical structure such as the hepatic vein, the intrahepatic cava or the portal structures are injured. In contrast, gunshot wounds, particularly high-energy injuries, and shotgun blasts can be devastating. Twenty-five per cent of penetrating injuries to the liver can be managed non-operatively. High-grade parenchymal liver injury (grades IV and V) or juxtahepatic caval injury from severe blunt trauma carry high mortality and continue to be the most challenging for the surgeon.

Richardson[1] and co-workers managed approximately 1200 blunt hepatic injuries over a 25-year period. Non-operative management was used in up to 80 per cent of cases. Deaths secondary to injury dropped from 8 to 2 per cent. They proposed four reasons for the decrease in mortality from liver injury: improved results with packing

Table 8.3.2 Evidence-Based Guidelines for Selective Non-Operative Management of Hepatic Injury [3]

Level of Evidence	Recommendation
I	Patients who have diffuse peritonitis or who are hemodynamically unstable after blunt abdominal trauma should be taken urgently for laparotomy.
II	1. A routine laparotomy is not indicated in the hemodynamically stable patient without peritonitis presenting with an isolated blunt hepatic injury.
	2. In the haemodynamically stable blunt abdominal trauma patient without peritonitis, an abdominal CT scan with intravenous contrast should be performed to identify and assess the severity of injury to the liver.
	3. The severity of hepatic injury (as suggested by CT grade or degree of haemoperitoneum), neurologic status, age >55 and/or the presence of associated injuries are not contraindications to a trial of non-operative management in a hemodynamically stable patient.
	4. Angiography with embolization should be considered in a haemodynamically stable patient with evidence of active extravasation (a contrast blush) on abdominal CT scan.
	5. Non-operative management of hepatic injuries should only be considered in an environment that provides capabilities for monitoring, serial clinical evaluations and an operating room available for urgent laparotomy.
III	1. After blunt hepatic injury, clinical factors such as a persistent systemic inflammatory response, increasing/persistent abdominal pain, or an otherwise unexplained drop in haemoglobin should prompt re-evaluation by CT scan.
	2. Contrast blush on CT scan alone is not an absolute indication for an operation or angiographic intervention. Factors such as patient age, grade of injury and presence of hypotension need to be considered in the clinical management of these patients.
	3. Interventional modalities, such as endoscopic retrograde cholangiopancreatography (ERCP) angiography, laparoscopy, or percutaneous drainage, may be required to manage complications (bile leak, biloma, bile peritonitis, hepatic abscess, bilious ascites and haemobilia), that arise as a result of non-operative management of blunt hepatic injury.
	4. Pharmacologic prophylaxis to prevent venous thromboembolism can be used for patients with isolated blunt splenic injuries without increasing the failure rate of non-operative management, although the optimal timing of safe initiation has not been determined.
Unanswered questions	1. Frequency of haemoglobin measurements
	2. Frequency of abdominal examinations
	3. Intensity and duration of monitoring
	4. Time to re-initiating oral intake
	5. Duration and intensity of restricted activity (both in hospital and after discharge)
	6. Optimum length of stay both for the intensive care unit and the hospital
	7. Timing of initiating chemical deep venous thrombosis (DVT) prophylaxis after a splenic injury

and re-operation (damage control), use of angiography and embolization, advances in operative techniques for major hepatic injury and decrease in the number of patients undergoing exploration for hepatic venous injury (surgeons were not exacerbating the injury).

8.3.5.1 **Non-operative Management (NOM)**

Nearly all children and 50 to 80 per cent of adults with blunt hepatic injuries can be treated without laparotomy[1,3–6]. See Table 8.3.2. This change in approach has been occasioned by the increasing availability of rapid ultrasound, helical CT scan and interventional radiology.

The primary requirement for non-operative therapy is haemodynamic stability. To confirm stability, frequent assessment of vital signs and monitoring of the haematocrit and lactate or base deficit are necessary, in association with CT scans as required. Continued haemorrhage occurs in 1 to 4 per cent of patients. Hypotension may develop, usually within the first 24 hours after hepatic injury, but sometimes several days later.

The presence of extravasation of contrast on CT denotes arterial haemorrhage; therapeutic angiography with embolization should be applied early in these patients. Otherwise, operative intervention will become necessary in these patients. Angiography/embolization may also be used post-operatively as a component of damage control for major liver injury.

A persistently falling haematocrit should be treated with packed red blood cell (PRBC) transfusions. If the haematocrit continues to fall after two or three units of pRBCs, embolization in the interventional radiology suite or laparotomy should be considered.

8.3.5.2 **Operative (Surgical) Management**

Most injuries requiring surgical intervention are managed simply by evacuating the free intraperitoneal blood, and washing out the peritoneal cavity; some will require drainage of the injury because of a possible bile leak. However, 25 per cent of liver injuries requiring surgical intervention require direct control of more major hepatic bleeding[6–10]. Most bleeding from hepatic injury is venous in nature and therefore can be controlled by direct compression and liver packs. Tissue sealants may be a useful adjunct[9]. Caution must be exercised since bile within the peritoneal cavity is not always well tolerated, and closed suction drainage should be routine in these patients.

8.3.6 **SURGICAL APPROACH**

During treatment of a major hepatic injury, ongoing haemorrhage may pose an immediate threat to the patient's life, and temporary control will give the anaesthesiologist time to restore the circulating volume before further blood loss occurs. This is best achieved immediately upon entry into the abdomen by direct manual compression of the liver. The goal is to restore the normal anatomy by manual compression and then maintain it with packing. Compress right and left halves of the liver back to normal anatomy and simultaneously push the liver posteriorly to tamponade potential retrohepatic venous bleeding.

Additionally, multiple bleeding sites beyond the liver are common with both blunt and penetrating trauma. Even if the liver is not the highest priority, temporary control of hepatic bleeding allows repair of other injuries without unnecessary blood loss:

- Perihepatic packing.
- Pringle manoeuvre.
- Tourniquet or liver clamp application.
- Electrocautery, or Argon beam coagulator.
- Haemostatic agents and glues.
- Hepatic suture.
- Hepatorrhaphy and non-anatomic re-section (resectional debridement).

8.3.6.1 **Incision**

- The patient is placed in the supine position.
- Warming devices are placed around the upper body and lower limbs.
- The chest and abdomen are surgically prepared and draped – prep the patient from chin to mid-thighs and table-to-table laterally.
- The instruments necessary to extend the incision into a sternotomy or thoracotomy must be available.
- A generous midline incision from pubis to xiphisternum is the minimum incision required. On rare occasion, for the patient 'in extremis', a combined sternotomy and midline laparotomy approach is recommended from the outset to allow access for internal cardiac massage and vena caval vascular control. Supradiaphragmatic intrapericardial inferior vena caval control is often easier than abdominal control adjacent to a severe

injury. However, this opens another body cavity and is uncommonly necessary.

- An 'Omnitract' or Bookwalter-type automatic retractor greatly facilitates access. The Rochard retractor is simpler and can be more quickly utilized in the unstable patient.

8.3.6.2 **Initial Actions**

Once the abdomen has been opened, intraperitoneal blood is evacuated and bleeding controlled, and if there is evidence of hepatic bleeding, the liver should be initially packed and the abdomen rapidly examined to exclude extrahepatic sites of blood loss. Autotransfusion should be considered. Once the anaesthetist has had an opportunity to restore intravascular volume and haemostasis has been achieved for any extrahepatic injury, the liver injury then can be approached.

In dealing with liver injury, be a minimalist – if the lesion has ceased bleeding, nothing more needs to done in most cases and above all, the non-bleeding lesion should *not* be explored further. If further surgery is required, adequate exposure and mobilization of the liver are necessary. Most injuries do not require formal mobilization of the injured lobe to permit repair or packing.

> *'Perfection is the enemy of good!'*
>
> *The non-bleeding liver should not be explored further.*
>
> *Call early for senior help for complex liver injuries which continue to bleed.*

8.3.6.3 **Techniques for Temporary Control of Haemorrhage**

- Perihepatic packing.
- Tract tamponade balloons.
- Pringle manoeuvre.
- Tractotomy and direct suture ligation.
- Mesh wrap.
- Hepatic artery ligation.
- Hepatic vascular isolation.
- Techniques to control retrohepatic caval bleeding.
- Moore-Pilcher balloon.
- Veno-venous bypass (uncommonly needed).

8.3.6.3.1 PERIHEPATIC PACKING

The philosophy of packing has altered, and packs are used to restore the anatomical relationship of the components, and secondarily to act as compressive agents. Packs for a liver wound should *not* be pushed into the wound itself as this worsens the injury and causes further bleeding. Do not pack tears with omentum - restore the anatomy.

Liver packing can also be definitive treatment, particularly with bilobar injury, or to buy time if the patient develops coagulopathy, hypothermia, or there are no blood resources. Liver packing is the method of choice where expertise in more sophisticated techniques is not available. If packing is successful, and the bleeding is controlled, then no further action may be required – this decision must be made early in the operation before the patient has received large numbers of red blood cells (RBCs) in transfusion. If simple actions fail to control bleeding, then a more complex operation will be necessary. Furthermore, surgical expertise and speed are essential to rapidly control the bleeding. Remember that mortality in trauma patients is 25 per cent after 10 units of RBCs and 50 per cent after 20 units of RBCs. Thus, bleeding should ideally be controlled prior to 10 units and certainly by 20 units of transfusion

> *This is your 'clock' when dealing with major hepatic injury.*

Packing is initially performed using large *dry* flat abdominal packs, placed laterally, inferiorly, medially and around the liver. Ideally it is not necessary to unfold these. Careful placement of packs is capable of controlling haemorrhage from the majority of hepatic venous injuries:

- Restore the anatomy of the liver by direct manual compression.
- Place the first pack(s) across the injury to stabilize the damaged tissue.
- Place additional packs, if necessary, between the liver and the diaphragm, posteriorly and laterally, and between the liver and the anterior chest wall.
- Note that there is no benefit in placing multiple packs between the dome of the liver and the diaphragm; this will only have the effect of raising the diaphragm.
- Pack the inferior surface of the liver from the porta hepatis laterally. This moves the right lobe of the liver laterally.

- Then pack the liver 'backward' between the subcostal margin and the anterior surface of the right lobe. The liver should not be packed so tightly as to cause compression of the vena cava which will reduce venous return.

If necessary, the liver can be mobilized by division of the hepatic ligaments until the bleeding has been controlled. Several packs may be required to control the haemorrhage from an extensive right lobar injury. The minimum number of packs to achieve haemostasis should be used (Figure 8.3.3).

8.3.6.3.2 FINAL PACKING

Packing is not as effective for injuries of the left lobe, because with the abdomen open, there is insufficient abdominal and thoracic wall anterior to the left lobe to provide adequate counter-compression. Fortunately, haemorrhage from the left lobe can be controlled by dividing the left triangular and coronary ligaments and

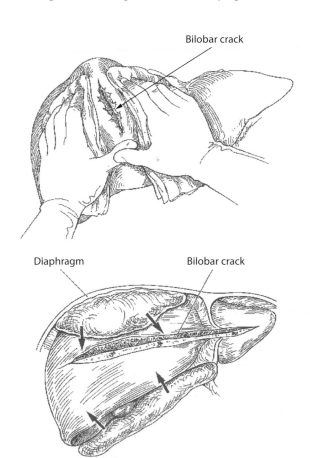

Figure 8.3.3 Packing of the liver.

compressing the lobe between the hands – segments II and III can be resected rapidly if needed.

Key factors for success are:

- Use dry abdominal swabs. Wet swabs are less absorbent and exacerbate hypothermia.
- Use them 'folded' as it is easier to layer them for even pressure.
- Ensure that they have radio-opaque markers included in their manufacture.
- Do *not* cover them with plastic as they will not hold position.
- Ongoing bleeding despite initial packing mandates repacking or other haemostatic procedure and consideration of embolization.

During the period of time that the packs are placed, it is important to establish more intravenous access lines and other monitoring devices as needed. Hypothermia should be anticipated and corrective measures taken. After haemodynamic stability has been achieved, the packs are removed, and the injury to the liver rapidly assessed. The control of haemorrhage is the first consideration, followed by control of contamination. If the bleeding has stopped, nothing further may be required.

If in doubt, apply damage control techniques, with definitive packing of the liver:

- Consider angiography and embolization with damage control surgery.
- Packs should preferably be removed within 24 to 72 hours. If removed too early, bleeding may recur. A higher risk of perihepatic infection results from packs remaining longer than 72 hours.
- The packs should be carefully removed to avoid precipitating further bleeding.
- If there is no bleeding, the packs can be left out and closed suction drains placed.
- Necrotic tissue should be resected.

Two complications may be encountered with the packing of hepatic injuries. First, tight packing compresses the inferior vena cava, decreases venous return and reduces right ventricular filling; hypovolaemic patients may not tolerate the resultant decrease in cardiac output. Second, perihepatic packing forces the right diaphragm to move superiorly and impairs its motion; this may lead to increased airway pressures and decreased tidal volume.

If compression and packing are unsuccessful, then it will be necessary to achieve direct access to the bleeding vessel and direct suture ligation. This will often necessitate extension of the wound to gain access and view the bleeding point. During this direct access, bleeding can be temporarily controlled by direct compression, which requires a capable assistant. Temporary clamping of the porta hepatis (Pringle manoeuvre) is also a useful adjunctive measure. Other adjunctive measures include interruption of the venous or arterial inflow to a segment or lobe (less than 1 per cent of all liver injuries), haemostatic agents such as crystallized bovine collagen, fibrin adhesives, gel foam and use of the argon laser or harmonic scalpel.

8.3.6.3.3 PRINGLE MANOEUVRE

The Pringle manoeuvre is often used as an adjunct to packing for the temporary control of haemorrhage. When encountering life-threatening haemorrhage from the liver, the hepatic pedicle should be compressed manually. The compression of the hepatic pedicle via the foramen of Winslow is known as the Pringle manoeuvre. The liver then should be packed as above. The hepatic pedicle is best clamped from the left side of the patient, by digitally dissecting a small hole in the lesser omentum, near the pedicle, and then placing a soft clamp over the pedicle from the left-hand side, through the foramen of Winslow. The advantage of this approach is the avoidance of injury to the structures within the hepatic pedicle, and the assurance that the clamp will be properly placed the first time. The pedicle can be left clamped for up to an hour. However, this is probably true only in the haemodynamically stable patient. In the hypotensive patient, intermittent clamping produces less ischemia than continuous clamping; leave the clamp on for 10 minutes at a time, with 5 minutes of reperfusion between clamp placement. The clamp should be replaced as soon as possible with a Rumel vascular sling.

The Pringle manoeuvre is both therapeutic and diagnostic. If bleeding within the liver stops with the Pringle manoeuvre, haemorrhage is from branches of the hepatic artery or the portal vein – these bleeding sites should be oversewn and controlled. If haemorrhage persists with the clamp on the porta hepatis, the source of bleeding is generally from the hepatic veins or the retrohepatic vena cava, or less commonly aberrant extrapedicular arterial supply to the left or right lobes.

8.3.6.3.4 HEPATIC TOURNIQUET

When faced with bleeding from the left lobe of the liver, once the bleeding lobe has been mobilized, Penrose tubing can be wrapped around the liver near the anatomic division between the left lobe and the right. The tubing is stretched until haemorrhage ceases, and tension is maintained by clamping the drain. Unfortunately, tourniquets are difficult to use, and they tend to slip off or tear through the parenchyma if placed over an injured area. An alternative is the use of a liver clamp; however, the application of such devices is hindered by the variability in the size and shape of the liver. Bleeding from the left lateral segment can be definitively and rapidly controlled with resection using the stapling devices.

8.3.6.3.5 ACCESS TO DEEPER BLEEDING WITHIN THE LIVER

At times, extension of the liver injury may be needed to gain access to deeper bleeding. Remember as you proceed more deeply within the liver, the vessels become larger.

8.3.6.3.6 FINGER FRACTURE

To provide the above access, 'finger fracture' through normal liver tissue, to get to the injured vessels deep in the parenchyma, may be necessary. The normal capsule is 'scored' using diathermy or scalpel. Then the normal liver tissue is gently compressed between thumb and forefinger, rubbing the normal parenchymal tissue away, leaving just the intact vessels for ligation or clipping. Avoid forceful pinching or crushing of the liver tissue, as this may disrupt the hepatic vasculature, increasing the haemorrhage.

8.3.6.3.7 STAPLING DEVICES

Stapling devices provide an even more rapid method to resect/divide liver parenchyma. Crushing staples with a vascular load are best. The Ligasure (Johnson & Johnson, Brunswick, NJ) or equivalent may also be used to quickly divide liver parenchyma.

As with any liver surgery, be certain to protect normal/non-injured vasculature and bile ducts as you perform these manoeuvers. Knowledge of hepatic anatomy is critical.

Do not cross the Cantlie's line as you resect a lobe or segment.

8.3.6.3.8 TRACT TAMPONADE BALLOONS

Tract tamponade balloons[11] can be useful in haemostasis of a tract, from stab or gunshot wounds. The balloon is threaded down the tract and inflated, to tamponade the bleeding from inside out. The balloon can be either manufactured by the surgeon using Penrose rubber tubing, or even a condom and a nasogastric tube. A Sengstaken-Blakemore tube for tamponade of oesophageal varices is ideal.

8.3.6.3.9 HEPATIC SUTURE

Suturing of the hepatic parenchyma is not routinely recommended to control more superficial lacerations which continue to bleed, but may be used if other methods are ineffective. If, however, the capsule of the liver has been stripped away by the injury, sutures which are tied over the capsule are far less effective.

The liver is usually sutured using a large curved, blunt-nosed needle with 0 or 2/0 resorbable sutures. The large diameter prevents the suture from pulling through Glisson capsule. At times, this may be life-saving. On the other hand, deeper injury may be present with resultant haemorrhage, abscess or biloma. For shallow lacerations, a simple continuous suture may be used to approximate the edges of the laceration. For deeper lacerations, interrupted horizontal mattress sutures may be placed parallel to the edges and tied over the capsule. The danger of suturing is that sutures tied too tight may cut off the blood supply to viable liver parenchyma, resulting in necrosis.

Most sources of venous haemorrhage can be managed with intraparenchymal sutures. An adjunct to parenchymal suturing or hepatotomy is the use of the omentum to fill large defects in the liver and to buttress hepatic sutures. The rationale for this use of the omentum is that it provides an excellent source for macrophages and fills a potential dead space with viable tissue. In addition, the omentum can provide a little extra support for parenchymal sutures, often enough to prevent them from cutting through the Glisson capsule.

8.3.6.3.10 MESH WRAP

A technique that may be attempted if packing fails is to wrap the injured portion of the liver with a fine porous material (e.g. polyglycolic acid mesh) after the injured lobe has been mobilized. Using a continuous suture or a linear stapler, the surgeon constructs a tight-fitting stocking that encloses the injured lobe. Blood clots beneath the mesh, which results in tamponade of the hepatic injury. It is best to secure this mesh to the falciform ligament once full mobilization is complete, in order to keep the mesh wrap from stripping off the liver.

8.3.6.3.11 HEPATIC RESECTION

In elective circumstances anatomic resection[12] produces good results, but in the uncontrolled circumstances of trauma, mortality has been recorded in excess of 50 per cent. Anatomic lobectomy should be reserved for patients with:

- Extensive injuries of the lateral segments of the left lobe where bimanual compression is possible
- Delayed lobectomy in patients where packing initially controls the haemorrhage, but where there is a segment of the liver that is non-viable
- Almost free segments of liver
- Devitalized liver at the time of pack removal

8.3.6.3.12 HEPATIC SHUNTS

The atriocaval shunt was designed to achieve hepatic vascular isolation while still permitting some venous blood from below the diaphragm to flow through the shunt into the right atrium. A shunt can be introduced from above via the left atrial appendage, or from below via the saphenofemoral junction.

The mortality remains high with this approach, and it is no longer in general use.

8.3.6.3.13 HEPATIC ISOLATION

Hepatic vascular isolation is accomplished by executing a Pringle manoeuvre, clamping the aorta at the diaphragm, and clamping the inferior vena cava above the right kidney (suprarenal) and above the liver (suprahepatic). The technique is not straightforward and is best achieved by those experienced in its use. In patients scheduled for elective procedures, this technique has enjoyed nearly uniform success, but in trauma patients, the results have been disappointing. The time limit for isolation is about 30 minutes.

8.3.6.3.14 HAEMOSTATIC AGENTS AND GLUES

Fibrin adhesive (see Section 8.1.4.3) has been used in treating both superficial and deep lacerations and appears to be the most effective topical agent. Some are suitable for injection deep into bleeding gunshot and stab wound tracts to prevent extensive dissection and blood loss. Others are more suitable for surface application. Fibrin adhesives are made by mixing concentrated human fibrinogen (cryoprecipitate) with a solution containing bovine thrombin and calcium. The resection is not necessarily anatomical. Resectional therapy almost invariably requires drainage of some type. A useful adjunctive measure is to use a pedicle of omentum over the cut surface.

8.3.6.4 Mobilization of the Liver

In general, and for most injuries, it is not necessary to mobilize the liver; injuries can be dealt with, without resorting to full mobilization. However, in some situations, particularly with injury to the superior or posterior aspects, mobilization is necessary.

Be certain that the self-retaining retractor (Omnitract, Bookwalter, Rochard, etc.) is lifting the costal margin in both a cephalad and anterior direction. Lifting the ribcage anteriorly (away from the table) is critical for adequate exposure. Access to the right lobe of the liver is restricted due to the right subcostal margin and the posterior attachments. If a self-retaining retractor is not immediately available, the costal margin can be elevated, initially with a Morris retractor, and then with a Kelly or Deaver retractor. The right triangular and coronary ligaments are divided with scissors or cautery. Be certain to avoid entering the diaphragm or liver parenchyma as you do so. This usually can be done under vision but in the larger subject it can be accomplished blindly from the patient's left side. The superior coronary ligament is divided, avoiding the lateral wall of the right hepatic vein. The inferior coronary ligament is divided, taking care not to injure the right adrenal gland (which is vulnerable because it lies directly beneath the peritoneal reflection) or the retrohepatic vena cava. When the ligaments have been divided, the right lobe of the liver can be rotated medially into the surgical field. Sudden onset or aggravation of bleeding during mobilization of the right liver attests to hepatic vein or retrohepatic caval injury and mandates immediate replacement of the mobilized liver and damage control packing.

The left lobe can be easily mobilized by dividing the left triangular ligament under vision, avoiding injury to the left inferior phrenic vein and the left hepatic vein.

In the event of a retrohepatic haematoma being evident, rotation of the right lobe of the liver should be avoided unless strong indications are present and adequate expertise is available. Packing and transport to a higher-level centre may be a safer option.

If exposure of the junction of the hepatic veins and the retrohepatic vena cava is necessary, the midline abdominal incision can be extended by means of a median sternotomy or a lateral subcostal extension. The pericardium and the diaphragm then can be divided in the direction of the inferior vena cava (IVC). In an unstable patient, a more rapid means to access the suprahepatic IVC is via the abdomen through the central diaphragm/pericardium (Figure 8.3.4).

8.3.6.5 Perihepatic Drainage

Several prospective and retrospective studies have demonstrated that the use of either Penrose or sump drains carries a higher risk of intra-abdominal infection than the use of either closed suction drains or no drains at all. It is clear that if drains are to be used, closed suction devices are preferred. Patients who are initially treated with perihepatic packing may also require drainage; however, drainage is *not* indicated at the initial damage control procedure, given that the patient will be returned to the operating room (OR) within the next 36–48 hours. The primary function is to drain bile, not blood.

The best treatment for a post-operative bile leak is prevention. As a routine part of the definitive operation for major hepatic injury (generally the re-look operation after damage control), obtain a cholangiogram. This defines the biliary anatomy and will identify major ductal injury while in the OR. Inject saline intermittently through the cholangiocatheter in the cystic duct remnant (cholecystectomy performed) to identify and oversew leaking bile ducts.

8.3.6.6 Subcapsular Haematoma

An uncommon but troublesome hepatic injury is subcapsular haematoma, which arises when the parenchyma of the liver is disrupted by blunt trauma but the Glisson capsule remains intact. Subcapsular haematomas range in severity from minor blisters on the surface

Even if hepatotomy with ligation is effective, one must still contend with diffuse haemorrhage from the large denuded surface, and packing may also be required. A haematoma that is expanding during operation (grade III) may have to be explored. Such lesions are often the result of uncontrolled arterial haemorrhage, and packing alone may not be successful. An alternative strategy is to pack the liver to control venous haemorrhage, close the abdomen and transport the patient to the interventional radiology suite for hepatic arteriography and embolization of the bleeding vessels. Ruptured grades III and IV haematomas are treated with exploration and selective ligation, with or without packing.

8.3.7 COMPLICATIONS

Overall mortality for patients with hepatic injuries is approximately 10 per cent. The most common cause of death is exsanguination, followed by multiple organ dysfunction syndrome (MODS) and intracranial injury.

- Morbidity and mortality increase in proportion to the injury grade and to the complexity of repair.
- Hepatic injuries caused by blunt trauma carry a higher mortality than those caused by penetrating trauma.
- Infectious complications occur more often with penetrating trauma.

Postoperative haemorrhage occurs in a small percentage of patients with hepatic injury. The source may be either a coagulopathy or a missed vascular injury (usually to an artery). In most instances of persistent post-operative haemorrhage, the patient is best served by return to the OR. Arteriography with embolization may be considered in selected patients. If coagulation studies indicate that a coagulopathy is the likely cause of postoperative haemorrhage, then correction of the coagulopathy must be a critical part of the strategy.

Perihepatic infections occur in fewer than 5 per cent of patients with significant hepatic injury. They develop more often in patients with penetrating injuries than in patients with blunt injuries, presumably because of the greater frequency of enteric contamination. An elevated temperature and a rising white blood cell count should prompt a search for intra-abdominal infection. In the absence of pneumonia, an infected line, or urinary tract infection, an abdominal CT with intravenous and upper gastrointestinal contrast should be obtained.

Figure 8.3.4 Access to the suprahepatic inferior vena cava (IVC) via the central tendon of the diaphragm.

of the liver to ruptured central haematomas accompanied by severe haemorrhage. They may be recognized either at the time of the operation or in the course of CT scanning. Regardless of how the lesion is diagnosed, subsequent decision making is often difficult. If a grade I or II subcapsular haematoma (i.e. a haematoma involving less than 50 per cent of the surface of the liver that is not expanding and is not ruptured) is discovered during an exploratory laparotomy, it should be left alone. If the haematoma is explored, hepatotomy with selective ligation may be required to control bleeding vessels.

Many perihepatic infections (but not necrotic liver) can be treated with CT or ultrasound-guided drainage. In refractory cases, especially for posterior infections, right 12th rib resection remains an excellent approach.

Bilomas are loculated collections of bile that may become infected. They are best drained percutaneously under radiological guidance. If a biloma is infected, it should be treated as an abscess; if it is sterile, it will eventually be resorbed.

Biliary ascites is caused by disruption of a major bile duct and requires reoperation and the establishment of appropriate drainage. Even if the source of the leaking bile can be identified, primary repair of the injured duct can be difficult to achieve. It is best to wait until a firm fistulous communication is established with adequate drainage. Adjunctive, transduodenal drainage by endoscopic retrograde cholangiopancreatography (ERCP) and papillotomy (ductotomy) or stent placement may be of benefit in selected cases.

Biliary fistulae occur in up to 15 per cent of patients with major hepatic injuries. They are usually of little consequence and generally close without specific treatment. In rare instances, a fistulous communication with intrathoracic structures forms in patients with associated diaphragmatic injuries, resulting in a bronchobiliary or pleurobiliary fistula. Because of the pressure differential between the biliary tract and the thoracic cavity, most of these fistulae must be closed operatively.

Haemorrhage from hepatic injuries is often treated without identifying and controlling each bleeding vessel individually, and arterial pseudoaneurysms may develop as a consequence. As the pseudoaneurysm enlarges, it may rupture into the parenchyma of the liver, into a bile duct or into an adjacent branch of the portal vein. Rupture into a bile duct results in haemobilia, which is characterized by intermittent episodes of right upper quadrant pain, upper gastrointestinal haemorrhage and jaundice; rupture into a portal vein may result in portal vein hypertension with bleeding varices. Both of these complications are rare and are best managed with hepatic arteriography and embolization.

8.3.8 INJURY TO THE RETROHEPATIC VENA CAVA

Approximately 2 per cent of all liver injuries are complex and represent injuries to major hepatic venous structures, portal triad, the intrahepatic cava, the injuries are bi-lobar or are difficult to control because of

hypothermia and coagulopathy. Injuries to the hepatic vein or retrohepatic cava can be approached in the following ways:

- Direct compression and definitive repair.
- Intracaval shunt.
- Temporary clamping of the porta hepatis, suprarenal cava and suprahepatic cava (vascular isolation).
- Veno-venous bypass.
- Packing.

Direct compression and control of hepatic venous injuries can be accomplished in some patients. Major liver injury requires manual compression and simultaneous medial rotation and retraction – a difficult manoeuvre. Ideally, two experienced surgeons are now in the operating room. In such a situation the most senior surgeon should be the one doing the direct compression and the assistant should do the actual suturing of the hepatic vein or cava.

Adequate exposure, experienced surgeons, good anaesthesia help and a deep blood bank are essential in salvaging these patients.

However, in many cases, especially with blunt injury, packing the liver against the cava secures haemostasis as part of damage control, and the definitive care can take place later.

Hepatic vascular isolation, by clamping of the porta hepatis, suprarenal cava and suprahepatic cava can be done on a temporary basis. This requires considerable experience by the anaesthesiologist and a surgeon capable of dealing with the problems rapidly.

Veno-venous bypass has been used successfully in liver transplant surgery, and with new heparin-free pumps and tubing may have a place in the trauma patient.

In some patients who have bilobar injuries with extensive bleeding, or in patients who have developed coagulopathy secondary to massive transfusions and hypothermia, it may be prudent to institute damage control procedures and return to surgery when physiological stability has been obtained. Packing may often be used as definitive treatment. Vicryl mesh and omental pedicles also have been advocated in controlling severe lacerations.

Injuries to the porta hepatis also can be exsanguinating. Right and left hepatic arteries usually can be managed by simple ligation as can injuries to the common hepatic artery. Remember that hepatic artery ligation or embolization is well tolerated by the liver parenchyma (via portal vein flow) but not by the bile ducts (depend on arterial flow).

Injury to the left or right portal vein can be ligated. Ligation of the main portal vein has been reported to be successful; however, shunting as part of damage control and subsequent repair are recommended whenever possible. The options for retrohepatic vein and cava injuries include direct compression and extension of the laceration as mentioned above, atrial caval shunt, non-shunt isolation (Heaney technique) and veno-venous bypass. Liver packing also can be definitive treatment, particularly when there is bilobar injury, or it can simply buy time if the patient develops a coagulopathy, hypothermia or there are no blood resources. Liver packing is the method of choice where expertise in more sophisticated techniques is not available, or when it is therapeutic in controlling the bleeding.

Packing should be removed in the standard damage control sequence (when the patient is warm, appropriately transfused and haemodynamic and respiratory parameters have been normalized). It is recommended that lateral and medial suction drains be placed after packs have been removed, as biliary leak is relatively common.

8.3.9 **INJURY TO THE PORTA HEPATIS**

If there is a haematoma in the porta hepatis,[13] there is a high probability of injury to the vessels of the portal triad, often in association with injury to the common bile duct.

The key is to obtain source control.

- Before entering the haematoma, perform a Pringle manoeuvre, preferably with a Rumel tourniquet.
- Control bleeding vessels in the porta, initially with finger compression, and subsequently with vascular clamps. *Do not clamp blindly.*
- Do *not* place sutures or ties until the common bile duct has been identified.
- When in doubt, *shunt* the portal vein.
- The hepatic artery can be ligated if necessary.

8.3.10 **INJURY TO THE BILE DUCTS AND GALLBLADDER**

Injuries to the extrahepatic bile ducts, although rare, can be caused by either penetrating or blunt trauma.[14,15] The diagnosis is usually made by noting the accumulation of bile in the upper quadrant during laparotomy for treatment of associated injuries.

Bile duct injuries can be divided into those below the confluence of the cystic duct and common duct and those above the cystic duct. Treatment of common bile duct (CBD) injuries after external trauma is complicated by the small size and thin wall of the normal duct.

For the lower ductal injuries (those injuries below the cystic duct), when the tissue loss is minimal, the lesion can be closed over a T-tube (as with exploration of the CBD for stones). A choledochoduodenostomy can be performed if the duodenum has not been injured. If the duodenum has been injured, or there is tissue loss, since the common duct is invariably small, a modification of the Carrel patch can be utilized. From blunt trauma, the common bile duct can be transected at the superior border of the pancreas. This is best treated with Roux-en-Y hepatojejunostomy.

In higher ductal injuries between the confluence of the cystic duct and the common duct and the hepatic parenchyma, a hepatojejunostomy with an internal splint is recommended. An adjunctive measure is to bring the Roux-en-Y end to the subcutaneous tissue so that access can be gained later if a stricture develops. Percutaneous intubation of the Roux-en-Y limb is then possible with dilatation of the anastomosis.

Treatment of injuries to the left or right hepatic duct is even more difficult. If only one hepatic duct is injured, a reasonable approach is to ligate it and deal with any infections or atrophy of the lobe rather than to attempt repair. If both ducts are injured, each should be intubated with a small catheter brought through the abdominal wall. Once the patient has recovered sufficiently, delayed repair is performed under elective conditions with a Roux-en-Y hepatojejunostomy.

REFERENCES

References

1. Richardson JD, Franklin GA, Lukan JK, et al. Evolution in the management of hepatic trauma: a 25-year perspective. *Ann Surg.* 2000;232:324–330.
2. Buckman RF Jr, Miraliakbari R, Badellino MM. Juxtahepatic venous injuries: a critical review of reported management strategies. J Trauma. 2000;48:978–984.
3. Stassen NA, Bhullar I, Cheng JD, et al. A non-operative management of blunt hepatic injury: an Eastern

Association for the Surgery of Trauma practice management guideline. *J Trauma Acute Care Surg.* 2012;73:5 Supplement 4:S289–300. Also available at http://www.east.org. doi:10.1097/TA.0b013e318270160d. Accessed January 2015.

4. Croce MA, Fabian TC, Menke PG, et al. Non-operative management of blunt hepatic trauma is the treatment of choice for haemodynamically stable patients. *Ann Surg.* 1995;221(6):744–753.

5. Pachter HL. Prometheus bound: evolution in the management of hepatic trauma — from myth to reality. *J Trauma.* 2012;72:321–329.

6. Badger SA, Barclay R, Campbell P, et al. Management of liver trauma. *W J Surg.* 2009;33:2522–2537.

7, Moore EE, Cogbill TH, Jurkovich GJ, et al. Organ injury scaling: spleen and liver (1994 revision). *J Trauma.* 1995;38:323–324.

8. Peitzman AB, Marsh JW. Advanced operative techniques in the management of complex liver injury. *J Trauma Acute Care Surg.* 2012;73:765–770.

9. Ochsner MG, Maniscalco-Theberge ME, Champion HR. Fibrin glue as a haemostatic agent in hepatic and splenic trauma. *J Trauma.* 1990;30:884–887.

10. Kozar RA, Feliciano DV, Moore EE, et al. Western Trauma Association/critical decision in trauma: operative management of blunt hepatic injury. *J Trauma.* 2011;71:1–5.

11. Poggetti RS, Moore EE, Moore FA, et al. Balloon tamponade for bilobar transfixing hepatic gunshot wounds. *J Trauma.* 1992;33:694-697.

12. Polanco P, Leon S, Pineda J, et al. Hepatic resection in the management of complex injury to the liver. *J Trauma.* 2008;651264–1270.

13. Sheldon GF, Lim RC, Yee ES, et al. Management of injuries to the porta hepatis. *Ann Surg.* 1985;202(5):539–545.

14. Bade PG, Thomson SR, Hirshberg A, et al. Surgical options in traumatic injury to the extrahepatic biliary tract. *Br J Surg.* 1989;76(3):256–258.

15. Feliciano DV, Bitondo CG, Burch JM, et al. Management of traumatic injuries to the extrahepatic biliary ducts. *Am J Surg.* 1985;150(6):705–709.

Recommended Reading

Ivatury RR, ed. *Operative Techniques for Severe Liver Injury.* New York, NY: Springer; 2015.

Moore EE. Critical decisions in the management of hepatic trauma. *Am J Surg.* 1984;148(6):712–716.

Piper GL, Peitzman AB. Current management of hepatic trauma. *Surg Clin North* Am. 2010;90:775–785.

Posner MC, Moore EE. Extrahepatic biliary tract injury: operative management plan. *J Trauma.* 1985;25:833–837.

8.4 Spleen

8.4.1 OVERVIEW

The conventional management of splenic injury used to be splenectomy. However, stimulated by the success of non-operative management (NOM) in children and the recognition of the importance of splenic function, there has been a shift in strategy. Today, the management of splenic injury should rely primarily on the haemodynamic status of the patient on presentation, although splenic injury grade, patient age, associated injuries and institutional specific resources must be taken into consideration.

8.4.2 ANATOMY

The splenic artery, a branch of the coeliac axis, provides the principal blood supply to the spleen. The artery gives rise to a superior polar artery, from which the short gastric arteries arise. The splenic artery also gives rise to superior and inferior terminal branches that enter the splenic hilum. The artery and the splenic vein are embedded in the superior border of the pancreas.

Three avascular splenic suspensory ligaments maintain the intimate association between the spleen and the diaphragm (splenophrenic ligament), left kidney (lienorenal/splenorenal ligament) and splenic flexure of the colon (splenocolic ligament). The gastrosplenic ligament contains the short gastric arteries.

These attachments place the spleen at risk of avulsion during rapid deceleration. The spleen is also relatively delicate and can be damaged by impact from the overlying ribs.

8.4.3 DIAGNOSIS

8.4.3.1 Clinical

The patient may complain of left upper quadrant pain or referred pain to the left shoulder, and there may be local tenderness. Signs of hypovolaemia (tachycardia or hypotension) might be present.

8.4.3.2 Computed Tomography (CT) Scan

In the haemodynamically stable patient with blunt abdominal trauma, computed tomography (CT) scanning is the preferred diagnostic modality to identify and grade splenic injury. Computed tomography will show the parenchymal lesions and any blood collection. Contrast blush on the CT scan will indicate whether there is still active bleeding. If so, angiography with embolization should be considered if available.

8.4.3.3 Ultrasound

Ultrasonic diagnosis has the great advantage that it can be performed in the emergency room during resuscitation.

Focussed abdominal sonography for trauma (FAST) ultrasound can detect free fluid around the spleen and in the paracolic gutter, indicating splenic injury. It will not show whether active arterial bleeding is taking place.

8.4.4 SPLENIC INJURY SCALE (TABLE 8.4.1)

The Organ Injury Scale[1] of the American Association for the Surgery of Trauma is based on the most accurate assessment of injury, whether it is by radiological study, laparotomy, laparoscopy or autopsy evaluation (Table 8.4.1).

8.4.5 MANAGEMENT

8.4.5.1 Non-operative Management

The approach of NOM[2] for blunt splenic injuries in the paediatric population is well described, with a splenic preservation rate of more than 90 per cent. Stimulated by the success of NOM in children, there has been a similar trend in haemodynamically stable adults with splenic injury. The advantages of NOM include the avoidance of non-therapeutic laparotomies with their associated cost and morbidity, a lower rate of intra-abdominal complications and reduced transfusion risk.

The risk of delayed re-bleeding of the spleen after NOM is acceptably low, reportedly in the range of 1 to 8 per cent. Rebleeding is considered more likely if a higher-grade injury (grade IV) has been managed non-operatively.

Table 8.4.1 Splenic Injury Scale (see also Appendix B: Trauma Scores and Scoring Systems)

Grade[a]	Injury Type	Description of Injury
I	Haematoma	Subcapsular <10% surface area
	Laceration	Capsular tear <1 cm parenchymal depth
II	Haematoma	Subcapsular 10%–50% surface area; intraparenchymal <5 cm in diameter
	Laceration	Capsular tear 1–3 cm parenchymal depth that does not involve a trabecular vessel
III	Haematoma	Subcapsular >50% surface area or expanding; ruptured subcapsular or parenchymal haematoma; intraparenchymal haematoma ≥5 cm or expanding
	Laceration	>3 cm parenchymal depth or involving trabecular vessels
IV	Laceration	Laceration involving segmental or hilar vessels producing major devascularization (>25% of spleen)
V	Laceration	Completely shattered spleen
	Vascular	Hilar vascular injury with devascularized spleen

[a]Advance one grade for multiple injuries up to grade III.

After resuscitation and completion of the trauma work-up, haemodynamically stable patients will undergo CT scan. Patients with grades I, II or III splenic injuries, who have no associated intra-abdominal injuries requiring surgical intervention, and no co-morbidities to preclude close observation, are obvious candidates for NOM[3-5]. Even haemodynamically stable patients with grades IV or V injury can be treated successfully with NOM, often with routine angiographic embolization as part of the treatment protocol. However, the failure rate of NOM for splenic injuries in adults increases with the grade of splenic injury. Patients with high-grade splenic injuries treated non-operatively should be monitored closely to detect any signs that indicate the need for intervention. Associated injuries must be excluded on admission[3]. However, there is less evidence to support the use of serial CT scans, without clinical indications, to monitor progress[4].

Table 8.4.2 Evidence-based Guidelines for Selective Non-operative Management of Splenic Injury[2]

Level of Evidence	Recommendation
I	Patients who have diffuse peritonitis or who are hemodynamically unstable after blunt abdominal trauma should be taken urgently for laparotomy.
II	1. A routine laparotomy is not indicated in the hemodynamically stable patient without peritonitis presenting with an isolated splenic injury.
	2. The severity of splenic injury (as suggested by CT grade or degree of haemoperitoneum), neurologic status, age >55 and/or the presence of associated injuries are not contraindications to a trial of non-operative management in a hemodynamically stable patient.
	3. In the hemodynamically normal blunt abdominal trauma patient without peritonitis, an abdominal CT scan with intravenous contrast should be performed to identify and assess the severity of injury to the spleen.
	4. Angiography should be considered for patients with American Association for the Surgery of Trauma (AAST) grade of greater than III injuries, presence of a contrast blush, moderate haemoperitoneum or evidence of ongoing splenic bleeding.
	5. Non-operative management of splenic injuries should only be considered in an environment that provides capabilities for monitoring, serial clinical evaluations and an operating room available for urgent laparotomy.
III	1. After blunt splenic injury, clinical factors such as a persistent systemic inflammatory response, increasing/persistent abdominal pain or an otherwise unexplained drop in haemoglobin should dictate the frequency of and need for follow-up imaging for a patient with blunt splenic injury.
	2. Contrast blush on CT scan alone is not an absolute indication for an operation or angiographic intervention. Factors such as patient age, grade of injury and presence of hypotension need to be considered in the clinical management of these patients.
	3. Angiography may be used either as an adjunct to non-operative management for patients who are thought to be at high risk for delayed bleeding or as an investigative tool to identify vascular abnormalities such as pseudoaneurysms that pose a risk for delayed haemorrhage.
	4. Pharmacologic prophylaxis to prevent venous thromboembolism can be used for patients with isolated blunt splenic injuries without increasing the failure rate of non-operative management, although the optimal timing of safe initiation has not been determined.
Unanswered questions	1. Frequency of haemoglobin measurements
	2. Frequency of abdominal examinations
	3. Intensity and duration of monitoring
	4. Is there a transfusion trigger after which operative or angiographic intervention should be considered?
	5. Time to reinitiate oral intake
	6. Duration and intensity of restricted activity (both in-hospital and after discharge)
	7. Optimum length of stay for both the intensive care unit (ICU) and hospital
	8. Necessity of repeated imaging
	9. Timing of initiating chemical deep venous thrombosis (DVT) prophylaxis after a splenic injury
	10. Should patients with severe injuries/or embolized injuries receive post-splenectomy vaccines?
	11. Is there an immunologic deficiency after splenic embolization?

Angiography with embolization, if available, is a useful adjunct to NOM[5,6]. The indications include evidence of ongoing bleeding with a significant drop in haemoglobin level and tachycardia or contrast extravasation outside or within the spleen on CT as well as formation of a pseudoaneurysm.

Patients with high-grade splenic injuries treated non-operatively should be monitored closely to detect any signs that indicate the need for intervention. There is, however, no evidence that bedrest or restricted activity is beneficial.

The advantages of NOM include the avoidance of non-therapeutic laparotomies (with associated cost and morbidity), fewer intra-abdominal complications and reduced transfusion risk. The risk of delayed re-bleeding of the spleen after non-operative management is acceptably low, reportedly in the range of 1 to 8 per cent. Re-bleed is considered more likely if a higher-grade injury (grade IV) has been managed non-operatively. However, prophylactic arterial embolization of the splenic artery in adults with grades IV and V injuries has been reported to result in a NOM success rate of 96 per cent[3].

8.4.5.2 Operative Management

If a patient with splenic injury is haemodynamically unstable, operative treatment is necessary. Although splenic preservation is desirable, most patients who require an operation due to splenic bleeding will have a splenectomy performed.

Non-operative management is contraindicated and urgent open surgical intervention is indicated[7] when there is:

- Haemodynamic instability.
- Risk of concurrent abdominal hollow organ injury, or associated intra-abdominal injury requiring surgery.
- Evidence of continued splenic haemorrhage.
- Replacement of greater than 50 per cent of the patient's blood volume.
- Age over 55 years.

8.4.6 SURGICAL APPROACH

Access to the spleen in trauma is best performed via a long midline incision. When indicated, the spleen is mobilized under direct vision. In paediatric patients, a midline incision should also be used, rather than a subcostal incision, since there is better access to the entire abdominal cavity if there is injury to other intra-abdominal structures.

The spleen is best approached by a surgeon standing on the patient's right-hand side. The spleen is mobilized under direct vision. Great care and gentle handling are necessary to avoid pulling on the spleen, avulsing the capsule, and making a minor injury worse and stripping the capsule off the lower pole.

Medial traction by the operator's non-dominant hand will give access to the lienophrenic, lienorenal and lienocolic ligaments.

- The spleen is gently pulled upwards and medially, and the lienorenal and lienocolic ligaments are divided.
- The spleen is then gently pulled downward, and the lienophrenic ligaments are divided with scissors, close to the spleen, between the spleen and the diaphragm.
- The short gastric vessels between the greater curvature of the stomach and the spleen must be divided between ligatures. These vessels must be divided away from the greater curvature, as there is a danger of avascular necrosis of the stomach if they are divided too close to the stomach itself.
- The spleen is pulled forward, and several packs can be placed in the splenic bed to hold it forward so that it can be inspected.

In the presence of other competing major injuries, haemodynamic instability or if the spleen has sustained damage at the hilum, a routine splenectomy should be performed. In the stable patient and in the absence of other life-threatening injuries, splenic preservation should be considered.

8.4.6.1 SPLEEN NOT ACTIVELY BLEEDING

If not actively bleeding, the spleen can be left alone.

8.4.6.2 SPLENIC SURFACE BLEED ONLY

These bleeds will usually stop with a combination of manual compression, packing, diathermy, argon beam or fibrin adhesives in combination with collagen fleece.

8.4.6.3 MINOR LACERATIONS

These may be sutured using absorbable sutures, with or without Teflon pledgets. Suturing is time-consuming and mostly not helpful in trauma patients. The superficial lacerations are best treated with fibrin adhesive and collagen tamponade. These measures are best taken at the beginning of the operation and the spleen packed; upon completion of the operation, the pack can be removed without displacing the collagen fleece.

8.4.6.4 SPLENIC TEARS

If the lacerations are deep and involve both the concave and convex surfaces, the spleen is best and most effectively preserved with a mesh splenorrhaphy. If the lacerations involve only one pole or one half of the organ, the respective vessels should be ligated and a partial splenectomy performed.

8.4.6.5 MESH WRAP

If the spleen is viable, it can be wrapped in an absorbable mesh to tamponade the bleeding.

The prerequisite for mesh splenorrhaphy is complete mobilization and elevation of the spleen. An absorbable mesh should be chosen (e.g. Vicryl). There are meshes that already include two or three purse-string sutures and can be used according to the size of the spleen. If one wants to make one's own purse-string pouch, it is advantageous to make an impression of the spleen and then to stitch in a circle exactly on the edges, using absorbable suture material. It is extremely important that the pouch should be slightly smaller than the spleen, so that the suture lies on the acute and obtuse margin when it has been pulled taut. The mesh is pulled laterally over the spleen like a headscarf; the suture is tied on the hilar side but without compressing the hilum. Mild bleeding through the holes in the mesh can be stopped with collagen tampons together with fibrin glue or, if possible, autologous fibrin.

8.4.6.6 PARTIAL SPLENECTOMY

This is rarely used in the trauma patient. Injuries involving only one pole of the spleen can be treated with partial resection. Prior to resection, the spleen should be mobilized. Stapler resection makes organ conservation possible in many cases, and it represents a valuable alternative to sutured partial splenectomy or splenorrhaphy. Its greatest advantages are simplicity of use, the practicality of the instrument itself and the reduction in time and blood transfusion.

8.4.6.7 SPLENECTOMY

In the presence of other major injuries, with haemodynamic instability or if the spleen has sustained damage at the hilum, a routine splenectomy should be carried out. Following careful mobilization of the spleen, the splenic vessels (artery and vein) should be isolated and tied separately, as there is a small risk of subsequent arteriovenous fistula formation.

Access to the splenic pedicle can be anterior or posterior. In the anterior approach, the short gastric vessels must be ligated away from the stomach to avoid the risk of avascular necrosis of the wall of greater curvature of the stomach. The posterior approach, more expedient, entails manual mobilization and rotation of the spleen medially, after opening the peritoneum lateral to the convex surface of the spleen. Care must be taken to avoid injuring the tail of the pancreas, which lies very close to the hilum of the spleen.

8.4.6.8 DRAINAGE

The splenic bed is *not* routinely drained after splenectomy. If the tail of the pancreas has been damaged, a closed suction drain should be placed in the area affected.

8.4.7 COMPLICATIONS

- Delayed splenic rupture[8] (This is probably not 'delayed' but 'contained'.)
- Left upper quadrant haematoma.
- Pancreatitis.
- Pleural effusion.
- Pulmonary atelectasis.
- Pseudoaneurysm of the splenic artery.
- Splenic arteriovenous fistula.
- Subphrenic abscess.
- Overwhelming post-splenectomy sepsis.
- Pancreatic injury/fistula/ascites.

8.4.8 OUTCOME

A large number of publications support NOM in the haemodynamically stable patient.

- Non-operative management is becoming more routine, with a high success rate in haemodynamically stable patients.

- The risk of delayed re-bleeding of the spleen after NOM is acceptably low, reportedly in the range of 1 to 8 per cent.
- Pleural effusion, pulmonary atelectasis and pneumonia are not uncommon in patients treated either non-operatively or operatively.
- Pseudoaneurysm development can be successfully treated with embolization.
- Subphrenic abscess can be seen in patients treated operatively but may be treated by percutaneous drainage.
- After splenectomy, there is a small but lifelong risk of overwhelming post-splenectomy sepsis. Patients should be informed of the defect in their immune system and be encouraged to keep their pneumococcus and influenza immunizations current. These patients are more susceptible to malaria than the rest of the population.

REFERENCES AND RECOMMENDED READING

References

1. Moore EE, Cogbill TH, Jurkovich GJ, Shackford SR, Malangoni MA, Champion HR. Organ injury scaling: spleen and liver (1994 Revision). *J Trauma.* 1995;38:323–324.
2. Stassen NA, Bhullar I, Cheng JD, et al. Practice Management Guidelines for the selective nonoperative management of blunt splenic injury. *J Trauma.* 2012;73(5):S294–S300. http://www.east.org. Accessed January 2015.
3. Skattum J, Naess PA, Eken T, Gaarder C. Refining the role of splenic angiographic embolization in high-grade splenic injuries. *J Trauma Acute Care Surg.* 2013;74(1):100–103; discussion 103–104.
4. Haan JM, Biffl W, Knudson MM, et al. Splenic embolization revisited: a multicenter review. *J Trauma.* 2004;56:542–547.
5. Raikhlin A, Baerlocher MO, Asch O, Myers A. Imaging and transcatheter arterial embolization for traumatic splenic injuries: review of the literature. *Can J Surg.* 2008;51:464–472.
6. Haan JM. Follow-up abdominal CT is not necessary in low-grade splenic injury. *Am Surg.* 2007;73:13–18.
7. Peizman AB, Harbrecht BG, Rivera L, Heil B. Failure of observation of blunt splenic injury in adults: variability in practice and adverse consequences. *J Am Coll Surg.* 2005;201:179–187.
8. Gamblin TC, Wall CE, Royer GM, Dalton ML, Asley DW. Delayed splenic rupture: case report and review of the literature. *J Trauma.* 2005;59:1231–1234.

Recommended Reading

Peizman AB, Heil B, Rivera L, et al. Blunt splenic injury in adults: multi-institutional study of the Eastern Association for the Surgery of Trauma. *J Trauma.* 2000;49:177–187.

Savage SA, Zarzaur BL, Magnotti LJ, et al. The evolution of blunt splenic injury: resolution and progression. *J Trauma.* 2008;64:1085–1092.

Smith J, Armen S, Cook CH, Martin LC. Blunt splenic injuries: have we watched long enough? *J Trauma.* 2008;64:656–665.

8.5 Pancreas

8.5.1 OVERVIEW

Pancreatic and combined pancreaticoduodenal injuries remain a dilemma for most surgeons and, despite advances and complex technical solutions, they still carry a high morbidity and mortality. The increase particularly in penetrating injuries, and the increase in wounding energy from gunshots, has made the incidence of pancreatic injury more common. Pancreatic injury must be suspected in all patients with abdominal injuries, even those who initially have few signs. Since the pancreas is retroperitoneal, it usually does not present with peritonitis. It requires a high level of suspicion and significant clinical acumen, as well as aggressive radiographic imaging to identify an injury early.

The pancreas and duodenum are difficult areas for surgical exposure and represent a major challenge for the operating surgeon when these organs are substantially injured. Although the retroperitoneal location of the pancreas means that it is commonly injured, its position also contributes to the difficulty in diagnosis as the organ is concealed, resulting in delay in diagnosis, with an attendant increase in morbidity.

Management varies from simple drainage to highly challenging procedures depending on the severity, the site of the injury and the integrity of the duct. Accurate intraoperative investigation of the pancreatic duct is particularly challenging. To compound this, pancreatic trauma is associated with a high incidence of injury to adjoining organs (duodenum, kidney, liver) and major vascular structures, which adds to the high morbidity and mortality[1]. A review of the English-language literature on pancreatic trauma from 1970 to 2006 states, among other things, that limited injuries affecting the head of the pancreas are best managed by simple external drainage, even if there is suspected pancreatic duct injury[2].

> *The surgeon must always be critically aware of the patient's changing physiological state, and be prepared to forsake the technical challenge of definitive repair for life-saving damage control.*

8.5.2 ANATOMY

The pancreas lies at the level of the pylorus and crosses the first and second lumbar vertebrae. It is about 15cm long from the duodenum to the hilum of the spleen, 3cm wide and up to 1.5cm thick. The head lies within the concavity formed by the duodenum, with which it shares its blood supply through the pancreaticoduodenal arcades.

The pancreas has an intimate anatomical relationship with the upper abdominal vessels. It overlies the inferior vena cava, the right renal vessels and the left renal vein. The uncinate process encircles the superior mesenteric artery and vein, while the body covers the suprarenal aorta and left renal vessels. The tail is closely related to the splenic hilum and left kidney, and overlies the splenic artery and vein, with the artery marking a tortuous path at the superior border of the pancreas.

There are a number of named arterial branches to the head, body and tail that must be ligated in spleen-sparing procedures. Studies have shown that between 7 and 10 branches of the splenic artery, and 13 and 22 branches of the splenic vein, run into the pancreas.

8.5.3 MECHANISMS OF INJURY

8.5.3.1 Blunt Trauma

The relatively protected location of the pancreas means that a high-energy force is required to damage it. Most injuries result from motor vehicle accidents in which the energy of the impact is directed to the upper abdomen – epigastrium or hypochondrium – commonly through the steering wheel of an automobile. This force results in crushing of the retroperitoneal structures against the vertebral column, which can lead to a spectrum of injury from contusion to complete transection of the body of the pancreas.

8.5.3.2 Penetrating Trauma

The rising incidence of penetrating trauma has increased the incidence of injury to the pancreas. A stab wound damages tissue only along the track of the knife, but in gunshot wounds the passage of the missile and its pressure wave will result in injury to a wider region. Consequently, the pancreas and its duct must be fully assessed for damage in any penetrating wound that approaches the substance of the gland. Injuries to the pancreatic duct occur in 15 per cent of cases of pancreatic trauma and are usually a consequence of penetrating trauma[3].

8.5.4 DIAGNOSIS

The central retroperitoneal location of the pancreas makes the investigation of pancreatic trauma a diagnostic challenge: the specific diagnosis is often unsuspected, or not clear until laparotomy, especially if there are other life-threatening vascular and other intra-abdominal organ injuries. In recent years, there has been debate about the need to accurately assess the integrity of the main pancreatic duct. Bradley et al.[4] showed that mortality and morbidity were increased when there was failure or delay in recognizing ductal injury. When these results are reviewed in conjunction with earlier work[5] that showed an increase in late complications if ductal injuries were missed, the importance of evaluating the duct is evident.

8.5.4.1 Clinical Evaluation

In a patient with an isolated pancreatic injury, even ductal transection may be initially asymptomatic or have only minor signs; the possibility must be kept in mind. Clinical examination is notoriously *unreliable*.

8.5.4.2 Serum Amylase and Serum Lipase

The level of the serum amylase and serum lipase is not related to pancreatic injury in either blunt or penetrating trauma. A summary of recent work on serum amylase in blunt abdominal trauma by Biffl[6] showed a positive predictive value of 10 per cent and a negative predictive value of 95 per cent for pancreatic injury, although more recent work has suggested that accuracy may be improved when the activity is measured more than 3 hours after injury[7]. At present, serum amylase has little value in the initial evaluation of pancreatic injury. There is increasing interest in the value of lipase in trauma but to date there are insufficient data to support this.

8.5.4.3 Ultrasound

The posterior position of the pancreas almost completely masks it from diagnostic ultrasound. In conjunction with its location, a post-traumatic ileus with loops of gas-filled bowel will mask it even further, and assessment of the pancreas is particularly difficult in obese patients.

8.5.4.4 Diagnostic Peritoneal Lavage (DPL)

Diagnostic peritoneal lavage (DPL) has been largely superseded and is infrequently performed. The retroperitoneal location of the pancreas renders diagnostic peritoneal lavage inaccurate in the prediction of isolated pancreatic injury. However, the numerous associated injuries that may occur with pancreatic injury may make the lavage diagnostic if the level of the amylase in the lavage fluid is checked.

8.5.4.5 Computed Tomography

Computed tomography (CT) scan has been advocated as the best investigation for evaluation of the retroperitoneum. In a haemodynamically stable patient, CT scanning with contrast enhancement has a sensitivity and specificity as high as 80 per cent[8]. However, particularly in the initial phase, CT scanning may miss

or underestimate the severity of a pancreatic injury[9], so normal findings on the initial scan do not exclude appreciable pancreatic injury, and a repeat scan in the light of continuing symptoms may improve its diagnostic ability.

8.5.4.6 Endoscopic Retrograde Cholangiopancreatography (ERCP)

There are two phases in the investigation of pancreatic injury in which endoscopic retrograde cholangiopancreatography (ERCP) may have a role[10].

8.5.4.6.1 ACUTE PRESENTATION

Patients with isolated pancreatic trauma occasionally have benign clinical findings initially. It must be stressed that these patients are a small number. In the investigation of pancreatic duct injury in the acute phase, ERCP has little practical role, as most patients will not be stable enough and their injuries will not allow positioning for ERCP. In those patients who do not settle with conservative management and there is suspicion of ductal injury, ERCP will give detailed information about the ductal system although cannulation of the pancreatic duct can itself cause pancreatitis.

8.5.4.6.2 DELAYED PRESENTATION

A small number of patients present with symptoms months to years after the initial injury potentially with a retroperitoneal collection or pancreatic fistula. Magnetic resonance cholangiopancreatography (MRCP) is likely to be the initial investigation; however, ERCP can be used to assess the integrity of the duct and consider pancreatic duct stenting.

8.5.4.7 Magnetic Resonance Cholangiopancreatography (MRCP)

In the non-acute setting, MRCP is the mainstay of evaluation of the pancreaticobiliary tree. There is no role in the initial evaluation of the injured patient but there is value in the assessment for ductal injury in those patients who have developed a complication such as a pseudocyst or pancreatic fistula[11]. The MRCP can allow better selection of patients with suspected injuries than can ERCP, because patients with an intact pancreatic duct or minor injury can be successfully treated conservatively. Some authors believe that it will have an increasing role in identifying patients who are unlikely to benefit from endoscopic intervention, those with an intact pancreatic duct or very minor injury, and those with severe duct strictures or obstruction. However, to date there has been little work done in acute pancreatic injuries.

8.5.4.8 Intraoperative Pancreatography

Intra-operative visualization of the pancreatic duct has been advocated in the investigation of the duct, particularly when it is not possible to assess its integrity by examination. Nevertheless, in the opinion of Subramanian et al., simple examination of the area of injury for several minutes with loupe magnification reveals clear pancreatic fluid leakage in most injuries that involve the pancreatic duct[12]. An accurate assessment of the degree of injury to the duct will reduce the complication rate[13], indicate the most appropriate operation and, when no involvement is found, allow a less aggressive procedure to be undertaken. However, the ductal system frequently cannot be found due to its small size in previously normal patients. Therefore, the invasive nature of intraoperative investigation by transduodenal pancreatic duct catheterization, distal cannulation of the duct in the tail or needle cholecystocholangiogram makes this unattractive and rarely indicated.

Intraoperative ultrasound can be used to help diagnose a parenchymal or ductal laceration[14].

8.5.4.9 Operative Evaluation

Operative evaluation of the pancreas necessitates complete exposure of the gland. A central retroperitoneal haematoma must be thoroughly investigated, and intra-abdominal bile staining makes a complete evaluation essential to find the pancreatic or duodenal injury. In this case, a ductal injury must be assumed until excluded.

If the sphincter of Oddi and the distal biliary tract are intact, it is wise to attempt to preserve the head and neck of the pancreas. A person can survive quite well with 10 per cent of the pancreas without pancreatic insufficiency or diabetes. Major injuries to the body of the pancreas are usually treated by a distal pancreatectomy with splenectomy. If the injury is to the head of the pancreas, involving the duct and sphincter, a Whipple procedure must be contemplated. Increasingly, there is a move toward lesser procedures since the mortality of a Whipple procedure continues to be significant in the severely injured trauma patient. These injuries continue to be a major challenge for the trauma surgeon. It is essential to understand the manoeuvres necessary for gaining complete control of the duodenum and pancreas in order to completely explore and identify any injuries.

8.5.5 PANCREAS INJURY SCALE

The organ injury scale developed by the American Association for the Surgery of Trauma (AAST)[15] has been accepted by most institutions that regularly deal with pancreatic trauma (Table 8.5.1).

Table 8.5.1 Pancreas Injury Scale (see Appendix B: Trauma Scores and Scoring Systems)

Grade[a]	Type of Injury	Description of Injury
I	Haematoma	Minor contusion without duct injury
	Laceration	Superficial laceration without duct injury
II	Haematoma	Major contusion without duct injury or tissue loss
	Laceration	Major laceration without duct injury or tissue loss
III	Laceration	Distal transection or parenchymal injury with duct injury
IV	Laceration	Proximal[b] transection or parenchymal injury involving the ampulla
V	Laceration	Massive disruption of the pancreatic head

[a]Advance one grade for multiple injuries up to grade III.

[b]The proximal pancreas is deemed to be that part of the pancreas to the *right* of the superior mesenteric artery and vein.

8.5.6 **MANAGEMENT**

8.5.6.1 **Non-operative Management**

In isolated blunt pancreatic injuries, exclusion of a major pancreatic duct injury with ERCP followed by expectant non-operative management is gaining popularity. Recent reports utilizing early ERCP to identify and sometimes treat blunt pancreatic injuries by transpapillary stent insertion are showing promising results[16,17] and can decrease the failure rate of non-operative management and incidence of pancreatic-related complications. A pancreatic duct stent appears useful for a proximal pancreatic fistula but may be complicated by a long-term stricture, whereas ductal stenting in the acute phase is potentially dangerous in that it may lead to a delay in necessary laparotomy and definitive repair of the pancreatic injury[18]. Because of the small size of the pancreatic duct distal to the ampulla, stenting is ordinarily not used in this location[19]. Recent evidence suggests that endoscopic interventions are more successful in managing pancreatic fistulae and pseudocysts than in managing patients with main pancreatic duct stricture.[12,19]

Non-operative management (NOM) of low-grade (grades I and II) blunt pancreatoduodenal injuries is safe despite occasional failures. Missed diagnosis continues to occur despite advances in CT scanning but does not seem to cause an adverse outcome in most patients[20].

8.5.6.2 **Operative Management**

Many pancreatic injuries will only be confirmed following a CT scan or actually at the time of surgery. The surgical approach is often for that of the presenting sign (e.g. peritonitis), and the pancreatic injury will be found at laparotomy. There are commonly associated injuries of the duodenum, bowel mesentery, etc.

8.5.7 **SURGICAL APPROACH**

8.5.7.1 **Incision and Exploration**

Access to the pancreas in trauma is gained via a long midline incision.

Penetrating pancreatic trauma should be obvious since the patient will almost invariably have been explored for an obvious injury. Once the retroperitoneum has been violated in penetrating trauma, it is imperative for the surgeon to do a thorough exploration of the central region.

Diagnosis of blunt pancreatic trauma is much more problematic. As the pancreas is a retroperitoneal organ, there may be no anterior peritoneal signs. The history can be helpful if information from the paramedics indicates that the vehicle's steering column was bent or if the patient can give a history of epigastric trauma. The physical examination, as stated above, is often misleading. However, a 'doughy' abdomen should make the clinician suspicious. Amylase level and full blood count are non-specific. Diagnostic peritoneal lavage and focused abdominal sonography for trauma (FAST) are unhelpful. Gastrografin swallow has fair sensitivity; CT scanning is at least 85 per cent accurate and remains the non-operative diagnostic modality of choice for blunt pancreatic injury. Endoscopic retrograde cholangiopancreatography can be helpful in selected patients.

For complete evaluation of the gland, it is essential to see the pancreas from both the anterior and posterior aspects. To examine the anterior surface of the gland, it is necessary to divide the gastrocolic ligament and open the lesser sac. An extended Kocher manoeuvre is required so that the duodenum can be mobilized and an adequate view gained of the pancreatic head, uncinate process and posterior aspect. Injury to the tail requires mobilization of the spleen and left colon to allow medial reflection of the pancreas and access to the splenic vessels. Division of the ligament of Treitz and reflection of the fourth part of the duodenum and duodenojejunal flexure give access to the inferior aspect of the pancreas. Any parenchymal haematoma of the pancreas should be thoroughly explored, including irrigation of the haematoma, to exclude possible injury of the duct.

8.5.7.1.1 ACCESS VIA THE LESSER SAC

The stomach is then grasped and pulled inferiorly, allowing the operator to identify the lesser curvature and the pancreas through the lesser sac. Frequently, the coeliac artery and the body of the pancreas can be identified through this approach. The omentum is then grasped and drawn upwards. An otomy is made in the omentum, and the operator's hand is passed into the lesser sac posterior to the stomach. This allows excellent exposure of the entire body and tail of the pancreas. Any injuries to the pancreas can be easily identified.

8.5.7.1.2 DUODENAL ROTATION (KOCHER MANOEUVRE)

If there is the possibility of an injury to the head of the pancreas, a Kocher manoeuvre is performed. The loose areolar of tissue around the duodenum is bluntly dissected, and the entire second and third portions of the duodenum are identified and mobilized medially. This dissection is carried all the way medially to expose the inferior vena cava and a portion of the aorta. By reflecting the duodenum and pancreas toward the anterior midline, the posterior surface of the head of the pancreas can be completely inspected.

8.5.7.1.3 RIGHT MEDIAL VISCERAL ROTATION

The inferior border of the proximal portion of the pancreas can be identified by performing a right medial visceral rotation. This is performed by taking down the ascending colon and then mobilizing the caecum, the terminal ileum and the mesentery toward the midline. The entire ascending colon and caecum are then reflected superiorly toward the left upper quadrant of the abdomen. This gives excellent exposure of the entire vena cava, the aorta and the third and fourth portions of the duodenum.

8.5.7.1.4 LEFT MEDIAL VISCERAL ROTATION

The descending colon on the left is mobilized, together with the spleen and the tail of the pancreas. These are rotated medially, allowing inspection of the tail and posterior and inferior aspects of the pancreas.

These manoeuvres allow for complete exposure of the first, second, third and fourth portions of the duodenum along with the head, neck, body and tail of the pancreas.

When pancreatic injury is suspected, extended exploration of the whole organ is imperative. Parenchymal lacerations that do not involve the pancreatic duct can be sutured when the tissue is not too soft and vulnerable. With or without the use of sutures, a worthwhile option in the treatment of such lacerations is fibrin sealing and collagen tamponade, and adequate drainage is essential.

8.5.7.2 Pancreatic Injury: Surgical Decision Making

When ductal injury to the body and/or the tail of the pancreas is suspected, the best and safest treatment is re-section. In the case of severe injuries, therapeutic options range from drainage alone to Whipple procedure. The latter is a rarely used option with a high incidence of morbidity and mortality. A good, effective and safe option is pyloric exclusion with drainage of the injured area.

Injuries to the tail and body of the pancreas that do not involve the duct can be drained. If there is obvious disruption to the pancreatic duct, it should be ligated with distal pancreatic resection with splenectomy in the unstable trauma patient. The results of all these treatment options can be improved by using fibrin adhesives and collagen fleece.

The injuries that vex the surgeon most, however, are those to the head of the gland, particularly those juxtaposed with or also involving the duodenum. Resection (Whipple procedure) is usually reserved for those patients who have destructive injuries or those in whom the blood supply to the duodenum and pancreatic head has been compromised. The remainder are usually treated with variations of drainage and pyloric exclusion. This includes extensive closed (suction) drainage around the injury site. Common duct drainage is not indicated.

8.5.7.2.1 DAMAGE CONTROL

Patients with severe pancreatic or pancreaticoduodenal injury (AAST grades IV and V) are not stable enough to undergo complex reconstruction at the time of initial laparotomy. Damage control with the rapid arrest of haemorrhage and bacterial contamination, and placement of drains and packing, is preferable. It may be helpful to place a tube drain directly into the duct, both for drainage and to allow easier isolation of the duct at the subsequent operation. The damage control laparotomy is followed by a period of intensive care and continued aggressive resuscitation to correct physiological abnormalities and restore reserve before the definitive procedure.

8.5.7.2.2 CONTUSION AND PARENCHYMAL INJURIES

Relatively minor pancreatic lacerations and contusions (AAST grades I and II) comprise most injuries to the pancreas. Nowak et al.[21] showed that these require simple drainage and haemostasis, and this has become standard practice. There is, however, debate about whether the ideal drainage system is a closed suction system or an open pencil drain. Suction drainage should be used, so that fewer intra-abdominal abscesses develop and that there is less skin excoriation with a closed suction system.[22]

Suturing of parenchymal lesions (AAST grades I and II) in an attempt to gain haemostasis simply leads to necrosis of the pancreatic tissue. Bleeding vessels should be ligated individually and a viable omental plug sutured into the defect to act as a haemostatic agent. Fibrin tissue sealants may have a use.

8.5.7.2.3 DUCTAL INJURIES: TAIL AND DISTAL PANCREAS

In most cases in which there is a major parenchymal injury of the pancreas to the left of the superior mesenteric vessels (AAST grades II or III), a distal pancreatectomy is the procedure of choice, independent of the degree of ductal involvement. Where there is concern over the involvement of the duct, an intraoperative pancreatogram can be done. After mobilization of the pancreas and ligation of the vessels, the pancreatic stump can be closed with sutures and the duct ligated separately, or it can be closed with a stapling device[23]. An external suction drain should be placed at the site of transection as there is a post-operative fistula rate of 14 per cent[24]. Suction drains are preferable.

Procedures associated with resection of greater than 80 per cent of the pancreatic tissue are associated with a risk of adult-onset diabetes mellitus. Most authors agree that a pancreatectomy to the left of the superior mesenteric vessels usually leaves enough pancreatic tissue to result in an acceptably low rate of insulin-dependent diabetes.

8.5.7.2.4 INTERNAL DRAINAGE OF THE DISTAL PANCREAS

Drainage of the distal pancreas with a Roux-en-Y pancreaticojejunostomy has been suggested in cases in which there is not enough proximal tissue for endocrine or exocrine function. Its popularity has greatly declined because of the high reported morbidity and mortality[25].

8.5.7.2.5 SPLENIC SALVAGE IN DISTAL PANCREATECTOMY

Splenic salvage has been advocated where possible, in *elective* distal pancreatectomy, and is possible occasionally in pancreatic trauma. However, this should be saved for the rare occasions when the patient is haemodynamically

stable and normothermic, and the injury is limited to the pancreas. The technical problems of dissecting the pancreas free from the splenic vessels and ligating the numerous tributaries make the procedure contraindicated in an unstable patient with multiple associated injuries[26]. When this operation is considered, the surgeon must clearly balance the extra time that it takes and the problems associated with lengthy operations in injured patients against the small risk of the development of overwhelming post-splenectomy infection (OPSI) post-operatively.

8.5.7.2.6 DRAINAGE ALONE

In most trauma units, simple drainage is reserved for minor injuries in which the pancreatic duct is not involved and injuries to both organs are slight[22].

8.5.7.2.7 DUCTAL INJURIES: COMBINED INJURIES OF THE HEAD OF THE PANCREAS AND DUODENUM

Severe combined pancreaticoduodenal injuries account for less than 10 per cent of injuries to these organs, and are commonly associated with multiple intra-abdominal injuries, particularly of the vena cava[27]. They are usually the result of penetrating trauma. The integrity of the distal common bile duct and ampulla on cholangiography, and the severity of the duodenal injury, will dictate the operative procedure. If the duct and ampulla are intact, simple repair and drainage or repair and pyloric exclusion will suffice.

8.5.7.2.8 DUODENAL DIVERSION

See Section 8.6.6 for a detailed discussion of the surgical approach to duodenal injuries.

8.5.7.2.9 PYLORIC EXCLUSION

Pyloric exclusion (Figure 8.5.1) has been widely reported for the management of severe combined pancreaticoduodenal injuries without major damage to the ampulla or the common bile duct[28,29]. The technique involves the temporary diversion of enteric flow away from the injured duodenum by closure of the pylorus. This is best achieved with access from the stomach through a gastrotomy and the use of a slowly absorbable suture. The

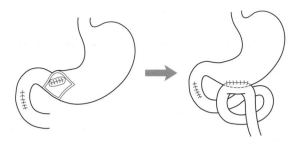

Figure 8.5.1 Pyloric exclusion and gastric bypass.

alternative is a TA stapler across the pylorus. (Note that the GIA type of staple cannot be used due to its integral guillotine.) Contrast studies have shown that the pylorus reopens within 2–3 weeks in 90–95 per cent of patients, allowing flow through the anatomical channel. The stomach is decompressed with a gastrojejunostomy.

There has been recent debate as to the need for a gastroenterostomy[30], since even with pyloric exclusion, a nasogastric tube will be effective. Once the pylorus is open, the gastrojejunostomy will probably close spontaneously. Pyloric exclusion has been adopted in many institutions for the treatment of grades III and IV combined pancreaticoduodenal injuries.

8.5.7.2.10 T-TUBE DRAINAGE

Some surgeons advocate closing the injury over a T-tube in combined injuries where the second part of the duodenum is involved. This ensures adequate drainage and allows the formation of a controlled fistula once the track has matured. Our preference in these injuries, however, is primary closure, pyloric exclusion and gastroenterostomy. Discussion continues and data are awaited.

8.5.7.2.11 INTERNAL AND EXTERNAL DRAINAGE

Although there is little controversy on the importance of external, periduodenal drainage of complex duodenal or pancreaticoduodenal injuries, the role of internal decompression via a nasogastroduodenal or retrograde jejunoduodenal tube, or tube duodenostomy, is more controversial. Delay in repairing a duodenal injury often results in duodenal leaks, emphasizing the importance of adequate external drainage that allows the formation of a controlled fistula once the track has matured. The preferred method of managing complex duodenal

injuries, however, is primary closure, pyloric exclusion and gastroenterostomy.

8.5.7.2.12 PANCREATICODUODENECTOMY (WHIPPLE PROCEDURE)

This is a major procedure to be practised in trauma only if no alternative is available[31]. In only 10 per cent of combined injuries will a pancreaticoduodenectomy, or Whipple procedure, be required. Damage control with control of bleeding and of bowel contamination, and ligation of the common bile and pancreatic ducts, should be the rule[32]. Indications for considering a pancreaticoduodenectomy are massive disruption of the pancreaticoduodenal complex, devascularization of the duodenum and sometimes extensive duodenal injuries of the second part of the duodenum involving the ampulla or distal common bile duct.

The Whipple procedure, as first described for carcinoma of the ampulla[33], is indicated only in the rare stable patient with this type of injury. The nature and severity of the injury and the coexisting damage to vessels are often accompanied by haemodynamic instability, and the surgeon must therefore control the initial damage and delay formal reconstruction until the patient has been stabilized. The results of this operation vary, and when patients with major retroperitoneal vascular injuries are included, mortality can approach 50 per cent. More recently in the largest series to date, with patients who underwent a damage control surgery (DCS) or staged Whipple procedure for complex pancreaticoduodenal trauma and the largest series with blunt trauma, in-hospital mortality was 13 per cent[34].

The role of pancreaticoduodenectomy in trauma is best summarized by Walt[35]:

> *Finally, to Whipple or not to Whipple, that is the question. In the massively destructive lesions involving the pancreas, duodenum and common bile duct, the decision to do a pancreaticoduodenectomy is unavoidable; and, in fact, much of the dissection may have been done by the wounding force. In a few patients, when the call is of necessity close, the overall physiologic status of the patient and the extent of damage become the determining factors in the decision. Though few in gross numbers, more patients are eventually salvaged by drainage, TPN [total parenteral nutrition] and meticulous overall care than by a desperate pancreaticoduodenectomy in a marginal patient.*

8.5.8 **ADJUNCTS**

8.5.8.1 **Somatostatin and Its Analogues**

Somatostatin and its analogue octreotide have been used to reduce pancreatic exocrine secretion in patients with acute pancreatitis. Despite meta-analysis, its role has not been clearly defined. Buchler et al.[36] reported a slight but not significant reduction in the complication rate in patients with moderate-to-severe pancreatitis, but this was not verified by Imrie's group in Glasgow[37], who found that somatostatin gave no benefit.

After pancreatic surgery, somatostatin can reduce the output from a pancreatic fistula[38]. Retrospective work on the role of octreotide in pancreatic trauma, however, differs. Somatostatin cannot be recommended in trauma on the current evidence, and a level I study is required.

8.5.8.2 **Nutritional Support**

Whether nutritional support is required should be considered at the definitive operation. Major injuries that precipitate prolonged gastric ileus and pancreatic complications may preclude gastric feeding. A feeding jejunostomy is ideal. Sometimes a long nasojejunal feeding catheter can be negotiated past the duodenojejunal flexure, providing a non-invasive alternative The creation of a percutaneous feeding jejunostomy via the abdominal wall, with the tip sited 15–30 cm distal to the duodenojejunal flexure, will allow early enteral feeding. We prefer elemental diets that are less stimulating to the pancreas and have no greater fistula output than total parenteral nutrition[39]. Total parenteral nutrition is far more expensive but may be used if enteral access distal to the duodenojejunal flexure is impossible.

8.5.9 **PANCREATIC INJURY IN CHILDREN**

The pancreas is injured in up to 10 per cent of cases of blunt abdominal trauma in children, usually as a result of a handlebar injury. Whether these children should be operated upon or managed conservatively (the current vogue for the management of solid organ injuries in children) is controversial. Shilyansky et al.[40] reported that non-operative management of pancreatic injuries in children was safe for both contusion and pancreatic transection, and a recent retrospective review of 31 cases

initially treated conservatively found that only 10 per cent needed secondary surgery.[41]

8.5.10 **COMPLICATIONS**

Pancreatic trauma is associated with up to 19 per cent mortality. Early deaths result from the associated intra-abdominal vascular and other organ injuries, and later deaths from sepsis and the systemic inflammatory response syndrome. Pancreatic injuries have post-operative complication rates of up to 42 per cent, and the number rises with increasing severity of injury; with combined injuries and associated injuries, the complication rate approaches 62 per cent[42,43].

Most complications are treatable or self-limiting, however, and could be avoided by an accurate assessment of whether the pancreatic duct was damaged. Pancreatic complications can be divided into those occurring early and those occurring late in the post-operative period.

8.5.10.1 **Early Complications**

8.5.10.1.1 PANCREATITIS

Post-operative pancreatitis may develop in about 7 per cent of patients. It may vary from a transient biochemical leak of amylase to a fulminant haemorrhagic pancreatitis. Fortunately, most cases run a benign course and respond to bowel rest and nutritional support.

8.5.10.1.2 FISTULA

The development of a post-operative pancreatic fistula is the most common complication; this increases when the duct is involved, and the rate may be as high as 37 per cent in combined injuries[43]. Most fistulas are minor (less than 200 mL of fluid per day) and self-limiting when there is adequate external drainage. However, high-output fistulas (>7000 mL per day) may require surgical intervention for closure or prolonged periods of drainage with nutritional support. Management is directed locally at adequate drainage, reduction of pancreatic output with octreotide and (recently) transpapillary pancreatic stenting of confirmed ductal injuries[44]. Systemic treatment includes treatment of the underlying cause (such as sepsis) and early adequate nutrition, preferably with distal enteral feeds through a feeding jejunostomy. If the fistula persists, the underlying cause should be investigated with ERCP, CT scanning and operation as necessary.

8.5.10.1.3 ABSCESS FORMATION

Most abscesses are peripancreatic and associated with injuries to other organs, specifically the liver and intestine. A true pancreatic abscess is uncommon and usually results from inadequate debridement of necrotic tissue. For this reason, simple percutaneous drainage is generally not enough, and further debridement is required.

8.5.10.2 Late Complications

8.5.10.2.1 PSEUDOCYST

Accurate diagnosis and surgical treatment of pancreatic injuries should result in a rate of pseudocyst formation of about 2–3 per cent[45], but Kudsk et al[46]. reported pseudocysts in half their patients who were treated non-operatively for blunt pancreatic trauma. Investigation entails imaging of the ductal system with either ERCP or magnetic resonance imaging (MRI). Accurate evaluation of the state of the duct will dictate management, and if the duct is intact, percutaneous drainage is likely to be successful. However, a pseudocyst together with a major ductal disruption will not be cured by percutaneous drainage, which will convert the pseudocyst into a chronic fistula. Current options include cystogastrostomy (open or endoscopic), endoscopic stenting of the duct or resection.

8.5.10.2.2 EXOCRINE AND ENDOCRINE DEFICIENCY

Pancreatic resection distal to the mesenteric vessels will usually leave enough tissue for adequate exocrine and endocrine function, as work has shown that a residual 10–20 per cent of pancreatic tissue is usually enough. Patients who have procedures that leave less functioning tissue will require exogenous endocrine and exocrine enzyme replacement.

8.5.11 Summary of Evidence-based Guidelines

Table 8.5.2 gives a summary of the evidence-based guidelines[47,48] for pancreatic trauma.

Table 8.5.2 Summary of EAST Evidence-Based Guidelines for Pancreatic Trauma

Level of Evidence	Recommendation
I	There are insufficient data to support a level I recommendation.
II	There are insufficient data to support a level I recommendation.
III	Delay in recognition of main pancreatic duct injury causes increased morbidity.
	Computed tomography scanning is suggestive, but not diagnostic, of pancreatic injury.
	Amylase/lipase levels are suggestive, but not diagnostic, of pancreatic injury.
	Grades I and II injuries can be managed by drainage alone.
	Grade III injuries should be managed with resection and drainage.
	Closed suction is preferred to sump suction.

Source: Bokhari F, Phelan H, Holevar M, et al., Eastern Association for the Surgery of Trauma Guidelines for the Diagnosis and Management of Pancreatic Trauma, http://www.east.org, accessed December 2014.

REFERENCES

References

1. Sims EH, Mandal AK, Schlater T, Fleming AW, Lou MA. Factors affecting outcome in pancreatic trauma. *J Trauma*. 1984;24:125–128.
2. Degiannis E, Glapa M, Loukogeorgakis SP, Smith MD. Management of pancreatic trauma. *Injury*. 2008;39:21–29.
3. Graham JM, Mattox K, Jordan G. Traumatic injuries of the pancreas. *Am J Surg*. 1978;136:744–748.
4. Bradley EL III, Young PR Jr, Chang MC, et al. Diagnosis and initial management of blunt pancreatic trauma: guidelines from a multi-institutional review. *Ann Surg*. 1998;227:861–869.
5. Leppaniemi A, Haapiainen R, Kiviluoto T, Lempinen M. Pancreatic trauma: acute and late manifestations. *Br J Surg*. 1988;75:165–167.
6. Biffl W. Injury to the duodenum and pancreas. In: Mattox KL, Moore EE, Feliciano DV, eds. *Trauma*, 7th ed. New York, NY: McGraw-Hill; 2013:603–619.
7. Takishima T, Sugimoto K, Hirata M, Asari Y, Ohwada T, Katika A. Serum amylase level on admission in the diagnosis of blunt injury to the pancreas: its significance and limitations. *Ann Surg*. 1997;226:70–76.

8. Peitzman AB, Makaraoun MS, Slasky BS, Ritter P. Prospective study of computed tomography in initial management of blunt abdominal trauma. *J Trauma.* 1986;26:585–592.

9. Ahkrass R, Kim K, Brandt C. Computed tomography: an unreliable indicator of pancreatic trauma. *Am Surg.* 1996;62:647–651.

10. Thomson DA, Krige JEJ, Thomson SR, Bornman PC. The role of endoscopic retrograde pancreatography in pancreatic trauma: a critical appraisal of 48 patients treated at a tertiary institution. *J Trauma Acute Care Surg.* 2014;76:1362–1366.

11. Bret PM, Reinhold C. Magnetic resonance cholangiopancreatography. *Endoscopy.* 1997;29:472–486.

12 Subramanian A, Dente CJ, Feliciano DV. The management of pancreatic trauma in the modern era. *Surg Clin N Am.* 2007;87:1515–1532.

13. Berni GA, Bandyk DF, Oreskovich MR, Carrico CJ. Role of intraoperative pancreatography in patients with injury to the pancreas. *Am J Surg.* 1982;143:602–605.

14. Hikida S, Sakamoto T, Higaki K, et al. Intra-operative ultrasonography is useful for diagnosing pancreatic duct injury and adjacent tissue damage in a patient with penetrating pancreas trauma. *J Hepatobiliary Pancreat Surg.* 2004;11:272–275.

15. Moore EE, Cogbill TH, Malangoni MA, et al. Organ injury scaling. II: pancreas, duodenum, small bowel, colon, and rectum. *J Trauma.* 1990;30:1427–1429.

16 Kong Y, Zhang H, He X, et al. Endoscopic management for pancreatic injuries due to blunt abdominal trauma decreases failure of nonoperative management and incidence of pancreatic-related complications. *Injury.* 2014;45:134–140.

16. Kim HS, Lee DK, Kim IW, et al. The role of endoscopic retrograde pancreatography in the treatment of traumatic pancreatic duct injury. *Gastrointest Endosc.* 2001;54:49–55.

17. Wolf A, Bernhardt J, Patrzyk M, Heidecke C-D. The value of endoscopic diagnosis and the treatment of pancreas injuries following blunt abdominal trauma. *Surg Endosc.* 2005;19:665–669.

18. Lin BC, Chen RJ, Fang JF, Hsu YP, Kao YC, Kao JL. Management of blunt major pancreatic injury. *J Trauma.* 2004;56:774–778.

19. Lin BC, Fang JF, Wong YC, et al. Blunt pancreatic trauma and pseudocyst: management of major pancreatic duct injury. *Injury.* 2007;38:588–593.

20. Velmahos GC, Tabbara M, Gross R, et al. Blunt pancreatoduodenal injury: a multicenter study of the Research Consortium of New England Centers for Trauma (ReCONECT). *Arch Surg.* 2009;144:413–419.

21. Nowak M, Baringer D, Ponsky J. Pancreatic injuries: effectiveness of debridement and drainage for non-transecting injuries. *Am Surg.* 1986;52:599–602.

22. Fabian TC, Kudsk KA, Croce MA, et al. Superiority of closed suction drainage for pancreatic trauma. A randomized prospective study. *Ann Surg.* 1990;211:724–728.

23. Andersen DK, Bolman RM, Moylan JA. Management of penetrating pancreatic injuries: subtotal pancreatectomy using the Auto-Suture stapler. *J Trauma.* 1980;20:347–349.

24. Cogbill T, Moore EE, Morris MD Jr, et al. Distal pancreatectomy for trauma: a multicentre experience. *J Trauma.* 1991;31:1600–1606.

25. Stone HH, Fabian TC, Satiani B, Turkleson ML. Experiences in the management of pancreatic trauma. *J Trauma.* 1981;21:257–262.

26. Pachter HL, Hofstetter SR, Liang HG, Hoballah J. Traumatic injuries to the pancreas: the role of distal pancreatectomy with splenic preservation. *J Trauma.* 1989;29:1352–1355.

27. Feliciano DV, Martin TD, Cruse PA, et al. Management of combined pancreatoduodenal injuries. *Ann Surg.* 1987;205:673–680.

28. Degiannis E, Krawczykowski D, Velmahos GC, et al. Pyloric exclusion in severe penetrating injuries of the duodenum. *World J Surg.* 1993;17:751–754.

29. DuBose JJ, Inaba K, Teixeira PG, et al. Pyloric exclusion in the treatment of severe duodenal injuries: results from the National Trauma Data Bank. *Am Surg.* 2008;74:925–929.

30. Ginzburg E, Carillo EH, Sosa JL, et al. Pyloric exclusion in the management of duodenal trauma: is concomitant gastrojejunostomy necessary? *Am Surg.* 1997;63:964–966.

31. Asensio JA, Petrone, Roldan G, Kuncir E, Demetriades D. Pancreaticoduodenectomy: a rare procedure for the management of complex pancreaticoduodenal injuries. *J Am Coll Surg.* 2003;197:937–942.

32. Kauder DR, Schwab SW, Rotondo MF. Damage control. In: Ivatury RR, Cayten CG, eds. *The Textbook of Penetrating Trauma.* Baltimore, MD: Williams & Wilkins; 1996:717–725.

33. Whipple A. Observations on radical surgery for lesions of the pancreas. *Surg Gynecol Obstet.* 1946;82:623.

34. Thompson CM, Shalhub SH, DeBoard ZM, Maier RV. Revisiting the pancreaticoduodenectomy for trauma: a single institution's experience. *J Trauma Acute Care Surg.* 2013;75:225–228.

35. Walt AJ. Pancreatic trauma. In: Ivatury RR, Gayten CG, eds. *The Textbook of Penetrating Trauma.* Baltimore, MD: Williams & Wilkins; 1996:641–652.

36. Büchler M, Friess H, Klempa I, et al. Role of octreotide in the prevention of postoperative complications following pancreatic resection. *Am J Surg.* 1992;163:125–130.

37. McKay C, Baxter J, Imrie C. A randomized, controlled trial of octreotide in the management of patients with acute pancreatitis. *Int J Pancreatol.* 1997;21:13–19.

38. Barnes SM, Kontny BG, Prinz RA. Somatostatin analogue treatment of pancreatic fistulas. *Int J Pancreatol.* 1993;14:181–188.

39. Kellum JM, Holland GF, McNeill P. Traumatic pancreatic cutaneous fistula: comparison of enteral and parenteral feeding. *J Trauma.* 1988;28:700–704.

40. Shilyansky J, Sena LM, Kreller M, et al. Non-operative management of pancreatic injuries in children. *J Pediatr.* 1998;33:343–349.

41. De Blaauw I, Rieu PN, van der Staak FH, et al. Pancreatic injury in children: good outcome of nonoperative treatment. *J Pediatr Surg.* 2008;43:1640–1643.

42. Skandalakis JE, Gray SW, Skandalakis LJ. Anatomical complications of pancreatic surgery. *Contemp Surg.* 1979;15:17–50.

43. Graham JM, Mattox KL, Vaughan GD III, Jordan GL. Combined pancreatoduodenal injuries. *J Trauma.* 1979;19:340–346.

44. Kozarek RA, Traverso LW. Pancreatic fistulas: etiology, consequences, and treatment. *Gastroenterologist.* 1996;4:238–244.

45. Wilson R, Moorehead R. Current management of trauma to the pancreas. *Br J Surg.* 1991;78:1196–1202.

45. Kudsk K, Temizer D, Ellison EC, Cloutier CT, Buckley DC, Carey LC. Post-traumatic pancreatic sequestrum: recognition and treatment. *J Trauma.* 1986;26:320–324.

47. Bokhari F, Phelan H, Holevar M, et al. Eastern Association for the Surgery of Trauma Guidelines for the Diagnosis and Management of Pancreatic Trauma. http://www.east.org. Accessed December 2014.

48. Biffl WL, Moore EE, Croce M, et al. Western Trauma Association critical decisions in trauma: management of pancreatic injuries. *J Trauma Acute Care Surg.* 2013;75:941–946.

8.6 Duodenum

8.6.1 OVERVIEW

Duodenal injuries can pose a formidable challenge to the surgeon, and failure to manage them properly can have devastating results. The total amount of fluid passing through the duodenum exceeds 6 L per day, and a fistula in this area can cause serious fluid and electrolyte imbalance. A large amount of activated enzymes liberated into a combination of the retroperitoneal space and the peritoneal cavity can be life-threatening.

Both the pancreas and the duodenum are well protected in the superior retroperitoneum deep within the abdomen. Since these organs are in the retroperitoneum, they usually do not present with peritonitis and are delayed in their presentation. Therefore, in order to sustain an injury to either one of them, there must be other associated injuries. If there is an anterior penetrating injury, the stomach, small bowel, transverse colon, liver, spleen or kidneys are frequently also involved. If there is a blunt traumatic injury, there are frequently fractures of the lower thoracic or upper lumbar vertebrae. It requires a high level of suspicion and significant clinical acumen as well as aggressive radiographic imaging to identify an injury to these organs this early in the presentation.

Pre-operative diagnosis of isolated duodenal injury can be very difficult to make, and there is no single method of duodenal repair that completely eliminates dehiscence of the duodenal suture line. As a result, the surgeon is frequently confronted with the dilemma of choosing between several pre-operative investigations and many surgical procedures. A detailed knowledge of the available operative choices and when each one of them is preferably applied is important for the patient's benefit[1].

8.6.2 MECHANISM OF INJURY

8.6.2.1 Penetrating Trauma

Penetrating trauma is the leading cause of duodenal injuries in countries with a high incidence of civilian violence. Because of the retroperitoneal location of the duodenum, and its close proximity to a number of other viscera and major vascular structures, isolated penetrating injuries of the duodenum are rare. The need for abdominal exploration is usually dictated by associated injuries, and the diagnosis of duodenal injury is usually made in the operating room.

8.6.2.2 Blunt Trauma

Blunt injuries to the duodenum are both less common and more difficult to diagnose than penetrating injuries, and they can occur in isolation or with pancreatic injury. These usually occur when crushing the duodenum between the spine and a steering wheel or handlebar, or when some other force is applied to the duodenum. These injuries can be associated with flexion/distraction fractures of the L1–L2 vertebrae – the Chance fracture. 'Stomping' and striking the mid-epigastrium are common. Less common in deceleration injury patterns are tears at the junction of the third and fourth parts of the duodenum (and less commonly, the first and second parts). These injuries occur at the junction of free (intraperitoneal) parts of the duodenum with fixed (retroperitoneal) parts. A high index of suspicion based on the mechanism of injury and physical examination findings may lead to further diagnostic studies.

8.6.2.3 Paediatric Considerations

A recent multi-institutional investigation found that child abuse is consistently associated with duodenal injuries in children younger than 2 years; also, the most common mechanism causing duodenal injuries in children younger than 5 years was non-accidental trauma.

8.6.3 DIAGNOSIS

8.6.3.1 Clinical Presentation

The clinical changes in isolated duodenal injuries may be extremely subtle until severe, life-threatening peritonitis develops. In the vast majority of the retroperitoneal perforations, there is initially only mild upper abdominal tenderness with a progressive rise in temperature, tachycardia and occasionally vomiting. After several hours, the duodenal contents extravasate into the peritoneal cavity, with the development of peritonitis. If the duodenal contents spill into the lesser sac, they are usually 'walled off' and localized, although they can occasionally leak into the general peritoneal cavity via the foramen of Winslow, with resultant generalized peritonitis.[2] Diagnostic difficulties do not arise in the cases in which the blunt injury causes intraperitoneal perforations.

8.6.3.2 Serum Amylase

Theoretically, duodenal perforations are associated with a leak of amylase and other digestive enzymes, and it has been suggested that determination of the serum amylase concentration might be helpful in the diagnosis of blunt duodenal injury[3,4]. However, the test lacks sensitivity[5,6]. The duodenum is retroperitoneal, the concentration of amylase in the fluid that leaks is variable and amylase concentrations often take hours to days to increase after injury. Although serial determinations of serum amylase are better than a single, isolated determination on admission, sensitivity is still poor, and necessary delays are inherent in serial determinations. If the serum amylase level is elevated on admission, a diligent search for duodenal rupture is warranted. The presence of a normal amylase level, however, does not exclude duodenal injury[7].

8.6.3.3 Diagnostic Peritoneal Lavage/Ultrasound

The duodenum, like the pancreas, lies in the retroperitoneum, so that neither ultrasound nor diagnostic peritoneal lavage (DPL) will be reliable. Although virtually all patients with blunt duodenal injury will eventually have increased white blood cell and amylase levels in DPL fluid, DPL has a low sensitivity for duodenal perforations[8]. If DPL is performed, amylase levels in the fluid must be checked.

8.6.3.4 Radiological Investigation

8.6.3.4.1 RADIOLOGICAL STUDIES

Radiological studies may be helpful in the diagnosis. Plain X-rays of the abdomen are useful, as gas bubbles may be present in the retroperitoneum adjacent to the right psoas muscle, around the right kidney or anterior to the upper lumbar spine. They can also show free intraperitoneal air, and, although rarely seen, air in the biliary tree also has been described[9]. Obliteration of the right psoas muscle shadow or fractures of the transverse processes in the lumbar vertebrae are indicative of forceful retroperitoneal trauma and serve as a predictor of duodenal trauma.

8.6.3.4.2 RADIOLOGICAL CONTRAST STUDIES

An upper gastrointestinal series using water-soluble contrast material can provide positive results in 50 per cent of patients with duodenal perforations. Meglumine (Gastrografin) should be infused via the nasogastric tube and then swallowed, and the study should be done under fluoroscopic control with the patient in the right lateral position. If no leak is observed, the investigation continues with the patient in the supine and left lateral positions. If the Gastrografin study is negative, it should be followed by administration of barium to allow for the detection of small perforations more readily. Upper gastrointestinal studies with contrast are also indicated in patients with a suspected intramural haematoma of the duodenum, because they may demonstrate the classic 'coiled-spring' appearance of complete obstruction by the haematoma[10].

8.6.3.4.3 COMPUTED TOMOGRAPHY

Computed tomography (CT) scan is the mode of choice for the investigation of subtle duodenal injuries. It is very sensitive to the presence of small amounts of retroperitoneal air, blood or extravasated contrast from the injured duodenum, especially in children[11,12]. Its reliability in adults is more controversial. The presence of periduodenal wall thickening or haematoma without extravasation of contrast material should be investigated with a gastrointestinal study with Gastrografin. If the result is normal, it should be followed by a barium study contrast, if the patient's condition allows this.

8.6.3.5 **Diagnostic Laparoscopy**

Unfortunately, diagnostic laparoscopy does not confer any improvement over more traditional methods in the investigation of the duodenum. In fact, because of its anatomical position, diagnostic laparoscopy is a poor modality to determine organ injury in these cases[13].

8.6.3.6 **Exploratory Laparotomy**

Exploratory laparotomy remains the ultimate diagnostic test if a high degree of suspicion of duodenal injury continues in the face of absent or equivocal radiographic signs[14].

8.6.4 **DUODENAL INJURY SCALE**

Grading systems have been devised to characterize duodenal injuries (Table 8.6.1).

Table 8.6.1 Duodenum Injury Scale (See also Appendix B: Trauma Scores and Scoring Systems)

Grade[a]	Type of Injury	Description of Injury
I	Haematoma	Involving a single portion of duodenum
	Laceration	Partial thickness, no perforation
II	Haematoma	Involving more than one portion
	Laceration	Disruption <50% of circumference
III	Laceration	Disruption 50%–75% of circumference of D2
		Disruption 50%–100% of circumference of D1, D3 or D4
IV	Laceration	Disruption >75% of circumference of D2
		Involving the ampulla or distal common bile duct
V	Laceration	Massive disruption of the duodenopancreatic complex
	Vascular	Devascularization of duodenum

[a]Advance one grade for multiple injuries up to grade III.

Note: D1, first portion of duodenum; D2, second portion of duodenum; D3, third portion of duodenum; D4, fourth portion of duodenum.

8.6.5 **MANAGEMENT**

While upper gastrointestinal radiological studies and CT scanning can lead to the diagnosis of blunt duodenal trauma, exploratory laparotomy remains the ultimate diagnostic test if a high suspicion of duodenal injury continues in the face of absent or equivocal radiographic signs.

The majority of duodenal injuries can be managed by simple repair. More complicated injuries require more sophisticated techniques. 'High-risk' duodenal injuries are followed by a high incidence of suture line dehiscence, and their treatment should include duodenal diversion. The management of all full-thickness duodenal lacerations should include adequate external periduodenal drainage. Pancreaticoduodenectomy is practised only if no alternative is available. 'Damage control' should precede the definitive reconstruction.

8.6.6 SURGICAL APPROACH

Although useful for research purposes, the specifics of the grading systems are less important than several simple aspects of the duodenal injuries:

- The anatomical relation to the ampulla of Vater.
- The characteristics of the injury (simple laceration versus destruction of duodenal wall).
- The circumference of the duodenum involved.
- Associated injuries to the biliary tract or pancreas, or major vascular injuries.

Timing of the operation is also very important as mortality rises from 11 to 40 per cent if the time interval between injury and operation is more than 24 hours[13]. (See also Section 8.5.7 on the surgical approach to the pancreas.)

In addition to the Kocher manoeuvre to visualize the second part of the duodenum, a medial visceral rotation can be used to expose the entire transverse part of the duodenum. Alternatively, the fourth part of the duodenum can be mobilized by dividing the ligament of Treitz and gently dissecting with the right index finger in the avascular plane behind the transverse duodenum. Combining this with the Kocher manoeuvre allows the index fingers to be brought together from both sides and thereby excluding a posterior perforation of the transverse part of the duodenum.

From a practical point of view, the duodenum can be divided into one 'upper' portion that includes the first and second parts, and another 'lower' portion that includes the third and fourth parts. The 'upper' portion has complex anatomical structures within it (the common bile duct and the sphincter) and the pylorus. It requires distinct manoeuvres to diagnose injury (cholangiogram and direct visual inspection), and complex techniques to repair them. The first and second parts of the duodenum are densely adherent and dependent for their blood supply on the head of the pancreas; therefore, the diagnosis and management of any injury are complex, and resection, unless involving the entire 'C' loop and pancreatic head, is impossible. The 'lower' portion involving the third and fourth parts of the duodenum can generally be treated like the small bowel, and the diagnosis and management of injury are relatively

simple, including debridement, closure, resection and reanastomosis.

8.6.6.1 Intramural Haematoma

This is a rare injury of the duodenum specific to patients with blunt trauma. It is most common in children with isolated force to the upper abdomen, possibly because of the relatively flexible and pliable musculature of the child's abdominal wall, and half of the cases can be attributed to child abuse.

The haematoma develops in the submucosal or subserosal layers of the duodenum. The duodenum is not perforated. Such haematomas can lead to obstruction. The symptoms of gastric outlet obstruction can take up to 48 hours to present. This is due to the gradual increase of the size of a haematoma as the breakdown of the haemoglobin makes it hyperosmotic, with resultant fluid shifts into it. The diagnosis can be made by double-contrast CT scan or upper gastrointestinal contrast studies that show the 'coiled spring' or 'stacked coin' sign[10].

Management of the injury is usually considered non-surgical, and best results are obtained by conservative treatment, if associated injuries can be ruled out[15]. Gastric residual volume will slowly decrease, eventually allowing normal feeding. If there is no improvement, the patient should undergo laparotomy to rule out the presence of duodenal perforation or injury of the head of the pancreas, which may be an alternative cause of duodenal obstruction.

The treatment of an intramural haematoma that is found at early laparotomy is controversial. One option is to open the serosa, evacuate the haematoma without violation of the mucosa and carefully repair the wall of the bowel. The concern is that this may convert a partial tear to a full-thickness tear of the duodenal wall. Another option is to carefully explore the duodenum to exclude a perforation, leaving the intramural haematoma intact and planning nasogastric decompression post-operatively.

8.6.6.2 Duodenal Laceration

The great majority of duodenal perforations and lacerations can be managed with simple surgical procedures. This is particularly true with penetrating injuries, when the time interval between injury and operation is normally short. On the other hand, the minority are 'high risk', for example with increased risk of dehiscence of the duodenal repair, with increased morbidity and sometimes mortality. These injuries are related to associated pancreatic injury, blunt or missile injury, involvement of more than 75 per cent of the duodenal wall, injury of the first or second part of the duodenum, a time interval of more than 24 hours between injury and repair and associated common bile duct injury. In these high-risk injuries, several adjunctive operative procedures have been proposed in an attempt to reduce the incidence of dehiscence of the duodenal suture line. The methods of repair of the duodenal trauma as well as the 'supportive' procedures against dehiscence are described.

Recently further evidence has supported a more simplified surgical approach to these injuries with improved outcomes compared to a complex technical solution.

8.6.6.3 Repair of the Perforation

Most injuries of the duodenum can be repaired by primary closure in one or two layers. The closure should be oriented transversely, if possible, to avoid luminal compromise. Excessive inversion should be avoided.

Longitudinal duodenostomies can usually be closed transversely if the length of the duodenal injury is less than 50 per cent of the circumference of the duodenum. If primary closure would compromise the lumen of the duodenum, several alternatives have been recommended. Pedicled mucosal graft, as a method of closing large duodenal defects, has been suggested, using a segment of jejunum or a gastric island flap from the body of the stomach. An alternative to that is the use of a jejunal serosal patch to close the duodenal defect[16]. The serosa of the loop of the jejunum is sutured to the edges of the duodenal defect. Although encouraging in experimental studies, the clinical application of both methods has been limited, and suture line leaks have been reported[17]. Laying a loop of jejunum onto the area of the injury so that the serosa of the jejunum buttresses the duodenal repair has also been suggested[18], although no beneficial results have been reported from this technique[19].

8.6.6.4 Complete Transection of the Duodenum

The preferred method of repair is usually primary anastomosis of the two ends after appropriate debridement and mobilization of the duodenum. This is frequently the case with injuries of the first, third or fourth part of the duodenum, where mobilization is technically not difficult. However, if a large amount of tissue is lost, approximation of the duodenum may not be possible without producing undue tension on the suture line. If this is the case and complete transection occurs in the first part of the duodenum, it is advisable to perform an antrectomy with closure of the duodenal stump and a Billroth II gastrojejunostomy. When such injury occurs distal to the ampulla of Vater, closure of the distal duodenum and Roux-en-Y duodenojejunal anastomosis is appropriate[20].

Mobilization of the second part of the duodenum is limited by its shared blood supply with the head of the pancreas. A direct anastomosis to a Roux-en-Y loop sutured over the duodenal defect in an end-to-side fashion is the procedure of choice. This also can be applied as an alternative method of operative management of extensive defects to the other parts of the duodenum when primary anastomosis is not feasible.

External drainage should be provided in all duodenal injuries because it affords early detection and control of the duodenal fistula. The drain is preferably a simple, soft silicone rubber, closed system placed adjacent to the repair.

8.6.6.5 Duodenal Diversion

In high-risk duodenal injuries, duodenal repair is followed by a high incidence of suture line dehiscence. In order to protect the duodenal repair, the gastrointestinal contents – with their proteolytic enzymes – can be diverted, a practice that would also make the management of a potential duodenal fistula easier.

8.6.6.6 Duodenal Diverticulation

This includes a distal Billroth II gastrectomy, closure of the duodenal wound, placement of a decompressive catheter into the duodenum and generous drainage of the duodenal repair[21]. Truncal vagotomy and biliary drainage could be added. The disadvantage of duodenal diverticulation is that it is an extensive procedure totally inappropriate for the haemodynamically unstable trauma patient or the patient with multiple injuries. Resection of a normal distal stomach cannot be beneficial to the patient, and should not be considered unless there is a large amount of destruction and tissue loss and no other course is possible. This procedure is not recommended.

8.6.6.7 Triple-Tube Decompression

'Tube decompression' was the first technique used for decompression of the duodenum and diversion of its contents in an attempt to preserve the integrity of the duodenorrhaphy. It was first described in 1954 as a method of management of a precarious closure of the duodenal stump after a gastrectomy[22]. To protect a duodenal repair, a tube duodenostomy can be used by inserting a tube through a separate incision through the lateral duodenal wall using the Witzel technique to ensure sealing of the hole after removing the tube. In trauma, the technique was introduced by Stone and Garoni as a 'triple ostomy'[23]. This consists of a gastrostomy tube to decompress the stomach, a retrograde jejunostomy to decompress the duodenum and an antegrade jejunostomy to feed the patient.

The initial favourable reports on the efficacy of this technique to decrease the incidence of dehiscence of the duodenorrhaphy have not, however, been supported by more recent reports[24]. The drawbacks of this technique are the formation of several new perforations in the gastrointestinal tract, the inefficiency of the jejunostomy tube to properly decompress the duodenum and the common scenario of finding that the drains have fallen out or been removed by the patient. Establishment of enteral feeding, preferably through a nasojejunal tube placed at the surgical procedure through the anastomoses, or if this is not feasible, placement of a feeding jejunostomy, is recommended at the final stage of damage control, when no further re-looks are planned.

8.6.6.8 Pyloric Exclusion

For more information on pyloric exclusion, see Section 8.5.7 on the surgical approach to pancreatic injury.

8.6.6.9 Pancreaticoduodenectomy (Whipple Procedure)

This is a major procedure to be practised in trauma only if no alternative is available. Damage control with control of bleeding and of bowel contamination, and ligation of the common bile and pancreatic ducts, should be the rule[25]. Reconstruction should take place within 48 hours or when the patient is stable. (See Section 8.5.7 for more information on the surgical approach to pancreatic injury.)

8.6.6.10 Specific Injuries

Simple combined injuries of the pancreas and duodenum should be managed separately. More severe injuries require more complex procedures. Feliciano et al. reported by far the largest experience of combined pancreaticoduodenal injuries,[26] and suggested the following:

- Simple duodenal injuries with no ductal pancreatic injury (grades I and II) should be managed with primary repair and drainage.
- Grade III duodenal and pancreatic injuries are best treated with repair or resection of both organs as indicated, pyloric exclusion, gastrojejunostomy and closure.
- Grades IV and V duodenal and pancreatic injuries are best treated by pancreaticoduodenectomy.

Extensive local damage of the intraduodenal or intrapancreatic bile duct frequently necessitates a staged pancreaticoduodenectomy. Less extensive local injuries can be managed by intraluminal stenting, sphincteroplasty or reimplantation of the ampulla of Vater[27,28].

REFERENCES AND RECOMMENDED READING

References

1. Boone DC, Peitzman AB. Abdominal injury – duodenum and pancreas. In: Peitzman AB, Rhodes M, Schwab SW, Wealy DM, eds. *The Trauma Manual*. Philadelphia, PA: Lippincott-Raven; 1998:242–247.
2. Carrillo EH, Richardson JD, Miller FB. Evolution in the management of duodenal injuries. *J Trauma*. 1996;40:1037–1046.
3. Levinson MA, Peterson SR, Sheldon GF, et al. Duodenal trauma: experience of a trauma centre. *J Trauma*. 1982;24:475–480.
4. Snyder WH III, Weigelt JA, Watkins WL, et al. The surgical management of duodenal trauma. *Arch Surg*. 1980;115:422–429.
5. Olsen WR. The serum amylase in blunt abdominal trauma. *J Trauma*. 1973;13:201–204.

6. Flint LM Jr, McCoy M, Richardson JD, et al. Duodenal injury: analysis of common misconceptions in diagnosis and treatment. *Ann Surg.* 1979;191:697–771.

7. Jurkovich GJ Jr. Injury to the pancreas and duodenum. In: Feliciano DV, Moore EE, Mattox KL, eds. *Trauma*, 3rd ed. Norwalk, CT: Appleton Lange; 1996:573–594.

8. Wilson RF. Injuries to the pancreas and duodenum. In: Wilson RF, ed. *Handbook of Trauma: Pitfalls and Pearls*. Philadelphia, PA: Lippincott Williams & Wilkins; 1999:381–394.

9. Ivatury RR, Nassoura ZE, Simon RJ, et al. Complex duodenal injuries. *Surg Clin North Am.* 1996;76:797–812.

10. Kadell BM, Zimmerman PT, Lu DSK. Radiology of the abdomen. In: Zimmer MJ, Schwartz SI, Ellis H, eds. *Maingot's Abdominal Operations*. Stanford, CT: Appleton & Lange; 1997:3–116.

11. Kunin JR, Korobkin M, Ellis JH, et al. Duodenal injuries caused by blunt abdominal trauma: value of CT in differentiating perforation from haematoma. *Am J Roentgenol.* 1993;163:833–838.

12. Shilyansky J, Pearl RH, Kreller M, et al. Diagnosis and management of duodenal injuries. *J Paed Surg.* 1997;32:229–232.

13. Brooks AJ, Boffard KD. Current technology: laparoscopic surgery in trauma. *Trauma.* 1999;1:53–60.

14. Degiannis E, Boffard K. Duodenal injuries. *Br J Surg.* 2000;87:1473–1479.

15. Toulakian RJ. Protocol for the nonoperative treatment of obstructing intramural duodenal haematoma during childhood. *Am J Surg.* 1983;145:330–334.

16. Jones SA, Gazzaniga AB, Keller TB. Serosal patch: a surgical parachute. *Am J Surg.* 1973;126:186–196.

17. Ordoñez C, García A, Parra MW, et al. Complex penetrating duodenal injuries: Less is better. *J Trauma Acute Care Surg.* 2014;76:1177–1183. doi:10.1097/TA.0000000000000214.

18. McInnis WD, Aust JB, Cruz AB, et al. Traumatic injuries of the duodenum: a comparison of 1° closure and the jejunal patch. *J Trauma.* 1975;15:847–853.

19. Ivatury RR, Gaudino J, Ascer E, et al. Treatment of penetrating duodenal injuries. *J Trauma.* 1985;25:337–341.

20. Purtill M-A, Stabile BE. Duodenal and pancreatic trauma. In: Naude GP, Bongard FS, Demetriades D, eds. *Trauma Secrets*. Philadelphia, PA: Hanley & Belfus; 1999:123–130.

21. Berne CJ, Donovan AJ, White EJ, et al. Duodenal 'diverticulation' for duodenal and pancreatic injury. *Am J Surg.* 1974;127:503–507.

22. Welch CE, Rodkey CV. Methods of management of the duodenal stump after gastrectomy. *Surg Gynecol Obstet.* 1954;98:376–380.

23. Stone HH, Garoni WJ. Experiences in the management of duodenal wounds. *South Med J.* 1966;59:864–868.

24. Cogbill TH, Moore EE, Feliciano DV, et al. Conservative management of duodenal trauma: a multicentre perspective. *J Trauma.* 1990;30:1469–1475.

25. Kauder DR, Schwab SW, Rotondo MF. Damage control. In: Ivantury RR, Cayten CG, eds. *The Textbook of Penetrating Trauma*. Baltimore, MD: Williams & Wilkins; 1996:717–725.

26. Feliciano DV, Martin TD, Cruse PA, et al. Management of combined pancreatoduodenal injuries. *Ann Surg.* 1987;205:673–680.

27. Jurkovich GJ, Hoyt DB, Moore FA, et al. Portal triad injuries. *J Trauma.* 1995;39:426–434.

28. Obeid FN, Kralovich KA, Gaspatti MG, et al. Sphincteroplasty as an adjunct in penetrating duodenal trauma. *J Trauma.* 1999;47:22–24.

Recommended Reading

Asensio JA, Demetriades D, Berne JD. A unified approach to surgical exposure of pancreatic and duodenal injuries. *Am J Surg.* 1997;174:54–60.

Asensio JA, Feliciano DV, Britt LD, et al. Management of duodenal injuries. *Curr Probl Surg.* 1993;30:1023–1092.

Seamon MJ, Pieri PG, Fisher CA, et al. A ten-year retrospective review: does pyloric exclusion improve clinical outcome after penetrating duodenal and combined pancreaticoduodenal injuries? *J Trauma.* 2007;62:829–833.

Velmahos GC, Constantinou C, Kasotakis G. Safety of repair for severe duodenal injuries. *World J Surg.* 2008;32:7–12.

8.7 Abdominal Vascular Injury

8.7.1 OVERVIEW

Abdominal vascular injury presents a serious threat to life where preparedness and anticipation are vital to a successful outcome. Consideration of both the possible injuries and the surgical approach to manage them is crucial. Adequate preparation is essential; an adequate incision will be required.

> *It is helpful to have available all the apparatus for massive transfusion, with adequate warming of all intravenous fluids. Autotransfusion should be considered in all cases.*

Major vessel injuries within the abdominal cavity primarily present as haemorrhagic shock that does not respond to resuscitation; thus, immediate surgery becomes a part of the resuscitative effort. In penetrating injury, this may necessitate an emergency department thoracotomy (EDT) and aortic cross-clamp. Consideration should also be given to resuscitative endovascular balloon occlusion of the aorta (REBOA) which has a role in controlling abdominal and pelvic haemorrhage in a similar but less invasive manner to that of EDT[1].

> *However, the emergency department thoracotomy is not indicated in the severely shocked patient with blunt abdominal trauma, as the survival rate is close to zero.*

Direct or proximal control of the vessel is mandatory for success. Injuries above the pelvic brim can be approached from the right side if the injury is thought to be below the renal artery, and from the left side for injuries between the renal artery and the hiatus. Vascular injuries in the pelvis following blunt trauma are best managed with an arteriogram. This will determine whether a direct operative approach or interventional radiology is appropriate.

8.7.2 INJURIES OF THE AORTA AND VENA CAVA

Aorta and caval injuries are primarily a problem of access (rapid) and control of haemorrhage. If the surgeon opens the abdomen and there is extensive retroperitoneal bleeding centrally, there are two options.

If the bleeding is primarily venous in nature, the right colon should be mobilized to the midline, including the duodenum and head of the pancreas. This will expose the infrarenal cava and infrarenal aorta. It will also facilitate access to the portal vein.

If the bleeding is primarily arterial in nature, it is best to approach the injury from the left. This includes taking down the left colon and mobilizing the pancreas and spleen to the midline. Access to the posterior aorta includes mobilizing the left kidney. By approaching the aorta from the left lateral position, it is possible to identify the plane of Leriche more rapidly than it is by approaching it through the lesser sac. The problem is the coeliac and superior mesenteric ganglion, which can be quite dense and hinder dissection around the origins of the coeliac and superior mesenteric artery. Additional exposure can be obtained simply by dividing the left crus of the diaphragm. This will allow proximal control of the abdominal aorta until complete dissection of the visceral vessels can be accomplished. The exception is in the area of the coeliac ganglion, which can contain aortic haemorrhage from significant injuries, and which may require short segmental graft replacement.

Treatment of aortic or caval injuries is usually straightforward. Extensive lacerations are not compatible with survival, and it is uncommon to require graft material to repair the aorta. Caval injuries below the renal veins, if extensive, can be ligated, although lateral repair is preferred. Injuries above the renal veins in the cava should be repaired if at all possible, including onlay graft of autogenous tissue.

8.7.3 RETROPERITONEAL HAEMATOMA

8.7.3.1 Central Haematoma

To expose the potential sites of arterial bleeding in the upper midline region of the retroperitoneum, medial visceral rotation is performed by mobilizing not only the left colon, but also the spleen, pancreas and stomach. The lienorenal and lienophrenic ligaments are divided, followed by an incision down the left paracolic gutter, and a blunt dissection to free the organs from the retroperitoneum towards the centre of the abdomen. An extended reflection of the abdominal structures from the left to the right will reflect the spleen, colon, tail of pancreas and fundus of the stomach towards the midline. This provides access to the aorta, the coeliac axis, the superior mesenteric artery, the splenic artery and vein and the left renal artery and vein. In order to reach the posterior wall of the aorta, the kidney should be mobilized as well and rotated medially on its pedicle, taking great care not to cause further injury.

8.7.3.2 Lateral Haematoma

If these are not expanding or pulsatile, blunt injuries are best left alone, as the damage is usually renal. Renal injuries can generally be managed non-operatively including the use of selective embolization. However, with penetrating injury, because of the risk of damage to adjacent structures such as the ureter, it is safer to explore lateral haematomas, even if they are not expanding. The surgeon must also be confident that there is no perforation of the posterior part of the colon in the paracolic gutters on either side.

8.7.3.3 Pelvic Haematoma

If the patient is stable, contrast-enhanced computed tomography (CT) in the emergency situation may demonstrate a large pelvic haematoma with a vascular 'blush' indicating ongoing arterial bleeding. In this case, it may be more appropriate to transfer the patient for immediate embolization.

> *This surgery is fraught with hazard, and exploration of such haematomas should be a last resort. Wherever possible, angiographic visualization and embolization of any arterial bleeding must be tried before surgery is commenced, if the patient is sufficiently stable. However, rapidly expanding or pulsating haematomas in this region may need exploration.*

The first concern should be to apply a binder to reduce pelvic volume. Stabilization of the pelvis using external fixators or a C-clamp in the emergency situation can be considered, but this does not always provide adequate posterior fixation, and may interfere with subsequent

visualization of vessels for embolization. If the patient is too unstable for angiography, damage control surgery with packing of the pelvis should provide initial control. The peritoneum is incised over the distal aorta or the iliac vessels, in order to control the arterial inflow, before attention is directed to the actual injury. However, it is best to leave pelvic haematomas undisturbed if they are not rapidly expanding or pulsatile, as they are most likely due to pelvic venous damage. These veins are notoriously fragile and unforgiving to any attempt at repair.

There is recent literature to support extraperitoneal pelvic packing as the most efficient damage control technique to control this type of bleeding[2]. After packing, the patient should be sent directly to the angiographic suite from the operating theatre, for embolization, without further exploration.

8.7.4 SURGICAL APPROACH

8.7.4.1 Incision

The patient must be prepared 'from sternal notch to knee'. It is critical to gain proximal and distal control, and patient preparation should include the need to extend to a left lateral thoracotomy to gain access to the thoracic aorta, a median sternotomy to control the intracardiac inferior vena cava (IVC) and groin incisions to gain control of the iliac vessels.

8.7.4.2 Aorta

Control of the aorta can be achieved at several different levels depending on the site of injury. The supracoeliac aorta can be exposed by incising the gastrohepatic ligament and retracting the left lobe of the liver superiorly and the stomach inferiorly. A window is then made in the lesser omentum, and the peritoneum overlying the crura of the diaphragm is divided. The fibres of the crura are separated by sharp or blunt dissection. Good assistance and retraction are necessary to facilitate this dissection. Identification of the oesophagus which lies to the left of the aorta is aided by the prior placement of a nasogastric tube. The aorta can be clamped or compressed at this point (Figure 8.7.1).

Exposure of the suprarenal aorta is not ideal with this anterior approach, and better exposure can be obtained by performing a left medial visceral rotation procedure. This entails mobilization of the splenorenal ligament

Figure 8.7.1 Control of the aorta by cross-clamping at the crura of the diaphragm.

and incision of the peritoneal reflection in the left para-colic gutter, down to the level of the sigmoid colon. The left-sided viscera are then bluntly dissected free of the ret-roperitoneum and mobilized to the right. Care should be taken to remain in a plane anterior to Gerota fascia. The entire abdominal aorta and the origins of its branches are exposed by this technique. This includes the coeliac axis, the origin of the superior mesenteric artery, the iliac vessels and the left renal pedicle. The dense and fibrous superior mesenteric and coeliac nerve plexuses, however, overlie the proximal aorta and need to be sharply dissected in order to identify the renal and superior mesenteric arteries.

The distal aorta can be approached transperitoneally by retracting the small bowel to the right, the transverse colon superiorly and the descending colon to the left. The aorta below the left renal vein can be accessed by incising the peritoneum over it and mobilizing the third and fourth parts of the duodenum superiorly. Both iliac vessels can be exposed by distal continuation of the dis-section. The ureters should be identified and carefully preserved, especially in the region of the bifurcation of the iliac vessels.

8.7.4.3 **Coeliac Axis**

The left colon is reflected to the right, together with the spleen and the tail of pancreas, to display the aorta and its branches. The coeliac trunk lies behind and inferior to the gastro-oesophageal junction. Injuries to this area

are commonly missed, particularly in patients with stab wounds. Major vascular injury is particularly likely if there is a central retroperitoneal haematoma. In this sit-uation, proximal vascular control prior to entering the haematoma is essential, either locally in the abdomen or via a left lateral thoracotomy. Division of the left trian-gular ligament and mobilization of the lateral segment of the left lobe of the liver are also helpful.

It is difficult to repair the coeliac axis. The artery can be tied off, provided that the tie is proximal to its main branches and the superior mesenteric artery is intact.

The left gastric and splenic arteries can be tied. The common hepatic artery can be safely tied provided that the injury is proximal to the gastroduodenal artery.

8.7.4.4 **Superior Mesenteric Artery**

The superior mesenteric artery is a vital artery for the via-bility of the small bowel, and should always be repaired, using conventional techniques. Proximally, the artery is accessible from the aorta at the level of the renal arteries, and is best approached with a left medial visceral rota-tion (Figure 8.7.2). More distally, the artery is accessed at the root of the small bowel mesentery.

If a period of ischaemia has elapsed, or the surgery is part of a damage control procedure, the artery should be shunted, using a plastic vascular shunt (e.g. Javid shunt, Bard Inc., Tempe, AZ), until repair can be effected[3].

If repair is not possible, and replacement of the artery with a graft is required, it is best to place the graft on the infrarenal aorta, away from the pancreas and areas of potential leak[4]. Placement of the proximal end of the graft too high can result in kinking and subsequent occlusion of the graft when the bowel is returned to the abdominal cavity. The graft must be tailored so that there is no tension, and the aortic suture line must be covered to prevent an aortoenteric fistula.

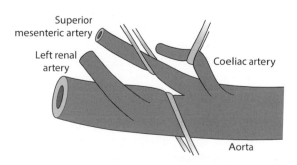

Figure 8.7.2 Anatomy of the superior mesenteric artery.

The survival rate with penetrating injuries of the superior mesenteric artery is approximately 58 per cent, falling to 22 per cent if a complex repair is required[4,5].

The superior mesenteric vein can be either shunted or simply ligated[6].

8.7.4.5 Inferior Mesenteric Artery

Injuries to the inferior mesenteric artery are uncommon, and the artery can generally be tied off. The viability of the colon should be checked before closure, with planned re-operation to evaluate viability of the colon.

8.7.4.6 Renal Arteries

Preliminary vascular control is best obtained by accessing the renal arteries on the aorta using a standard infrarenal aortic approach. Access can also be obtained by mobilizing the viscera medially.

Repair is done using standard vascular techniques. However, the kidney tolerates warm ischaemia poorly, and its viability after 45 minutes is in doubt. Therefore, if there has been complete transection of the artery, and the kidney is of doubtful viability, preservation may not be in the best interest of the patient.

8.7.4.7 Iliac Vessels

Proximal and distal control may be required, and distal control via a separate groin incision should be considered.

The iliac vessels are exposed by lifting the small bowel upwards, out of the pelvis. On the left, the sigmoid colon and its mesentery can be mobilized, and on the right, division of the peritoneal attachments over the caecum and mobilization of the caecum to the midline will aid exposure of the vessels.

The ureters must be formally identified as they cross the iliac bifurcation.

The common iliac veins are often adherent to the back wall of the common iliac artery, and attempts to mobilize the veins for control may result in torrential bleeding. A vascular clamp, applied proximally from above to the hypogastric and iliac veins, may be preferable to direct control.

8.7.4.8 Inferior Vena Cava (IVC)

8.7.4.8.1 SUPRAHEPATIC IVC

Access to the suprahepatic IVC can be obtained by incising the central tendon of the diaphragm or by performing a median sternotomy and opening the pericardium.

8.7.4.8.2 INFRAHEPATIC IVC

The infrahepatic vena cava can be exposed by means of a right medial visceral rotation procedure (Figure 8.7.3). (See also right medial visceral rotation in Section 8.1.2.5.)

The right colon is mobilized by taking down the hepatic flexure and incising the peritoneal reflection down the length of the right paracolic gutter. The colon is then reflected medially in a plane anterior to Gerota fascia. If more exposure is required, the root of the mesentery can be mobilized by dividing the inferior mesenteric vein. Performance of a Kocher manoeuvre and medial mobilization of the duodenum and head of the pancreas will reveal the segment of vena cava immediately below

Figure 8.7.3 Right medial visceral rotation to expose the inferior vena cava.

the liver, and also provide excellent exposure of the right renovascular pedicle.

Control is best achieved by direct pressure on the IVC[7] above and below the injury, utilizing swabs (Figure 8.7.4).

If more definitive control is required, a combination of vascular clamps to the renal arteries and Rumel[8] tourniquets placed above the renal vessels (suprarenal), or above and below the injury, should be used (Figure 8.7.5).

Injuries to the posterior part of the IVC should always be expected with penetrating injury to the anterior part of the IVC. Not all bleeding posterior wounds need to be repaired.

It is very difficult to 'roll' the IVC to approach it posteriorly, due to multiple lumbar veins, so all injuries should be approached transcavally. Not all non-bleeding posterior wounds require repair.

Provided it is infrarenal, ligation of the IVC is acceptable.

8.7.4.9 **Portal Vein**

The portal vein[9] lies in the free edge of lesser omentum, together with the common bile duct and the hepatic artery (Figure 8.7.6).

The portal vein generally can be controlled with a Pringle manoeuvre. If the injury is more proximal, it may be necessary to reflect the duodenum medially, or divide the pancreas.

The portal vein should be shunted early to avoid venous hypertension of the bowel, which will make access to the area increasingly difficult. The stent can be left in place as part of a damage control procedure, or repaired. Portocaval shunting is a possibility, and ligation is a last resort, which, however, carries a high mortality.

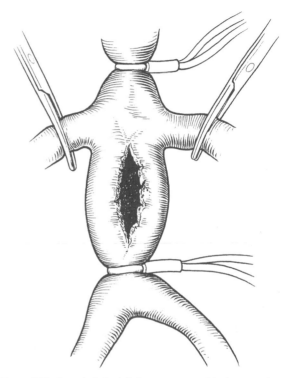

Figure 8.7.5 Control of the inferior vena cava with clamps and two Rumel tourniquets.

Figure 8.7.4 Control of the inferior vena cava using swab pressure.

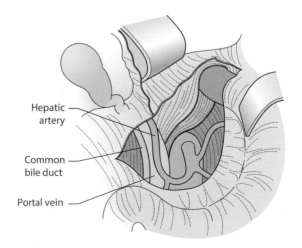

Hepatic artery

Common bile duct

Portal vein

Figure 8.7.6 Access to the portal vein.

8.7.5 SHUNTING

If repair is not possible, or the procedure is being abbreviated, vascular shunting will restore circulation. It can be performed atraumatically and rapidly.

If Javid or other proprietary shunts are available, these can be used. However, if they are not, a shunt can be fashioned from a suitable size of plastic tube, for example nasogastric tube, endotracheal tube, chest tube, etc.:

- The length required is three times the length of the defect.
- The diameter should be two-thirds of the diameter of the vessel to be shunted.

The shunt is fashioned as follows (Figure 8.7.7):

- Choose a plastic tube with the correct diameter.
- Cut the tube to length, as described above, bevelling the edges so that they can be passed into the vessel.
- Tie a length of silk around the tube, dividing it into a one-third to two-thirds ratio.
- Once the vessel has been controlled, using either clamps or Rumel tourniquets:

  · Clamp one end of the shunt to prevent leakage.
  · Pass the 'long' (two-thirds) end of the shunt up the vessel until the shunt is lying inside the vessel lumen or proximally, releasing the tourniquet to allow it to pass through.
- Using the silk as a 'handle', pull the shunt distally into the other end of the vessel.
- Secure it with ties.

There is no need for anticoagulation as the patients are often coagulopathic, and the rate of flow itself should prevent clot formation. The shunt can be left in place for 48–72 hours.

REFERENCES AND RECOMMENDED READING

References

1. Brenner ML, Moore LJ, DuBose JJ, et al. A clinical series of resuscitative endovascular balloon occlusion of the aorta for hemorrhage control and resuscitation. *J Trauma Acute Care Surg.* 2013;75:506–511.
2. Smith WR, Moore EE, Osborn P, et al. Retroperitoneal packing as a resuscitation technique for haemodynamically unstable patients with pelvic fractures: report of two representative cases and a description of technique. *J Trauma.* 2005;59:1510–1514.
3. Reilly PM, Rotondo MF, Carpenter JP, Sherr SA, Schwab CW. Temporary vascular continuity during damage control: intraluminal shunting for proximal superior mesenteric artery injury. *J Trauma.* 1995;39:757–760.
4. Accola KD, Feliciano DV, Mattox KL, Burch JM, Beall AC Jr, Jordan GL Jr. Management of injuries to the superior mesenteric artery. *J Trauma.* 1986;26:313–319.
5. Asensio JA, Britt LD, Borzotta A, et al. Multi-institutional experience with the management of superior mesenteric artery injuries. *J Am Coll Surg.* 2001;193:354–365; discussion 365–366.
6. Donahue TK, Strauch GO. Ligation as definitive management of injury to the superior mesenteric vein. *J Trauma.* 1988;28:541–543.
7. Feliciano DV, Burch JM, Mattox K, Edelman M. Injuries of the inferior vena cava. *Am J Surg.* 1988;156:548–552.
8. Welling DR, Rich NM, Burris DG, Boffard KD, Devries WC. Who was William Ray Rumel? *World J Surg.* 2008;32:2122–2157.
9. Stone HH, Fabian TC, Turkleson ML. Wounds of the portal venous system. *World J Surg.* 1982;6:335–341.

Figure 8.7.7 'Manufacture' and placement of a vascular shunt.

8.8 Urogenital System

8.8.1 **OVERVIEW**

Urogenital trauma refers to injuries to the kidneys, ureters, bladder and urethra, the female reproductive organs in the pregnant and non-pregnant state, and the penis, scrotum and testes.

Death from penetrating bladder trauma was mentioned in Homer's *Iliad*, as well as by Hippocrates and Galen, while Evans and Fowler in 1905 demonstrated that the mortality from penetrating intraperitoneal bladder injuries could be reduced from 100 per cent to 28 per cent with laparotomy and bladder repair. Ambroise Paré observed death following a gunshot wound of the kidney, with haematuria and sepsis, and it was only in 1884 that nephrectomy became the recommended treatment for renal injury.

Haematuria is the hallmark of urological injury, but may be absent even in severe trauma, and a high index of suspicion is then needed, based on the mechanism of injury and the presence of abdominal and pelvic injury.

8.8.2 **RENAL INJURIES**

Injury to the kidney is seen in up to 10 per cent of patients with blunt or penetrating abdominal injuries; however, most cases involve blunt rather than penetrating injury. Serious renal injuries are frequently associated with injuries to other organs, with multiorgan involvement in 80 per cent of patients with penetrating trauma and in 75 per cent of those with blunt trauma.

Haematuria, defined as more than five red blood cells per high-power field, is present in over 95 per cent of patients who sustain renal trauma; however, the absence of haematuria does not preclude significant renal injury.

8.8.2.1 **Diagnosis**

The first investigation is to look for gross haematuria, followed by urinalysis to check for microscopic haematuria.

Up to 30 per cent of patients with serious renal trauma will have no haematuria whatsoever, while the majority of patients with significant abdominal trauma will have microscopic haematuria, often in the absence of relevant renal injury.

The haemodynamic status of the patient will then determine the subsequent steps, for both blunt and penetrating trauma.

8.8.2.1.1 **UNSTABLE PATIENT**

The investigation of choice in unstable patients is immediate surgery.

8.8.2.1.2 **STABLE PATIENT**

Computed tomography (CT) has replaced intravenous urography as the primary modality for the assessment of suspected renal injuries. The investigation of choice is the multiphase, double- or triple-contrast CT scan, but this can misgrade the renal injury. More commonly, however, it does allow grading of renal injuries, and forms the basis for non-operative treatment, possibly up to, and inclusive of, non-vascular grade IV injuries and blunt renal artery thrombosis.

It has been shown that the size of the haematoma can be related to the grade of renal injury, which is a useful correlation in suboptimal studies and where older machines are used.

Contrast-enhanced ultrasound can also allow the visualization of active intrarenal bleeds.

In addition, duplex Doppler ultrasound can allow visualization of arteriovenous fistulas and active intrarenal bleeds.

8.8.2.1.3 **PENETRATING TRAUMA**

The individual trauma centre's accepted method of evaluation of penetrating torso trauma must be used, the renal visualization being provided by an intravenous pyelogram (IVP)/tomogram, followed by angiography if suspicious, or multiphase contrast-enhanced CT scanning of the abdomen as a stand-alone investigation.

8.8.2.1.4 BLUNT TRAUMA

Investigations as above are reserved for children irrespective of urinalysis and adults with frank haematuria or a systolic blood pressure below 90 mm Hg.

8.8.2.2 Renal Injury Scale

Table 8.8.1 outlines the renal injury scale.

8.8.2.3 Management

8.8.2.3.1 UNSTABLE PATIENT

At laparotomy, it will become apparent whether or not the kidneys are the source of the shock. Should a large retroperitoneal haematoma be present in the region of the kidney, the options are to leave the kidney alone at first and perform a single-shot on-table IVP, to assess the functionality of both kidneys, explore the injured kidney immediately or pack the area around the kidney and get out, if in a damage control situation.

A 'single-shot' intravenous urogram can be performed in the emergency room (the patient by definition is too unstable for formal CT scan) by injecting 2 mL/Kg of radiographic contrast medium, followed by a single plain X-ray film of the abdomen, taken 10 minutes after the contrast was injected.

8.8.2.3.2 STABLE PATIENT

8.8.2.3.2.1 Non-operative Management

In recent years, it has been recognized that many renal injuries can be managed without operation, and

angioembolization is a worthwhile option, if the skills are readily available.

In a recent review, 97 patients sustained a kidney injury, 72 from blunt force trauma and 25 from penetrating injury. Of the 72 blunt trauma patients, only 5 patients (7 per cent) underwent urgent nephrectomy, 3 (4 per cent) had repair and/or stenting, and 89 per cent were observed despite a 29 per cent laparotomy rate for associated intra-abdominal injuries. Of the 25 patients with penetrating trauma, 8 (31 per cent) underwent a nephrectomy, 1 had a partial nephrectomy, and 2 underwent renal repairs. Nephrectomy was more likely to be required after penetrating injury and was most likely in severely injured patients with ongoing haemorrhage.

An on-table IVP should be obtained even in the absence of a large haematoma to exclude renal artery thrombosis, followed by exploration with repair or nephrectomy in the persistently unstable patient.

Up to half of renal stab injuries, and up to one-third of gunshot in one series, can be treated non-operatively, as long as excellent diagnostic methods can visualize the injuries.

In principle, management can be guided by the severity of injury, and many patients can be treated non-operatively[1,2].

8.8.2.3.2.1.1 *Grades 1 and 2*

These comprise the majority of renal injuries and can usually be treated non-operatively.

8.8.2.3.2.1.2 *Grade 3*

These comprise major lacerations through the cortex extending to the medulla or collecting system with

Table 8.8.1 Kidney Injury Scale (See also Appendix B: Trauma Scores and Scoring Systems)

Grade[a]	Type of Injury	Description of Injury
I	Contusion	Microscopic or gross haematuria, urological studies normal
	Haematoma	Subcapsular, non-expanding without parenchymal laceration
II	Haematoma	Non-expanding perirenal haematoma confined to the renal retroperitoneum
	Laceration	<1.0-cm parenchymal depth of renal cortex without urinary extravasation
III	Laceration	>1.0-cm parenchymal depth of renal cortex without collecting system rupture or urinary extravasation
IV	Laceration	Parenchymal laceration extending through the renal cortex, medulla and collecting system
	Vascular	Main renal artery or vein injury with contained haemorrhage
V	Laceration	Completely shattered kidney
	Vascular	Avulsion of renal hilum that devascularizes the kidney

[a]Advance one grade for bilateral injuries up to grade III.

Source: Moore EE, Shackford SR, Pachter HL, et al., *J Trauma*, 29(12), 1664–1666, 1989. With permission.

or without urinary extravasation. Drainage may be necessary.

8.8.2.3.2.1.3 *Grade 4*

These are 'catastrophic' injuries, and include multiple renal lacerations and vascular injuries involving the renal pedicle. These injuries often require surgery and may need nephrectomy. The most significant vascular injury following blunt trauma is thrombosis of the main renal artery, caused by deceleration with intimal tear and propagation of thrombus in the renal artery.

> *Partial nephrectomy should not be contemplated in the patient with competing injuries, or potential or actual haemodynamic instability.*

8.8.2.3.2.1.4 *Grade 5*

Pelviureteric junction injuries are a rare consequence of blunt trauma, and are caused by sudden deceleration, which creates tension on the renal pedicle. The diagnosis may be delayed because haematuria is absent in one-third of patients. Pelviureteric junction injuries are classified into two groups: avulsion (complete transection) and laceration (incomplete tear). Nephrectomy is usually required.

8.8.2.4 **Surgical Approach**

Access should be by midline laparotomy, even if isolated renal injury is suspected, since the likelihood of other injuries is always present.

The kidneys are usually explored after dealing with the intra-abdominal emergencies. Ideally, control of the renal pedicle should be obtained before opening Gerota fascia.

A direct approach to suspected peripheral penetrating injuries is advocated by some as being faster and equally safe. A left medial visceral rotation on the left, including division of Gerota fascia and medial rotation of the left kidney, or an extended Kocher manoeuvre on the right can also afford good control of the aorta, inferior vena cava (IVC) and renal vessels, if required.

The right renal artery can be found by dissecting posteriorly between the aorta and the IVC (Figure 8.8.1). Dissection lateral to the IVC may lead to inadvertent isolation of a segmental branch of the right renal artery. The vessels are then controlled by loops to allow rapid occlusion should bleeding occur on opening Gerota

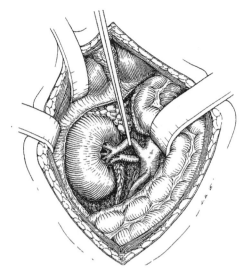

Figure 8.8.1 Access to the right kidney.

fascia. The right renal vein is easily controllable after reflection of the right colon and duodenum, and has to be mobilized to expose the artery. It always should be repaired if possible, because of the lack of collateral venous drainage.

The peritoneum over the aorta is opened, and the anterior wall of the aorta followed up to the left renal vein. After exposing the retroperitoneum from the right or the left, the left renal artery is identified by dissecting upwards on the lateral aspect of the aorta above the inferior mesenteric vein. The left renal vein crosses the aorta just below the level of the origin of the renal arteries (Figures 8.8.2 and 8.8.3).

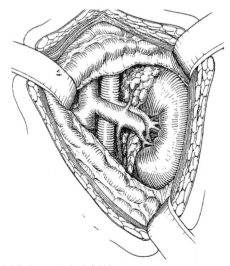

Figure 8.8.2 Access to the left kidney.

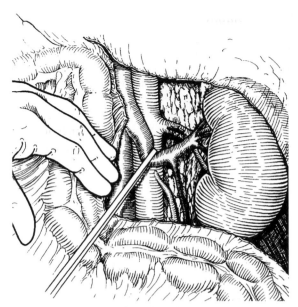

Figure 8.8.3 Access to the left renal vessels.

Access to the left renal artery may also be improved by one of two manoeuvres:

- Ligation of the adrenal, gonadal and lumbar tributaries of the left renal vein will enhance the mobilization of the vein to expose the renal artery.
- Ligation of the distal renal vein at the IVC can improve exposure of the origin of the renal artery. The collateral drainage via the lumbar gonadal and adrenal vessels will be sufficient to deal with the venous drainage on the left (Figure 8.8.4).

After control of the renal pedicle has been obtained, Gerota fascia can be opened or debrided as necessary. Care must be taken not to strip the renal capsule from the underlying parenchyma, as this may bleed profusely. The mobilized kidney now can be examined, debrided, trimmed and sutured with drainage (Figure 8.8.5).

The kidney tolerates a single ischaemic event much better than repeated ischaemic times. However, the maximum

Figure 8.8.4 Division of the left renal vein.

Figure 8.8.5 Techniques of renal repair.

warm ischaemic time that the kidney will tolerate is less than 1 hour, although this can be prolonged by ice packing.

With complete vascular isolation for up to 30 minutes, Gerota fascia is then opened, and the injured kidney debrided by sharp dissection, and sutured or partially amputated. The renal pelvis collecting system should be closed with a running absorbable suture to provide a watertight seal. Nephrectomy will be required in less than 10 per cent of stable patients.

Cover can then be effected using the renal capsule, omentum, meshes, etc., replacing the kidney within Gerota fascia and draining the area with a suction drain until it is draining minimally and urine collections have been excluded.

Nephrostomy tubes or ureteric stents can be used either immediately or at some later time in cases of major renal trauma with extravasation.

8.8.2.5 Adjuncts

- Pledgets: The kidney does not hold sutures well. Care should be taken that the suture is not over-tightened, as it will cut through. The use of pledgets, though not essential, may be helpful.
- Sealants: Urine leakage is common. Tissue sealants can be a useful additional means of sealing the suture line.
- Drains: Whether a nephrectomy or a repair is performed, the high incidence of fluid (urine or blood) mandates the use of a suction drain.

8.8.2.6 Post-operative Care

Urinomas, infected urinomas, perinephric abscesses and delayed bleeding are the most common complications of conservative management and are often amenable to imaging and percutaneous, transureteric or angiographic management. Even when the kidney appears to be shattered into several pieces, drainage of the surrounding urinomas seems to encourage healing and avoid sepsis.

Hypertension (Page kidney) is a rare late complication[3].

8.8.3 URETERIC INJURIES

Significant ureteric injuries are often missed or not picked up until late, after the onset of complications or deterioration in renal function.

8.8.3.1 Diagnosis

Patients with ureteric injury present without even microscopic haematuria in up to 50 per cent of cases, and the injuries are mostly associated with penetrating trauma, although ureteric avulsion and rupture can happen in blunt trauma, especially in the paediatric population. Ureteric injuries may even be missed by high-dose IVP, and a high index of suspicion is essential. Intraoperative recognition may be facilitated by the intravenous or intraureteral injection of indigo carmine or methylene blue.

8.8.3.2 Surgical Approach

The procedures described for access to the retroperitoneal great vessels allow perfect exposure to both ureters. Ureteric injuries are rare, usually due to penetrating trauma, so that local exploration and mobilization of part of the ascending or descending colon alone may be sufficient, depending on the site of injury. Minimal dissection of the periureteric tissues should take place, except at the precise level of injury, in order to preserve the delicate blood supply. Ureteric injuries close to the kidney are accessed by left or right medial visceral rotation as described above. Ureteric injuries near the bladder may be accessed by opening the peritoneal layer in the region and mobilizing the bladder.

8.8.3.2.1 UNSTABLE PATIENTS

Unstable patients require immediate surgery and exploration of the ureter after life-threatening injuries have been dealt with, ideally preceded by one-shot on-table IVP.

If the patient requires an abbreviated laparotomy, the ureteric injury can be safely left alone, stented or ligated until the patient returns to the operating theatre for definitive procedures; indeed, successful repair has frequently been affected after delayed or missed presentation. Percutaneous nephrostomy can be used as a post-operative adjunct for the ligated ureter.

In unstable patients with associated colonic injuries, especially those requiring colectomy, even nephrectomy can be justified.

8.8.3.2.2 STABLE PATIENTS

Stable patients with fresh injuries between the pelvi-ureteric junction and the pelvic brim are treated by end uretero-ureterostomy with spatulation and interrupted suturing over a double-J stent (Figure 8.8.6).

The stent can be safely left *in situ* for 4–6 weeks. It has been suggested that stents can be omitted in injuries requiring minimal debridement, such as stab wounds, but not in gunshot wounds, where stenting results in significantly fewer leaks.

Injuries to the pelviureteric junction and its vicinity are treated in the same fashion, but a tube nephrostomy should be added.

Injuries around the pelvic brim are best treated by uretero-neocystostomy, with an antireflux reimplantation.

More advanced repair methods include the retrocolic transuretero-ureterostomy and the creation of a Boari flap with attached uretero-neocystostomy.

In the case of loss of long segments where anastomosis to the contralateral ureter is not possible, an end-ureterostomy could be brought out, or nephrectomy done in rare cases of serious associated injuries in the area.

Figure 8.8.6 Technique of ureteric repair.

After surgery, the bladder is drained transurethrally, or ideally suprapubically, and closed suction drains can be placed retroperitoneally in proximity to the repaired ureter; these can be expected to drain for a number of days.

8.8.3.3 Complications

Complications comprise stricture with hydronephrosis, leakage from the anastomosis and infected urinomas, especially in late diagnosis, most of which are amenable to percutaneous management.

8.8.4 BLADDER INJURIES

Bladder injuries are mainly due to blunt trauma, and are found in about 8 per cent of pelvic fractures. Penetrating trauma is due to gunshot, stabs, impalement or iatrogenic injuries, mostly in relation to orthopaedic pelvic fixation.

8.8.4.1 Diagnosis

Signs and symptoms vary from inability to void and frank haematuria, to vague abdominal or suprapubic tenderness without haematuria in a small percentage of cases.

Intraperitoneal injuries may be associated with a higher serum creatinine and urea, and low sodium, but this biochemical derangement takes some time to develop. Elevated serum creatinine levels are due to absorption of urine through the peritoneum.

Ultrasound and CT scanning can be of use to demonstrate free fluid in the abdomen, the presence of clots in the bladder and a change in bladder filling and shape (with sonar probe compression). A CT cystogram can be done as part of an abdominal CT study and can differentiate between intra- and extraperitoneal bladder injuries.

Retrograde cystography is the method of choice in the emergency room, as it is very accurate as long as a large enough volume of contrast (about 7 mL/kg) is instilled and at least two separate projections (anteroposterior and lateral views) are obtained. Postmicturition films are essential. A minimum of 350 mL dilute contrast medium should be instilled.

Contrast extravasation will delineate loops of bowel and the peritoneal contours in intraperitoneal ruptures, while it will track along the pelvic bones, scrotum, obturator areas, etc. in extraperitoneal ruptures.

8.8.4.2 Management

Urgent operative treatment is indicated in all intraperitoneal, and some types of extraperitoneal, injuries, while others require delayed surgery upon failure of non-operative methods. The greatest majority of penetrating injuries require immediate surgery.

8.8.4.2.1 NON-OPERATIVE MANAGEMENT

Urethral or suprapubic catheter drainage with a large-bore catheter, for up to 2 weeks, will allow most extraperitoneal injuries from blunt trauma to heal; surgery will be needed only if a cystogram at that stage shows ongoing leakage. Contraindications to non-operative management are bladder neck injury, the presence of bony fragments through the bladder wall, infected urine and associated female genital injuries.

Extraperitoneal bladder repair during a laparotomy for other trauma is often easily accomplished, but may be dangerous if it requires opening into a tamponaded pelvic haematoma, and is inappropriate in the context of damage control.

8.8.4.3 Surgical Approach

Bladders can be repaired easily and with few complications with absorbable sutures.

All repairs should to be carried out through an intraperitoneal approach, from within the lumen of the bladder, after performing an adequate longitudinal incision on the anterior surface in order to avoid entering lateral pelvic haematomas.

The presence and patency of both ureteric orifices must be confirmed in all cases. If suturing in the vicinity, these should be cannulated with a size 5 feeding tube or ureteric catheter.

In cases of gunshot wound, *both* wounds to the bladder must be sought and identified. In some situations, it will be necessary to open the bladder widely, explore and repair from within.

Single-layer mass suturing is indicated in extraperitoneal ruptures, but for intraperitoneal ruptures closure should be in separate layers.

A large-bore transurethral or suprapubic catheter, or both, can be used, the latter being fed extraperitoneally into the bladder, and a drain left in the Retzius space. A cystogram will be done in most cases after 10 days to 2 weeks, followed by removal of the suprapubic catheter.

8.8.5 URETHRAL INJURIES

Urethral injuries can have the most disastrous consequences of all genitourinary trauma, such as incontinence, long-lasting impotence and strictures.

8.8.5.1 Diagnosis

The mechanism of injury, a pelvic fracture and blood at the meatus must alert the surgeon to the possibility of a urethral rupture, mainly of the posterior urethra from blunt trauma.

Rectal examination is mandatory before urethral catheter insertion, and a high-riding prostate will suggest that the urethra is disrupted. Rupture of the female urethra is, fortunately, very uncommon.

Once rupture is suspected, two completely different approaches are practised and acceptable:

- Retrograde urethrography is performed by placing a small Foley catheter in the fossa navicularis, with the patient in the oblique position.
- The preferable approach, however, is not to intervene with an emergency procedure at all. This is particularly important if a pelvic haematoma is present, due to the risk of effectively causing a compound injury. It is preferable to place a suprapubic catheter (it will be necessary to allow the bladder to fill until it is palpable) prior to the insertion of the suprapubic catheter. A cystogram and, if necessary, cystoscopy can then be done under controlled circumstances at a later stage.

8.8.5.2 Management

8.8.5.2.1 SUPRAPUBIC CYSTOSTOMY

The mainstay of immediate treatment is the placement of a suprapubic catheter for urinary drainage. This can be done as an isolated open procedure, as an open procedure during a laparotomy, or using a percutaneous method. The isolated open method requires a lower midline laparotomy incision, and an intra-peritoneal approach to the bladder to avoid entering a pelvic haematoma. Suprapubic placement during a laparotomy done for other reasons follows the same principles.

Percutaneous placement is done using specifically designed trochar and catheter kits.

The procedure requires a full bladder, as identified clinically or on ultrasound. If this is not the case, and the patient is not in a condition to produce a lot of urine, a small intravenous catheter can be placed under ultra-sonic guidance using the Seldinger technique, and the bladder can then be distended with saline until a standard percutaneous method can be used.

8.8.5.3 **Ruptured Urethra**

Urethral injuries are most often associated with pelvic fractures, especially anterior arch fractures with displacement. Although blood at the urethral meatus, gross haematuria and displacement of the prostate are signs of urethral disruption, their absence does not exclude urethral injury.

The male urethra is divided into two portions:

- The *posterior urethra* is made up of the *prostatic* urethra and the *membranous* urethra, which courses between the prostatic apex and the perineal membrane.

  The membranous urethra is prone to injury from pelvic fracture because the puboprostatic ligaments fix the apex of the prostate gland to the bony pelvis, and shearing forces are applied to the urethra when the pelvis is disrupted.

- The *anterior urethra* is distal to that point. It is susceptible to blunt force injuries along its path in the perineum (such as from direct blows or fall-astride injuries).

The conventional treatment for urethral injury is to divert the urinary stream with a suprapubic catheter and refer to a specialist centre for delayed reconstruction of the urethral injury. Early endoscopic realignment (within 1 week of injury) using a combined transurethral and percutaneous transvesical approach is advocated by some experts.

Anterior urethral trauma may present late, with symptoms of urethral stricture.

8.8.5.3.1 URETHRAL REPAIR

Immediate surgical intervention is recommended for the following conditions:

- All penetrating injuries of the posterior urethra and most of the anterior urethra.
- Posterior urethral injuries associated with rectal injuries and bladder neck injuries.
- Where there is wide separation of the ends of the urethra.
- Penile fracture.

Accurate approximation and end-to-end anastomosis are recommended for injuries to the anterior urethra, while for membranous urethra injuries, realignment and stenting over a Foley catheter for 3 or 4 weeks may be sufficient. This can be achieved by an open lower midline laparotomy and passage of Foley catheters from above and below, with ultimate passage into the bladder, or via flexible cystoscopy and manipulation.

Patients managed with a suprapubic catheter alone should have their definitive urethral repair after about 3 months from the injury.

> *Primary realignment may have better results than delayed repair, but delayed primary repair (day 8 to 10) is recommended when there is a large haematoma.*

8.8.6 **INJURY TO THE SCROTUM**

8.8.6.1 **Diagnosis**

Ultrasound of the scrotum is indicated in evaluation of blunt trauma to the testicle, and can differentiate between torsion, disruption and haematoma.

8.8.6.2 **Management**

The blood supply to the scrotum is so good that penetrating trauma usually can be treated by debridement and suturing.

If the tunica vaginalis of the testis is disrupted, the extruding seminiferous tubules should be trimmed off and the capsule closed as soon as possible, in order to minimize host reaction against the testis.

Loss of scrotal skin with exposed testicle, a well-described occurrence after burns and other trauma, often can be remedied by the creation of pouches in the proximal thigh skin and subsequent approximation, with little effect on the testicles.

8.8.7 GYNAECOLOGICAL INJURY AND SEXUAL ASSAULT

Any evidence of gynaecological injury requires external and internal examination using a speculum, and exclusion of associated urethral and anorectal injuries. If rape is suspected or reported, the official sexual assault evidence collection kit should be used, and detailed clinical notes should be made. The patient must be counselled, and informed consent must, where possible, be obtained for *all* examinations.

Reporting of all cases of sexual assault should be carried out by the treating physician, in order to minimize under-reporting by the already traumatized patient.

8.8.7.1 Management

Lacerations of the external genitalia and vagina can be sutured under local or general anaesthesia, and a vaginal pack left in for 24 hours to minimize the swelling.

Intrapelvic organs are dealt with at laparotomy by suturing, hysterectomy or oophorectomy. Oxytocin is used to minimize uterine bleeding and colostomy to avoid soiling.

Additional supportive care for the psychological effects of sexual assault should be made available.

Antiretroviral treatment is more effective if instituted within 3 hours of injury, and sexually transmitted disease and pregnancy prophylaxis should be given according to standard protocols. Baseline blood tests required include human immunodeficiency virus (HIV) status, hepatitis B, full blood count, and liver and renal function; follow-up arrangements must be made to monitor medication and HIV status.

8.8.8 INJURY OF THE PREGNANT UTERUS

Aggressive resuscitation of the mother and the fetus must be carried out in keeping with Advanced Trauma Life Support recommendations. Midline laparotomy always should be used when surgery is necessary, but simple intra-uterine death is best managed by induced labour at a later stage.

REFERENCES AND RECOMMENDED READING

References

1. Armenakas NA. Duckett CP, McAninch JW. Indications for nonoperative management of renal stab wounds. *J Urol.* 1999;16:768–771.
2. Velmahos GC, Demetriades D, Cornwell EE 3rd, et al. Selective management of renal gunshot wounds. *Br J Surg.* 1998;85:1121–1124.
3. Montgomery RC, Richardson JD, Harty JI. Posttraumatic renovascular hypertension after occult renal injury. *J Trauma.* 1998;45:106–110.

Recommended Reading

Morey AF, Brandes S, Dugi III DD, et al. Urotrauma: AUA Guideline. Linthicum, MD: American Urological Association Education and Research Inc; 2014.

Santucci RA, Bartley JM. Urologic trauma guidelines: A 21st century update. *Nat Rev Urol.* 2010;7:510–519.

Santucci RA, Wessels H, Bartsch G, et al. Evaluation and management of renal injuries: consensus statement of the Renal Trauma Subcommittee. *Br J Urol Int.* 2004;93:937–954.

RENAL INJURIES

Coburn M. Genitourinary trauma. In: Mattox KL, Moore EE, Feliciano DV, eds. *Trauma*, 7th ed. New York, NY: McGraw-Hill; 2013:669–708.

El Khader K, Bouchot O, Mhidia A, Guille F, Lobel B, Buzelin JM. Injuries of the renal pedicle: is renal revascularization justified? *Prog Urol.* 1998;8:995–1000.

Gonzales RP, Falimirski M, Holevar MR, Evankovich C. Surgical management of renal trauma: is vascular control necessary? *J Trauma.* 1999;47:1039–1044.

Hammer CC, Santucci RA. Effect of an institutional policy of non-operative treatment of grades I–IV renal injuries. *J Urol.* 2003 May:169(5):1751–1753.

Meng MV, Brandes SB, McAnich JW. Renal trauma: indications and techniques for surgical exploration. *World J Urol.* 1999;17:71–77.

Velmahos GC, Constantinou C, Tilou A, et al. Abdominal computed tomographic scan for patients with gunshot wounds to the abdomen selected for non-operative management. *J Trauma.* 2005 Nov;59(5):1156–1160; discussion 1160–1161.

Velmahos GC, Degiannis E. The management of urinary tract injuries after gunshot wounds of the anterior and posterior abdomen. *Injury.* 1997;28:535–538.

URETERIC INJURIES

Armenakas NA. Current methods of diagnosis and management of ureteral injuries. *World J Urol.* 1999;17:78–83.

Velmahos GC, Degiannis E, Wells M, Souter I. Penetrating ureteral injuries: the impact of associated injuries on management. *Am Surg.* 1996;62:461–468.

BLADDER

Haas CA, Brown SL, Spirnak JP. Limitations of routine spiral computerized tomography in the evaluation of bladder trauma. *J Urol.* 1999;162:50–52.

Volpe MA, Pachter EM, Scalea TM, Macchia RJ, Mydlo JH. Is there a difference in outcome when treating traumatic intraperitoneal bladder rupture with or without a suprapubic tube? *J Urol.* 1999;161:1103–1105.

SCROTUM

Chang AJ, Brandes SB. Advances in diagnosis and management of genital injuries. *Urol Clin North Am.* 2013;40:427.

Cline KJ, Mata JA, Venable DD, Eastham JA. Penetrating trauma to the male external genitalia. *J Trauma.* 1998;44:492–494.

Munter DW, Faleski EJ. Blunt scrotal trauma: emergency department evaluation and management. *Am J Emerg Med.* 1989;7:227–234.

The Pelvis 9

9.1 INTRODUCTION

Fractured pelvis is a surgical problem, since 65 per cent of patients with a fractured pelvis suffer associated injuries, and mortality is largely due to haemorrhage and infections in pelvic soft tissues. Both can lead to multiple organ failure.

Although mortality following severe pelvic fractures has decreased dramatically with better methods of controlling haemorrhage, these patients still represent a significant challenge to every link of the treatment chain. Mortality rates exceeding 40 per cent have recently been reported. Further, pelvic bleeding as one of the 'hidden bleeding sources' is still underestimated or missed as retrospective charts analyses of potentially preventable death are revealed. Extreme force is required to disrupt the pelvic ring, and associated injuries and extrapelvic bleeding sources are common. The haemodynamically unstable patient with severe pelvic fracture has a 90 per cent risk of associated injuries, a 50 per cent risk of extrapelvic bleeding sources and a 30 per cent risk of intra-abdominal bleeding.

To save these patients, three questions need to be addressed:

- Is the patient at high risk of massive bleeding?
- What are the sources of bleeding?
- How can the bleeding be stopped?

All sources of bleeding need to be identified and controlled. The decisions are made on an individual basis, taking into account the patient's status, the injury pattern, the available resources and the surgeon's experience in dealing with these complex injuries. Identification of a pelvic injury as bleeding source is a mandatory step in the primary survey of the Advanced Trauma Life Support (ATLS). The identification of an unstable pelvic fracture and the compression of the pelvis by an external compression device ('reduce the pelvic volume') are potentially life-saving procedures that have to be done in the emergency room. Severe pelvic injuries require a multidisciplinary team involving trauma-trained general surgeons and interventional radiologists, as well as orthopaedic surgeons. If adequate orthopaedic experience is unavailable, consideration should be given towards early transfer of this patient to an institution with the necessary expertise, as soon as the patient's condition allows.

9.2 ANATOMY

The surgical anatomy of the pelvis is key to the pathogenesis of pelvic injuries:

- The pelvic inlet is circular, a structure that is immensely strong, but routinely gives way at more than one point should sufficient force be applied to it. Therefore, isolated fractures of the anterior or posterior pelvic ring are rather uncommon – look for the disruption of the posterior pelvic ring.
- The forces required to fracture the pelvic ring do not respect the surrounding organ systems.
- The pelvis has a rich collateral blood supply, especially across the sacrum and posterior part of the ileum. The cancellous bone of the pelvis also has an excellent blood supply. Most pelvic haemorrhage emanates from venous injury and fracture sites. However, in the haemodynamically unstable patient with severe pelvic injury, arterial bleeding is frequent (50–80 per cent). Important for the treatment is that the surgeon has to deal with arterial *and* venous bleeding.
- Post-mortem examination has shown that the pelvic peritoneum that 'should' tamponade pelvic haematomas can accommodate more than 3000 mL. However, in case of severe pelvic fractures where the retroperitoneal compartment

is disrupted, and the external bony barrier is not stable, haematoma may extend upward toward the mediastinum ('chimney effect') or downward into the medial thigh in case of rupture of the pelvic floor.

- All iliac vessels, the sciatic nerve roots, including the lumbosacral nerve, and the ureters that cross the sacroiliac joint and disruption of this joint may cause severe haemorrhage, and sometimes causes arterial obstruction of the iliac artery and nerve palsy. Fortunately, injuries to the ureters are rare.
- The pelvic viscera are suspended from the bony pelvis by condensations of the endopelvic fascia. Shear forces acting on the pelvis will transmit these to pelvic viscera, leading to avulsion and shearing injuries.
- The pelvis also features the acetabulum, a major structure in weight transfer to the leg. Inappropriate treatment will lead to severe disability.

9.3 CLASSIFICATION

The different classification systems are all based on grade of fracture stability, and close correlation with risk of bleeding has been shown. However, no fracture pattern can exclude significant haemorrhage. Pelvic ring fractures can be classified into three types, using the Tile classification[1,2], based on their severity.

9.3.1 Type A

This involves isolated fracture of the iliac wing or pubic rami, mostly caused by direct compression (Figure 9.1). These are stable fractures, to be treated conservatively.

9.3.2 Type B

These fractures (Figure 9.2) are subdivided into the following:

- *Type B1*: This occurs less commonly, and is a lateral compression-type injury, which results in an intrinsically stable fracture of the pelvic ring, with an impression of the posterior complex in the sacral bone and mostly a fracture of the pubic arch. Perforation of the bladder can be caused by the anterior fracture, as can hypovolaemic shock due to severe disruption of the soft tissues of the pelvic

Figure 9.1 Tile classification: type A fracture.

Figure 9.2 Tile classification: type B fracture.

diaphragm; organ injury to the lower urogenital tract and rectum can be seen in these cases.

- *Type B2*: This is the most common type of fracture, also known as an 'open book' fracture. There is horizontal (rotational) instability due to an anterior lesion (disruption of the symphysis and/or fracture of the superior and inferior pubic rami) combined with a posterior disruption of the anterior *or* posterior ligaments of the sacroiliac joint. It can result in bleeding in an enlarged pelvic cavity. Injury of the lower urogenital tract, rectum and vagina and severe soft tissue damage due to the rotation are frequently seen in these cases. Internal or external stabilization is required.

9.3.3 Type C

In this type (Figure 9.3), there is complete horizontal and vertical instability, due to anterior and posterior fractures and/or disruptions (complete sacroiliac disruption or displaced vertical sacral fracture). A fall from height and anteroposterior shearing forces in a dashboard

Figure 9.3 Tile classification: type C fracture.

impact in a motor vehicle accident result in this type of fracture. Type C fracture is the result of major mechanical forces and is associated with major blood loss and related injuries within the pelvis (bladder, urethra, rectum, vagina, sciatic and femoral nerve, and iliac vein and artery).

In both types B and C pelvic injuries, there is a high risk of associated abdominal injuries (bowel perforation or mesenteric laceration) and laceration of the diaphragm.

9.4 CLINICAL EXAMINATION AND DIAGNOSIS

Pelvic fractures should be easily identified if ATLS guidelines are followed (i.e. clinical palpation of the pelvic brim from the sacroiliac [SI] joint to pubic symphysis and a routine chest X-ray and pelvic X-ray for any blunt injury in a patient unable to walk). In the absence of X-ray facilities, a clinical examination can be performed with gentle bimanual palpation of the brim of the pelvis from the SI joints to the pubic symphysis. Any palpable defect or boggy swelling is indicative of a pelvic disruption. In the absence of these signs, gentle bimanual lateral and anteroposterior compression (not distraction) of the pelvis can be performed. Any instability felt indicates the presence of major pelvic instability, associated with life-threatening blood loss, requiring appropriate measures. The absence of clinical instability does not, however, preclude an unstable pelvic fracture. One-third of such trauma victims with pelvic ring fractures sustain circulatory instability on arrival. Focussed abdominal sonography for trauma (FAST) may be unreliable as it does not exclude intra-abdominal bleeding in these patients. Upon recognition of an unstable pelvis, immediate external compression by pelvic sheeting is mandatory.

Inspection of the skin may reveal lacerations in the groin, perineum or sacral area, indicating an open pelvic fracture, the result of gross deformation. Evidence of perineal injury or haematuria mandates radiological evaluation of the urinary tract from below upward (retrograde urethrogram followed by cystogram or computed tomography [CT] cystogram, followed by an excretory urogram as appropriate) when the physiology allows. Inspection of the urethral meatus may reveal a drop of blood, indicating urethral rupture. There seems to be little evidence to support the fear of converting partial urethral rupture into a complete rupture by gently trying to insert a Foley catheter. Urological tract imaging is mandated if you cannot pass a catheter easily with the return of clear urine. Blood at the meatus or a high riding prostate should have raised the alert and the most highly skilled person available utilized to insert an indwelling catheter with great care. Inability to pass the catheter easily mandates a cystourethrogram to define the suspected urethral injury. If there is resistance, the patient should have a suprapubic catheter inserted.

Inspection of the anus may reveal lacerations of the sphincter mechanism. Diligent rectal examination may reveal blood in the rectum, and/or discontinuity of the rectal wall, indicating a rectal laceration. In male patients, the prostate is palpated; a high-riding prostate indicates a complete urethral avulsion. A full neurological examination is performed of the perineal area, sphincter mechanism and femoral and sciatic nerves.

The CT scanner is the diagnostic modality of choice in the haemodynamically stable patient, and CT angiography is particularly helpful.

9.5 RESUSCITATION

The priorities for resuscitating patients with pelvic fractures are no different from the standard. These injuries produce a real threat to the circulation, and management is geared towards controlling this threat.

Management is based on haemodynamic status. The patient is either haemodynamically normal, haemodynamically stable (maintaining output due to ongoing resuscitation) or haemodynamically unstable. Because of the capacity of the pelvis to continue to bleed, these patients require urgent control of haemorrhage. These patients tend to exsanguinate rapidly, and immediate measures are required to control bleeding. Most contemporary treatment protocols rely on stabilization and interventional radiology, alone or in combination. Other (damage control) options are needed for the unstable exsanguinating patient and when angiography is unavailable.

The treatment options also depend on the resources available in the individual trauma system. Interventional angiography has to be available within 30 minutes for such cases which cannot be guaranteed even in all modern trauma systems.

Since pelvic bleeding is commonly associated with traumatic coagulopathy, early blood and coagulation factor substitution is mandatory. Volume resuscitation should be based on blood and blood products to prevent further dilutive coagulopathy.

9.5.1 Haemodynamically Normal Patients

There is usually an isolated injury possibly requiring external or internal (open) reduction and fixation to limit future instability and disability. The management is not critically urgent and can be done either as immediate surgery in cases of isolated injury or in a delayed fashion with the first week after trauma.

9.5.2 Haemodynamically Stable Patients

Patients responding to initial volume resuscitation need external stabilization of the pelvic ring. Three principal methods for external stabilization of the pelvic ring exist:

- External compression by circumferential wrap with standard hospital draw sheets or special devices such as the SAM Sling or traumatic pelvic orthotic device (T-POD). Such devices are applied in the emergency room (ER) or in some trauma systems even in a preclinical setting. It is important to centre the compression at the level of the greater trochanters.
- External compression devices such as sheets or T-Pod are easy to place; however, they give less stability to the bony pelvis than external fixator or a C-clamp. In addition, access to the abdomen or the femoral vessels is limited. Also intensive care unit (ICU) nursing is hampered by such devices. Therefore, the surgeon should consider replacing the sheet or T-Pod in the operating room (OR) with, for example, an external fixator.
- External fixators can be applied over the iliac crest or in the supra-acetabular region of the iliac bone. The latter may be technically more difficult to apply; however, it gives significantly more stability to the pelvic ring. An external fixator on the iliac crest may even dislodge a sacral fracture. Therefore the supra-acetabular external fixator should be preferred.
- The pelvic C-clamp, applied close to the level of the sacroiliac joint, is most effective in providing pelvic compression. The application may be more difficult and cannot be performed in cases with dorsal iliac bone fractures. A pelvic X-ray needs to be done before application of a C-clamp.

If patients continue to bleed after external fixation in the OR, additional bleeding control needs to be done either by interventional angiography or pelvic packing, as described below.

9.5.3 Haemodynamically Unstable Patients

Severely disrupted pelvic fracture may present as the classical non-responder to any volume or blood restoration. Because of the capacity of the pelvis to bleed, these patients require urgent control of haemorrhage. These patients tend to exsanguinate rapidly, and immediate measures are required to control bleeding. Applying a pelvic binder or sheet at the level of the greater trochanters is often effective and less time-consuming than using the external fixator or the C-clamp, immediately followed by bleeding control. In a type C fracture, any vertical displacement should be reduced by applying and maintaining traction to the leg on the side of the cranially displaced hemipelvis before binding the pelvis together.

Depending on the available resources either external fixation and extra peritoneal pelvic packing or interventional angioembolization is the next choice for bleeding control. Angioembolization is only a choice if any other bleeding sources are excluded or do not need surgical interventions. Angioembolization normally demands access to the femoral artery on the contralateral side of the main fracture. This access is limited by some external fixation devices and their removal in the angiography suite is not possible. Under these considerations, extra peritoneal packing is a reasonable alternative especially since it can be performed independently of special resources. Principally both techniques for bleeding control do not exclude each other but rather may complement each other. Persistent bleeding after packing may require angioembolization and vice versa.

Interventional balloon occlusion of the infra-renal aorta has been performed in clinical studies. However, so far clinical results are not encouraging.

9.5.4 Laparotomy

If the patient is exsanguinating or requires surgery for other injuries, or angiography is delayed or unavailable, it is prudent to perform a laparotomy to treat or exclude intra-abdominal bleeding. If a major source of bleeding is the pelvis, consider extraperitoneal pelvic packing, which should preferably be performed *first* (i.e. before the laparotomy). Packing of the pelvis will be most effective against a stabilized pelvis. If pelvic bleeding persists, direct exploration with suturing or ligature of lacerations of major blood vessels may be required.

In the exsanguinating patient, immediate control of any arterial haemorrhage can be achieved by aortic clamping. However, 85 per cent of bleeding is venous in origin, and can generally be controlled with packing. In the unstable patient, consider damage control surgery (DCS). Other sources of intra-abdominal bleeding must be excluded. Most can wait until the patient has been physiologically corrected.

- Temporary closure of the abdominal wall is preferable, ideally using a negative-pressure (sandwich) technique.
- Angiography should be performed after DCS for control of any remaining pelvic bleeding by embolization of the bleeding vessels. Extraperitoneal pelvic packing should be considered.

In the more stable patient, if bleeding persists, explore the pelvis and tamponade the area, with suturing or ligature of lacerations of the major blood vessels, repair of anatomical structures (bladder and rectum) where possible and cystostomy and/or colostomy with rectal wash-out as required. If it is required and possible at this stage, undertake internal fixation of the pelvic ring.

After the initial haemorrhage has been controlled, general DCS principles apply, and the patient is returned to the operating room for definitive surgery when physiology has been restored (36–48 hours). Making a plan for definitive surgery and further wound management is a multidisciplinary task. A caveat of pack removal is that the longer the packs are left in, the greater the risk of pelvic sepsis. Definitive internal fixation of the pelvis is ideally performed early, but timing will obviously depend on the physiology.

Formal treatment protocols for pelvic injuries have been shown to decrease mortality and should be developed in every hospital treating pelvic injuries.

Requirements for blood average 15 units for open pelvic fractures. To avoid dilutional coagulopathy, protocols for massive transfusion should be instituted. Volume replacement is ultimately only an adjunct to the treatment of haemorrhagic shock – stopping the bleeding. Thromboelastography is invaluable in monitoring and correcting any coagulopathies that may arise.

9.6 **PELVIC PACKING**

A total of 85 per cent of pelvic bleeding is venous, arising from the multiple venous plexuses around the pelvis.

This bleeding is usually not controllable by embolization. However, pelvic packing, if performed properly with a stabilized pelvic ring, will be able to control venous and arterial bleeding.

Extraperitoneal packing was first described in 1985 by Pohleman[2], and the technique was further described by Ertel in 2001[3] and Smith in 2005[4]. The original technique was more aggressive, but the current technique stops below or medial to the external iliac vessels at the pelvic brim.

European guidelines recommend pelvic packing as a first choice (although with a low level of recommendation)[5] with the actual Eastern Association for the Surgery of Trauma (EAST) guideline suggesting angio-embolization as the treatment of choice for the bleeding pelvis[6]. Comparative studies will not contribute further evidence to this debate. Therefore, the availability of the necessary resources in the local trauma system will influence the surgeon's decision in this context.

If the source of the bleeding is in doubt, or FAST or diagnostic peritoneal lavage (DPL) results are positive, it is wise to perform an exploratory laparotomy to treat or rule out intra-abdominal bleeding. In the presence of a large or expanding pelvic haematoma, extraperitoneal pelvic packing should be performed by grabbing the edges of the peritoneum and entering the preperitoneal space from the midline.

If other sources of bleeding have been ruled out, the extraperitoneal pelvic packing can be done without entering the abdomen via a lower midline suprapubic incision.

9.6.1 **Technique of Extraperitoneal Packing**

- The patient is positioned supine, and, if necessary, to provide a firm surface to pack against, an anterior external fixator with bilateral single supra-acetabular pins and external fixator or C-clamp is applied.
- A 5-cm midline suprapubic incision is made, and the fascia anterior to the rectus muscle is exposed.
- The fascia is divided until the symphysis can be palpated directly (the pre-peritoneal plane has been reached). The fascia is divided in the midline, protecting against urinary bladder damage. From the symphysis, the pelvic brim is followed laterally and posterior to the sacroiliac joint (first bony irregularity felt), first on the side of major bleeding (most often the side of sacroiliac joint disruption).

- The bladder and rectum are then held to the opposite side while the plane is opened bluntly down to the pelvic floor, avoiding injury to vascular and nerve structures in the area.
- The space is then packed with vascular or abdominal swabs, starting posteriorly and distal to the tip of the sacrum, and building the packs cranially and anteriorly.
- The procedure is then repeated on the opposite side.
- Packing a pelvis efficiently implies also addressing arterial bleeding. This requires applying force while packing. In an unbroken pelvis with an intact pelvic floor, one should be able to accommodate three large abdominal swabs on each side. In severe pelvic fractures, efficient packing might require much more (over 10 packs not being unusual). The number of packs needed is defined by the available space and the appropriate force applied.
- Closure is by using standard DCS techniques including negative-pressure dressings.

As in the abdomen, the packs should be removed after 24–48 hours.

9.7 ASSOCIATED INJURIES

Associated injuries can only be managed once the patient is haemodynamically stable. Procedures for damage control may be the only available option.

9.7.1 Head Injuries

These are the most commonly associated major injuries. It is worthwhile remembering that 'C' precedes 'D' during resuscitation and management: the CT scan and neurosurgical procedures have to wait for haemodynamic stability, and haemodynamic stability may be achieved only after DCS.

9.7.2 Intra-abdominal Injuries

These are frequently masked by pelvic pain. Retroperitoneal haematomas may break through into the peritoneal cavity, causing a false-positive result on FAST or DPL. In the presence of a pelvic fracture, CT scanning is the diagnostic modality of choice in the stable patient. In all other patients, diagnostic ultrasound is preferred. If open diagnostic peritoneal lavage is performed, the entry point should be above the umbilicus

to avoid entering extraperitoneal haematomas tracking up the anterior abdominal wall. A low threshold should be maintained for laparotomy because of associated intraperitoneal injury.

9.7.3 Bladder Injuries

Bladder injuries (see also Section 8.8.4) are the most common accompanying injury of pelvic fractures. It is important to distinguish between extraperitoneal and intraperitoneal bladder injuries. While intraperitoneal bladder injuries demand primary surgical repair, extraperitoneal bladder injuries can be handled nonsurgically only by suprapubic catheters.

9.7.4 Urethral Injuries

Urethral injuries (see also Section 8.8.5) should be managed conservatively. Primary urethral repair by cystoperineal traction sutures results in minimal disability in the hands of experts when performed immediately in stable patients. For the majority, suprapubic cystostomy (preferably under ultrasonic guidance) and delayed urethral repair are required.

9.7.5 Anorectal Injuries

Injuries of the anus and rectum are managed according to the degree of damage to the sphincters and anorectal mucosa. Injuries superficial to these require only debridement and dressings. Deep injuries require colostomy and drainage (presacral drainage is *not* required and may disrupt the nervous plexuses). There is doubt about the benefit of prograde wash-out of the rectum due to the risk of pelvic infection introduced by washing faeces into the pelvic cavity. Careful mechanical cleansing of the rectum, wash-out via a wide-bore tube after gentle anal dilatation and adequate debridement performed in a stable patient makes common sense. Sphincter repair is best left for the experts, but repeated debridement and early approximation of mucosa to skin should limit infection and scarring.

9.8 COMPOUND PELVIC INJURIES

Complex pelvic fractures with open pelvic injury can be the most difficult of all injuries to treat. Initially, they can cause devastating haemorrhage and may later be associated with overwhelming pelvic sepsis and distant multiple organ failure.

9.8.1 **Diagnosis**

For those patients who present with compound pelvic fractures and are haemodynamically stable, diagnostic studies such as plain films of the pelvis, three-dimensional CT scans and CT angiography should be rapidly carried out.

9.8.2 **Surgery**

All patients with open (compound) pelvic fractures should be taken to the operating room as soon as the necessary diagnostic studies have been carried out. Stabilization of pelvic bleeding can be temporarily achieved by packing the open wound and then making the decision of whether or not to obtain a pelvic arteriogram (which will be positive in 15 per cent of cases), or to move rapidly to external fixation of the anterior pelvis and consideration for posterior stabilization as well. These decisions are made on an individual basis, taking into account the patient's status, the injury pattern and the surgeon's experience in dealing with these complex injuries.

Based on location of the injury, colostomy may be required in order to prevent contamination of the wound in the post-injury period. In general, all injuries involving the perineum and perianal area should have a diverting colostomy. However, in the damage control situation, contamination must be controlled (if necessary by temporary occlusion), but establishment of a colostomy should be postponed until the patient's physiology has returned to normal.

All vaginal injuries should be explored under a general anaesthetic. Vaginal lacerations should be managed as follows:

- High lesions should be repaired and closed.
- Lower lesions should be packed.

9.9 **SUMMARY**

In summary, a haemodynamically normal patient can be safely transferred for stabilization of unstable fractures within hours after injury and following control of the associated damage:

- Associated injuries can only be managed once the patient is haemodynamically stable.
- Procedures for damage control may be the only available option.
- External stabilization of the pelvic ring is the basis of all treatments.
- Correction coagulopathy and blood restoration is the second step and a prerequisite for the creation of a stable clot in the retroperitoneum.
- If necessary further bleeding control can be achieved either by angioembolization or extraperitoneal packing.
- Packing controls both venous and arterial bleeding, while angioembolization only addresses arterial bleeders.
- Most associated injuries can be managed once the patient is haemodynamically stable.
- Extraperitoneal packing should be performed prior to opening the abdomen, where possible.

REFERENCES AND RECOMMENDED READING

References

1. Tile M. Acute pelvic fractures: causation and classification. *J Am Acad Orthop Surg.* 1996;4:143–151.
2. Pohleman T, Gänsslen A, Bosch U, Tscherne H. The technique of packing for control of haemorrhage in complex pelvic fractures. *Tech Orthop.* 1995;9:267–270.
3. Ertel W, Keel M, Eid K, Platz A, Trentz O. Control of severe haemorrhage using C-clamp and pelvic packing in multiply injured patients with pelvic ring disruption. *J Orthop Trauma.* 2001;15:468–474.
4. Smith WR, Moore EE, Osborn P, et al. Retroperitoneal packing as a resuscitation technique for haemodynamically unstable patients with pelvic fractures: report of two representative cases and a description of technique. *J Trauma.* 2005;59:1510–1514.
5. Cullinane DC, Schiller HJ, Zielinski MD et al. Eastern Association for the Surgery of Trauma Practice management guidelines for haemorrhage in pelvic fracture - update and systematic review. *J Trauma.* 2011;71(6):1850-68.

6. Cullinane DC, Schiller HJ, Zielinski MD, et al. Eastern Association for the Surgery of Trauma Practice Management Guidelines for hemorrhage in pelvic fracture—update and systematic review. *J Trauma*. 2011;71(6):1850–1868.

Recommended Reading

Brohi K, Management of exsanguinating pelvis injuries. An algorithm for the management of exsanguinating pelvic trauma. London, UK; May 20, 2008. http://www.trauma.org/index.php/main/article/668/.

Fry RD. Anorectal trauma and foreign bodies. *Surg Clin North Am*. 1994;74:1491–1506.

Velmahos GC. The pelvis. In: Mattox KL Moore EE, Feliciano DV, eds. *Trauma*, 7th ed. New York, NY: McGraw-Hill; 2004:655–668.

Extremity Trauma **10**

10.1 OVERVIEW

Extremity injuries often look dramatic and occur in 85 per cent of patients who sustain blunt trauma, but they rarely cause a threat to life or limb. However, in some circumstances, the relevance of such injuries assumes major importance.

Fractures of the bony skeleton may occur in isolation or as part of multiple injuries. Catastrophic external bleeding, mostly in the military setting due to gunshot wounds (GSWs) and explosive devices, will lead directly to hypovolaemic shock. In the c-A-B-C concept, circulation control ('c') will be applied by a combat applied tourniquet (CAT) in the prehospital setting, even before airway control.

Multiple fractures, especially femoral shaft fractures, contribute to hypovolaemia as well. The possibility must be borne in mind when there are multiple long bone fractures associated with vascular damage, and non-visible but ongoing bleeding is occurring. Where this is the case, and direct control of the bleeding is not possible, a timely and appropriately applied tourniquet may buy time to stabilize the patient and treat other life-threatening injuries.

10.2 MANAGEMENT OF SEVERE INJURY TO THE EXTREMITY

The primary survey and resuscitation must take priority.

10.2.1 Life-saving Measures

- Notice ongoing external bleeding and control it (pressure bandage, tourniquet).
- Exclude or detect other bleeding sources.

10.2.2 Limb-saving Measures

- Rapidly assess limb injuries, making careful note of distal perfusion.
- Involve the orthopaedic and plastic surgeons early.
- Restore impaired circulation.
- Cover open wounds with a sterile dressing, and give tetanus toxoid and antibiotic prophylaxis.
- Debride non-viable tissue.
- Restore skeletal stability.
- Achieve wound closure and commence rehabilitation.

A fracture is a soft tissue injury in which broken bone is present. (Unknown)

It is important to remember that a fracture is not a separate entity from the soft tissue damage that accompanies it – it is simply an extension of the soft tissue injury that involves bone, and the principles of management are the same.

During the past two decades, a better understanding of the individual injuries, and technical advances in diagnostic evaluation and surgery (allowing revascularization of the extremity, stabilization of the complex fracture and reconstruction of the soft tissues), medicine and rehabilitation have led to an increased frequency of attempts at limb salvage. In some of these patients, however, limb salvage may have subsequent deleterious results, being associated with a high morbidity and a poor prognosis and often requiring late amputation (27–70 per cent) despite initial success. In these, early or primary ablation might even be beneficial. Especially in the elderly, significant co-morbidity (diabetes, pre-existent limb ischaemia, smoking) should be included in decision making as well.

The management of the mangled limb remains a vexing problem and should thus be multidisciplinary and involve the combined skills of the orthopaedic, vascular, plastic and reconstructive surgeons, as well as the rehabilitation specialist. Poorly coordinated management often results in more complications, increased duration of treatment and a less favourable outcome for the patient. Ultimately, the decision to amputate or repair is often a difficult one, and best shared, if possible, with a senior colleague. The cost of rehabilitation is often less – and the time shorter – if a primary amputation is performed than if lengthy and repeated operations are undertaken, and persistent painful debility or an insensate or flail limb is still the outcome. A successful limb salvage is defined by the overall function and satisfaction of the patient.

10.3 MANAGEMENT OF VASCULAR INJURY OF THE EXTREMITY

Vascular injuries are present in 25–35 per cent of all penetrating trauma to the extremities. More recently, duplex scanning has been found to play a useful screening role. Except for inconsequential intimal injuries and distal artery injuries, most extremity vascular injuries should be repaired.

Extremity arterial injury after penetrating trauma is common in military conflict or civilian trauma centres. Most peripheral arterial injuries occur in the femoral and popliteal vessels of the lower extremity. Loss of distal pulse and unilateral cool or pale extremities are the most significant hard signs of vascular impairment. It can be confirmed by Doppler ultrasound and supported by lack of signal on pulse oximetry. In severe hypovolaemic shock (SBP <60 mm Hg), however, it is not always easy to evaluate vascular impairment in the acute phase. After primary survey and resuscitation the extremity should be assessed again. Other more soft signs of vascular injury include an expanding or pulsating haematoma, a false aneurysm, continuous murmurs of arteriovenous fistulae, progressive swelling of an extremity and unexplained ischaemia or dysfunction. A significant percentage of these patients have no physical findings suggesting vascular trauma; thus, routine further investigation has been advocated.

The most common cause of peripheral vascular injury is penetrating trauma, which includes a spectrum from simple puncture wounds to wounds resulting from high-velocity missiles. Normal pulses do not rule out vascular injuries: 10 per cent of significant and major vascular injuries have no physical findings. Penetrating trauma also includes iatrogenic injuries such as those following percutaneous catheterization of the peripheral arteries

for diagnostic procedures or access for monitoring. When a needle or catheter dislodges an arteriosclerotic plaque or elevates the intima, a vessel may thrombose, leading to acute ischaemia in a limb.

The key, therefore, is to maintain a high index of suspicion based on the mechanism of injury and the proximity of vascular structures.

Recently, duplex scanning of blood vessels has been shown to be a useful adjunct in determining if an arteriogram is indicated. A positive duplex scan is valuable, but a negative one does not exclude vascular injury. A positive duplex scan, or an ankle-brachial index of less than 0.9 in a distal pulse, is a mandatory indication for arteriogram and possible operation.

The gold standard for confirming a suspected vascular injury remains the arteriogram. However, arteriography should not be performed in the patient who is unstable and needs emergency laparotomy or thoracotomy. The arteriogram should be delayed until after resuscitation and treatment of the life-threatening emergency.

If doubt exists, an angiogram should be obtained.

Blunt trauma also may cause peripheral vascular injuries, with shear injuries as the most common cause. Contusions or crushing injuries may produce transmural or partial disruption of arteries, resulting in elevation of the intima and the formation of intramural haematomas. Blunt trauma such as posterior dislocation of the knee may cause total disruption of a major vessel. Blunt trauma may also indirectly contribute to vascular occlusion by creating large haematomas in proximity to the vessel. These haematomas may lead to arterial spasm, distortion or compartment syndromes that interfere with arterial flow.

In principle, it is wise to fix the bony skeleton before embarking on vascular repair. However, this can be catastrophic if ischaemia is present. The following protocol should be used:

- Initial assessment for ischaemia.
- Exploration of the vessels.
- Fasciotomy if required and in case of any doubt.
- Temporary stenting of the vein and artery.
- Temporary orthopaedic fixation of the skeletal damage.
- Definitive repair of the vascular damage.

Damage control of the extremity injury should take place in the same fashion as in the abdomen. If there is doubt regarding viability, the wound should not be closed.

There are five options open to the surgeon when vascular damage is encountered: vessels may be repaired, replaced (grafted), ligated (and bypassed), stented or shunted.

Intraluminal shunts may be manufactured out of intravenous tubing, nasogastric tubing, biliary T- tubes or even chest drain tubing, depending on the size of the vessel to be shunted. Commercially made shunts (as used routinely in carotid surgery) are on the market, and others are now being made specifically for trauma. Essentially, the shunt is tied into the damaged vessel and ligated securely proximally and distally – there is no need for heparinization – and this allows time for other damage control procedures to take precedence while maintaining perfusion of the limb. Where possible, both artery and vein should be shunted if both are damaged. If not possible, the vein should be tied off. The shunts may safely be left in place for 24 hours and probably longer; there are no controlled trials reporting on this.

Some injury complexes should raise a specific suspicion of vascular damage, for example a supracondylar fracture of the humerus or femur, and posterior dislocation of the knee. The presence of palpable pulses does not exclude arterial injury, and a difference of 10 per cent in the measured Doppler pressure compared with the opposite uninjured limb mandates urgent angiography. This is not hard to do, and the technique is well described elsewhere. An absent pulse mandates exploration if the level of injury is known and angiography if it is not.

Repairs, particularly graft replacements of injured vessels, should only be attempted by those competent to do them, and only in limbs where the viability of the soft tissues is not in doubt (i.e. after fasciotomy). Ligation may be done as a measure of desperation in the exsanguinating patient, and limb survival is often surprising. Claudication pain may be dealt with at a later date. Extra-anatomical bypass has no place in the setting of damage control and trauma surgery. Endovascular stenting is rapidly becoming a procedure of choice in some areas (e.g. traumatic aortic rupture), but requires facilities and expertise that may not always be available.

The Eastern Association for the Surgery of Trauma (EAST) first published guidelines for evaluation and treatment of such trauma in 2002. Since that time there have been advancements in the management of penetrating lower extremity arterial trauma. The current guidelines are presented in Table 10.1[1].

10.3.1 **Chemical Vascular Injuries**

The frequency of chemical injury to blood vessels has increased secondary to iatrogenic injury and the intra-arterial injection of illicit drugs. These agents may cause intense vasospasm or direct damage to the vessel wall, often associated with intense pain and distal ischaemia.

Chemical vascular injuries may be treated with intra-arterial or intravenous administration of 10 000 units heparin to prevent distal thrombosis. Reserpine (0.5 mg) also has been recommended, although its only effect experimentally has been to protect against the release of catecholamines from the vessel walls. Other vasodilators and thrombolytic enzymes have been tried, with variable results. A reliable combination is 5000 units heparin in 500 mL Hartmann solution (Ringer lactate) to which is added 80 mg papaverine to combat arterial spasm. This is administered in boluses of 20–30 mL intra-arterially every 30 minutes, or intravenously at the rate of 1000 units heparin per hour.

10.4 **CRUSH SYNDROME**

Badly injured limbs will all have an element of crush syndrome associated with them unless one is dealing with a traumatic amputation by a sharp instrument such as a chain saw or machete. As such, a watch must be kept for the development of a compartment syndrome and/or myoglobinuria.

10.5 **MANAGEMENT OF OPEN FRACTURES**

Sepsis is a constant threat to the healing of open fractures. Risk factors for infection are:

- Severity of injury (especially the injury to the soft tissue envelope of a limb).
- Type of contamination.
- Delay from injury to surgical care (>6 hours).
- Failure to use prophylactic antibiotics.
- Inappropriate wound toilet.
- Lack of coverage of bony structures.
- Inappropriate wound closure (including primary wound closure in contaminated and contused wounds).

Table 10.1 EAST Guidelines for the Management of Lower Extremity Arterial Injury

Level of Evidence	Recommendation
I	1. Computed tomographic angiography (CTA) may be used as a primary diagnostic study for evaluation of penetrating lower extremity vascular injury when imaging is required.
II	1. Patients with hard signs of arterial injury (pulse deficit, pulsatile bleeding, bruit, thrill, expanding haematoma) should be surgically explored. There is no need for arteriogram in this setting unless the patient has an associated skeletal or shotgun injury. Restoration of perfusion to an extremity with an arterial injury should be performed in less than 6 hours to maximize limb salvage.
	2. Patients (without hard signs of vascular injury) who have abnormal physical examination findings and/or ankle brachial index (ABI) <0.9 should have further evaluation to rule out vascular injury.
	3. Patients with normal physical examination findings and an ABI >0.9 may be discharged (in the absence of other injuries requiring admission).
III	1. In cases of haemorrhage from penetrating lower extremity trauma in which manual compression is unsuccessful, tourniquets may be used as a temporary adjunct for haemorrhage control until definitive repair.
	2. The use of temporary intravascular shunts may be indicated to restore arterial flow in combined vascular orthopaedic injuries (Gustilo IIIC fractures) to facilitate limb perfusion during orthopaedic sterilization.
	3. Temporary intravascular shunts may be indicated in damage control situations to facilitate limb perfusion when the physiological status of the patient or operative capabilities prevent definitive repair.
	4. There are no data to support the routine use of endovascular therapies following infra-inguinal trauma.
	5. Embolization of profunda branches tibial vessels is acceptable, and there are no data to support preferential use of coils or n-butyl-2-cyanoacrylate glue.
	6. The role of non-invasive Doppler pressure monitoring with duplex ultrasonography to confirm or exclude arterial injury is not well defined. There may be a role for these studies in patients with soft signs of vascular injury or with proximity injuries.
	7. Non-operative observation of asymptomatic non-occlusive arterial injuries is acceptable.
	8. Repair of occult and asymptomatic non-occlusive arterial injuries managed non-operative league, and subsequently require repair, can be done without significant increase in morbidity.
	9. Simple arterial repairs fare better than grafts. If complete repair is required, vein graft seems to be the best choice. Polytetrafluoroethylene (PTFE), however, is also an acceptable conduit.
	10. PTFE may be used in a contaminated field. Effort should be made to obtain soft tissue coverage.
	11. Tibial vessels may be navigated if there is no documented flow distally.
	12. Early four-compartment lower legs fasciotomy should be applied liberally when there is an associated injury or where there has been prolonged ischaemia. If not performed, compartment pressures should be closely monitored.
	13. Arteriography for proximity is indicated only in patients with shotgun injuries.
	14. Completion arteriogram should be performed after arterial repair.
Unanswered questions	None

Source: Fox N, Rajani RR, Bokhari F, et al., *J Trauma Acute Care Surg.*, Supplement 4, 73(5), 315–320, 2012. With permission.

10.5.1 Severity of Injury (Gustilo Classification)

Table 10.2 outlines the Gustilo classification[2] of injury.

10.5.2 Sepsis and Antibiotics

Sepsis is a constant threat to the healing of open fractures, and the main risk factors include the severity of the injury, the delay from injury to surgical care, failure to use prophylactic antibiotics and inappropriate wound closure.

The early use of prophylactic antibiotics is important, but it must be recognized that antibiotics are an adjunct to appropriate wound care. The introduction of the Thomas splint and improved understanding of the need for surgical wound care are credited with reducing the mortality rate for open fractures of the femur from 80 per cent to 16 per cent during World War I[3]. During the Spanish Civil War, Truetta reported a septic mortality

Table 10.2 Gustilo Classification of Injury

Fracture Grade	Description
Grade I	Wound less than 1 cm with minimal soft tissue injury. Wound bed is clean.
	Bone injury is simple with minimal comminution.
	With intramedullary nailing, average time to union is 21–28 weeks.
Grade II	Wound is greater than 1 cm with moderate soft tissue injury.
	Wound bed is moderately contaminated.
	Fracture contains moderate comminution.
	With intramedullary nailing, average time to union is 26–28 weeks.
Grade III	Following fracture, automatically results in classification as type III:
	• Segmental fracture with displacement
	• Fracture with diaphyseal segmental loss
	• Fracture with associated vascular injury requiring repair
	• Farmyard injuries or highly contaminated wounds
	• High-velocity gunshot wound
	• Fracture caused by crushing force from a fast-moving vehicle
Grade IIIA	Wound is greater than 10 cm with crushed tissue and contamination.
	Soft tissue coverage of bone is usually possible.
	Wound sepsis rate is ±4%.
	With intramedullary nailing, average time to union is 30–35 weeks.
Grade IIIB	Wound is greater than 10 cm with crushed tissue and contamination; there is periosteal stripping and bone exposure, usually associated with contamination.
	Soft tissue injury is extensive – cover is inadequate and requires a regional or free flap
	Wound sepsis rate is ±52%
	With intramedullary nailing, average time to union is 30–35 weeks.
Grade IIIC	A fracture in which there is a major vascular injury requiring repair for limb salvage; major soft tissue injury is not necessarily significant.
	Wound sepsis rate is ±42%.
	Fractures can be classified using the Mangled Extremity Severity Score.
	In some cases, it will be necessary to consider below-knee amputation.

Source: Gustilo RB, Mendoza RM, Williams DN, *J Trauma*, 24, 742–746, 1984. With permission.

rate of 0.6 per cent in 1069 open fractures with a policy of aggressive wound excision and debridement, reduction of the fracture, stabilization with plaster and leaving the traumatic wound open[4].

Secondary soft tissue management with coverage of the bone by reconstructive surgery, including free flaps, has the best results if completed within the first week.

Recent consensus guidelines (Eastern Association for the Surgery of Trauma Guidelines) recommend that antibiotics be discontinued 24 hours after wound closure for grades I and II fractures. For grade III wounds, the antibiotics should be continued for only 72 hours after the time of injury, or for not more than 24 hours after soft tissue coverage of the wound is achieved, whichever occurs first. Agents effective against *Staphylococcus aureus* appear to be adequate for grades I and II fractures; however, the addition of broader Gram-negative coverage may be beneficial for grade III injuries[5,6]. In fractures classified by the Gustilo grading, grades I and II patients may be given agents effective against *S. aureus*, but for grade III injuries, broader Gram-negative cover is advisable.

10.5.3 Venous Thromboembolism

Deep venous thrombosis prophylaxis remains an integral part of management of patients with severe limb injury. Ideally, both mechanical and chemical prophylaxis should be used[7].

10.5.4 Timing of Skeletal Fixation in Polytrauma Patients

Most comparative studies have shown a reduction in the risk of post-traumatic respiratory compromise after early, definitive fixation of fractures (within 48 hours) both for isolated injuries and for multisystem trauma. There is also evidence of reduction in mortality, duration of mechanical ventilation, thromboembolic events and cost in favour of early fixation. There is no evidence that early fixation alters the outcome in those with concomitant head injury. The advantages of early fixation of fractures in patients with multiple injuries have been challenged.

The acute stabilization by early external fixation as part of damage control by orthopaedics may obviate some of the risks[8,9]. In cases where damage control surgery is indicated a phased approach by temporary fixation is taken in the acute phase, followed by definitive reconstruction as a secondary procedure.

Specific areas of risk are described here.

10.5.4.1 RESPIRATORY INSUFFICIENCY

Episodes of respiratory insufficiency[10] often occur after orthopaedic injury. Extremity injury may occur as part of a multisystem insult, with associated head, chest and other injuries. Hypoxia, hypotension and tissue injury provide an initial 'hit' to prime the patient's inflammatory response; operative treatment of fractures constitutes a modifiable secondary insult. In addition, post-traumatic fat embolism has been implicated in the respiratory compromise that appears after orthopaedic injury, especially following intramedullary nailing.

Nevertheless, most comparative studies have shown a reduction in risk of post-traumatic respiratory compromise after early, definitive fixation of fractures (i.e. within 48 hours), both for isolated injuries and multisystem trauma. There is also evidence of reduction in mortality, duration of mechanical ventilation, thromboembolic events and cost in favour of early fixation.

In case of severe thoracic trauma, even in haemodynamically stable cases, damage control by external fixation should be considered.

10.5.4.2 HEAD INJURY

In approximately 5 per cent of long bone fractures of the leg, the patient is physiologically unstable due to haemodynamic instability, raised intracranial pressure or other problems. Temporary methods of fixation are attractive in this setting. Although some studies have suggested that early nailing of a femoral fracture may be harmful in patients with a concomitant head injury, there is no compelling evidence that early long bone stabilization in mildly, moderately or severely brain-injured patients either enhances or worsens the outcome.[11] However, time-consuming procedures should be avoided and early transfer to the ICU environment with a staged approach to the orthopaedic trauma should be considered.

10.6 MASSIVE LIMB TRAUMA: LIFE VERSUS LIMB

Certain skeletal injuries by their nature indicate significant forces sustained by the body and should prompt the treating surgeon to look for other associated injuries. Other limb injuries, presenting with crush injury with extensive soft tissue damage, concomitant vascular or nerve injury and major bony disruption, pose other threats to either life or limb, and it is on these that this topic concentrates.

Despite huge advances in the management of these injuries, and the resultant decrease in amputation rates associated with them, there remains a small group of patients who present with 'mangled limbs', produced by mechanisms of high-energy transfer or crush in which there is vascular disruption in combination with severe open comminuted fractures and moderate loss of soft tissue. These injuries most frequently affect healthy individuals during their prime years of gainful employment and can result in varying degrees of functional and emotional disability.

There are many ways to classify major limb injuries and their complications, and these scoring systems can be found toward the end of this chapter.

The salvage of severe lower extremity fractures can be extremely challenging.[12] Even if the surgical team is successful in preserving the limb, the functional result may be unsatisfactory because of residual effects of injuries to muscle and nerve, bone loss and the presence of chronic infection. Failed efforts at limb salvage consume resources and are associated with increased patient mortality and high hospital costs.

Many lower extremity injury severity scoring systems[13] have been developed to assist the surgical team with the initial decision to amputate or salvage a limb. Scores such as the mangled extremity severity score (MESS)[14] can be used to facilitate identification of the irretrievably injured lower extremity. Recent prospective studies have, however, sounded a note of caution about relying exclusively on a scoring system to make these important decisions.

10.6.1 Scoring Systems

10.6.1.1 MANGLED EXTREMITY SYNDROME INDEX

Gregory et al.[14] retrospectively reviewed 17 patients with severe injuries (12 of the lower extremity) and proposed a Mangled Extremity Syndrome Index (Table 10.3). The injury was categorized according to the integument, nerve, vessel and bone injury. A point system quantified injury severity, delay in revascularization, ischaemia, age of the patient, pre-existing disease and whether the patient was in shock.

10.6.1.2 PREDICTIVE SALVAGE INDEX SYSTEM

Howe et al.[15] reviewed 21 patients with pelvic or lower extremity trauma with vascular injuries and proposed

Table 10.3 Mangled Extremity Syndrome Index

Criterion	Score
Injury Severity Score	
<25	1
25–50	2
>50	3
Integument Injury	
Guillotine	1
Crush/burn	2
Avulsion/degloving	3
Nerve Injury	
Contusion	1
Transection	2
Avulsion	3
Vascular Injury	
Vein transected	1
Artery transected	1
Artery thrombosed	2
Artery avulsed	3
Bone Injury	
Simple	1
Segmental	2
Segmental comminuted	3
Bone loss <6 cm	4
Articular	5
Articular with bone loss >6 cm	6
Delay in time to operation	1 point per hour >6 hours
Age (Years)	
<40	0
40–50	1
50–60	2
>60	3
Pre-existing disease	1
Shock	2

Note: Score <20: functional limb salvage can be expected; score >20: limb salvage is improbable.

Source: Reproduced from Gregory RT, Gould RJ, Peclet M, et al., *J Trauma*, 25, 1147–1150, 1985. With permission.

Table 10.4 Predicted Salvage Index System

Criterion	Score
Level of Arterial Injury	
Suprapopliteal	1
Popliteal	2
Infrapopliteal	3
Degree of Bone Injury	
Mild	1
Moderate	2
Severe	3
Degree of Muscle Injury	
Mild	1
Moderate	2
Severe	3
Interval from Injury to Operating Room (Hours)	
<6	0
6–12	2
>12	4

Note: Salvage: score <7. Amputation: score >8.

Source: Reproduced from Howe HR Jr, Poole GV Jr, Hansen KJ, et al., *Am Surg.*, 53, 205–228, 1987. With permission.

a predictive index incorporating the level of the arterial injury, degree of bony injury, degree of muscle injury and interval for warm ischaemia time (Table 10.4). Variables such as additional injuries and the presence of shock were not felt to be predictive of amputation. Of the patients, 43 per cent underwent amputation, infrapopliteal injuries being associated with the highest amputation rate (80 per cent).

The MESS, which characterizes the skeletal and soft tissue injury, warm ischaemia time, shock and age of the patient, has also been proposed as a means of solving this dilemma.

10.6.1.3 MANGLED EXTREMITY SEVERITY SCORE

Johansen et al.[11] described the MESS (Table 10.5), which characterizes the skeletal and soft tissue injury, warm ischaemia time, presence of shock and age of the patient, as a means of solving the dilemma of which patient needs amputation. A MESS value greater than 7 predicted amputation.

10.6.1.4 NISSSA SCORING SYSTEM

McNamara et al.[16] and others have, subsequently, retrospectively evaluated the MESS in 24 patients with severely injured tibias. Attempts have been made to address criticisms of the MESS by including nerve injury

Table 10.5 Mangled Extremity Severity Score

Factor	Score
Skeletal/Soft Tissue Injury	
Low energy (stab, fracture, civilian gunshot wound)	1
Medium energy (open or multiple fracture)	2
High energy (shotgun or military gunshot wound)	3
Very high energy (above plus gross contamination)	4
Limb Ischaemia	
Pulse reduced or absent but perfusion normal	1[a]
Pulseless, diminished capillary refill	2[a]
Patient is cool, paralyzed, insensate, numb	3[a]
Shock	
Systolic blood pressure always >90 mm Hg	0
Systolic blood pressure transiently <90 mm Hg	1
Systolic blood pressure persistently <90 mm Hg	2
Age (Years)	
<30	0
30–50	1
>50	2

[a]Double the value if the duration of ischaemia is over 6 hours.

Note: Score >7 predicted amputation.

Source: Reproduced from Johansen K, Daines M, Howey T, Helfet D, Hansen ST Jr., *J Trauma*, 30, 568–572, 1990. With permission.

Table 10.6 NISSSA Scoring System

Factor	Score
Nerve Injury	
Sensate	0
Loss of dorsal	1
Partial plantar	2
Complete plantar	3
Ischaemia	
None	0
Mild	1[a]
Moderate	2[a]
Severe	3[a]
Soft Tissue Injury/Contamination	
Low	0
Medium	1
High	2
Severe	3
Skeletal Injury	
Low energy	0
Medium energy	1
High energy	2
Very high energy	3
Shock/Blood Pressure	
Normotensive	0
Transient hypotension	1
Persistent hypotension	2
Age (Years)	
<30	0
30–50	1
>50	2

[a]Double the value if the duration of ischaemia exceeds 6 hours.

Note: Score >11 predicted amputation.

Source: Reproduced from McNamara MG, Heckman JD, Corley FG, *J Orthop Trauma*, 8, 81–87, 1994. With permission.

in the scoring systems and by separating the soft tissue and skeletal injury components of the MESS. The result is the NISSSA (**n**erve injury, **i**schaemia, **soft tissue** injury/contamination, **s**keletal injury, **s**hock/blood pressure, **a**ge) scoring system (Table 10.6), which is thus more sensitive and more specific than the MESS.

Scoring systems clearly have their limitations when the resuscitating surgeon is faced with an unstable polytrauma patient. Thus, these scoring systems are not universally accepted. They have shortcomings with respect to reproducibility, prognostic value and treatment-planning in this context. These factors can lead to inappropriate attempts at limb salvage when associated life- and limb-threatening injuries might be overlooked if attention is focused mainly on salvage of the mangled limb, or to an amputation when salvage may have been possible. While experience with these scoring systems is generally limited, they may provide some objective parameters on which clinicians can base difficult decisions regarding salvage of life or limb, but it must be stressed that any recommendations derived

from them must be judged in terms of available technology and expertise.

In summary, the decision of whether to amputate primarily or to embark on limb salvage and continue with planned repetitive surgeries is complex. Prolonged salvage attempts that are unlikely to be successful should be avoided, especially in patients with insensate limbs and predictable functional failures. Scoring systems should be used only as a guide for decision making. The relative importance of each of the associated trauma parameters (with the exception of prolonged, warm isch-aemia time or risking the life of a patient with severe, multiple organ trauma) is still of questionable predictive value. A good understanding of the potential complica-tions facilitates the decision-making process in limb sal-vage versus amputation.

10.7 **COMPARTMENT SYNDROME**

Compartment syndrome[17,18] may occur after extremity injury, with or without vascular trauma. Increasing pres-sure within the closed fascial space of a limb compromises the blood supply of muscle. Early clinical diagnosis and treatment is important to prevent significant morbidity.

Compartment syndrome occurs relatively commonly, following trauma or ischaemia to an extremity, with or without vascular injury. It is important to emphasize that reperfusion probably plays a major role. As such, the classical clinical findings may be absent prior to vascu-lar repair. Once the diagnosis of compartment syndrome is made, urgent fasciotomy is indicated. This applies to both upper[19] and lower[20] limbs

10.7.1 **Measurement**

The measurement[21] of intra-compartment pressure is invaluable when doubt exists about the diagnosis. This can be particularly helpful in cases not accessible for physical examination such as the unconscious patient and the patient in intensive care, sedated and ventilated. It must be emphasized that a pulse still may be palpable, or recordable on the Doppler, even though a compart-ment syndrome exists. It is important that measure-ments be taken on both lower legs, at the same place (e.g. in the tibialis anterior muscle 2 cm below and lateral to the tibial tubercle) for comparison.

10.7.2 **Technique**

It is critically important that the fasciotomy is compre-hensive and adequate[22], releasing all four lower limb com-partments (Figure 10.1). Key components are as follows:

- Medial incision
  · The medial incision commences 2 cm medial to, and below, the tibial tuberosity, running down the entire lower leg, 2–3 cm behind the posterior

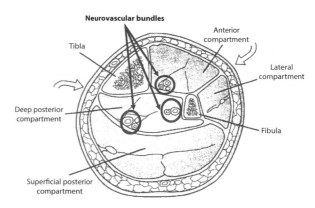

Figure 10.1 Intramuscular compartments.

border of the tibia, as far as 2 cm above the medial malleolus. Care must be taken to protect the great saphenous vein.
- Lateral incision (Figure 10.2)
  · The lateral incision starts anterolaterally over the fibula, 2–3 cm below the head, so as not to damage the common peroneal nerve, running down the entire lateral side as far as 2 cm above the lateral malleolus.
  · Retract skin.
  · Make a transverse incision at mid-point across the septum.
- Cut on either side of the septum using curved scissors.

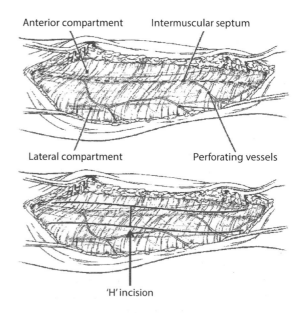

Figure 10.2 Technique of 'H' incision for lateral fasciotomy.

10.8 FASCIOTOMY

Two techniques have been described:

- Two-incision, four-compartment fasciotomy
- Fibulectomy

The skin must be opened widely, in order to allow a good view of the underlying fascia. It is critical that the fascia is split over its entire length, and this can only be done under direct vision. Care must be taken not to damage the saphenous veins, which may constitute the major system of venous return in such an injured leg. On the lateral side, the common peroneal nerve branches should be identified and preserved.

In trauma, there is no place for subcutaneous fasciotomy.

10.8.1 Four-compartment Fasciotomy

For four-compartment fasciotomy[22], two long incisions are made:

1. A long incision is made, anterolaterally, 2 cm anterior to the shaft of the fibula. The anterior and lateral fascial compartments are opened separately.
2. A long posteromedial incision is made 2 cm posterior to the medial border of the tibia. The subcutaneous tissue is pushed away by blunt dissection, and the superficial and deep posterior compartments are opened separately.

Fasciotomy must be performed *before* arterial exploration when an obvious arterial injury exists or where there is a suspicion of high intra-compartmental pressures.

Should there be doubt over whether or not the compartment syndrome is significant, a fasciotomy should be performed.

10.8.2 Fibulectomy

This is a difficult procedure, leading to extensive blood oozing, and may well result in damage to the peroneal artery.

It should not be practised in the trauma situation.

10.9 COMPLICATIONS OF MAJOR LIMB INJURY

Table 10.7 outlines fracture complications.

In a review of 53 mangled lower extremities, Bondurant et al. compared primary with delayed amputation in terms of morbidity and cost.[23] Patients undergoing delayed ablation had longer periods of hospitalization (53.4 versus 22.3 days) and more surgical procedures (6.9 versus 1.6) at greater cost ($53 462 versus $28 964). Six patients with delayed amputation developed sepsis from the injured lower extremity and died, while no patient with a primary amputation developed sepsis or died. Georgiadis et al.[24] indicated that patients with limb salvage at an average of 3 years follow-up had more complications, more procedures and a longer hospital stay than patients with early below-knee amputation. Slow recuperation and decreased motivation toward gainful

Table 10.7 Complications of Fractures

Skin and soft tissue	Skin and tissue loss, wound slough, coverage failure
Bone and fracture site	Compartment syndrome with necrosis of muscle/nerve injury
	Deep infection – acute/chronic
	Bone loss, delayed union, malunion/loss of alignment, non-union fixation problems – failure of hardware
	Bone refracture
Nerve	Direct injury or ischaemic damage
	Reflex sympathetic dystrophy
Vascular	Arterial occlusion, venous insufficiency
	Deep vein thrombosis, compartment syndrome
Joint motion	Associated joint surface fracture
	Contracture, late arthritis
Secondary	Ototoxicity, nephrotoxicity, myonecrosis from antibiotics
	Secondary spread of infection, sepsis/multiple organ failure/death
Psychosocial	Depression, loss of self-worth
	Economic hardship, questionable employment status, marital problems
Functional	Chronic pain
	Disability – muscle strength/endurance
	Decrease in activities of daily function
	Loss of ability to return to work, inability to participate in recreational activities
Cosmesis	Scars, bulky flaps

employment were also noted. The cost of initial hospitalization was lower with early amputation.

The decision to amputate primarily is difficult. At the initial examination, the extent of the eventual loss of soft tissue can never be fully appreciated, distal perfusion is also difficult to assess (many patients are shocked), and the neurological evaluation is often unreliable (as a result of associated head injury or ischaemia and soft tissue disruption). Any thoughts of limb salvage should take into consideration the Advanced Trauma Life Support protocols, always maintaining the priority of life over limb, and thus minimizing systemic complications and missed injuries. In an attempt to facilitate this early decision making, a number of systems have been devised providing objective criteria using a grading score to predict which injuries might eventually require amputation[25].

10.10 SUMMARY

It seems preferable to perform early, definitive long bone stabilization in polytrauma patients. Recent consensus guidelines suggest that, for patients with dominant head or chest injuries, the timing of long bone stabilization should be individualized according to the patient's clinical condition. Damage control orthopaedics has a real place in limb salvage[26].

REFERENCES AND RECOMMENDED READING

References

1. Fox N, Rajani RR, Bokhari F, et al. Evaluation and management of penetrating lower extremity arterial trauma: An Eastern Association for the Surgery of Trauma practice management guideline. *J Trauma Acute Care Surg.* 2012;Supplement 4, 73(5):315–320.
2. Gustilo RB, Mendoza RM, Williams DN. Problems in the management of type III (severe) open fractures: a new classification of type III open fractures. *J Trauma.* 1984;24:742–746.
3. Gustilo RB, Anderson JT. Prevention of infection in the treatment of one thousand and twenty-five open fractures of long bones: retrospective and prospective analyses. *J Bone Joint Surg.* 1976;58A:453–458.
4. Truetta J. War surgery of extremities: treatment of war wounds and fractures. *Br Med J.* 1942;1:616.
5. Luchette FA, Bone LB, Born CT, et al. Practice management guidelines for prophylactic antibiotic use in open fractures. In: *Eastern Association for the Surgery of Trauma. Practice Management Guidelines.* http://www.east.org. Accessed December 2014.
6. Hoff WS, Bonadies JA, Cachecho R, Dorlac WC. EAST Practice Management Guidelines Work Group: update to Practice Management Guidelines for prophylactic antibiotic use in open fractures. In: *Eastern Association for the Surgery of Trauma. Practice Management Guidelines.* http://www.east.org. Accessed December 2014.
7. Rogers FB, Cipolle MD, Velmahos G, Rozycki G. Practice management guidelines for the management of venous thromboembolism (VTE) in trauma patients. *J Trauma.* 2002;53:142–164.
8. Scalea TM, Boswell SA, Scott JD, Mitchell KA, Kramer ME, Pollak AN. External fixation as a bridge to intramedullary nailing for patients with multiple injuries and with femur fractures: damage control orthopedics. *J Trauma.* 2000;48:613–621.
9. Dunham CM, Bosse MJ, Clancy TV, et al. The EAST Practice Management Guidelines Work Group. Practice management guidelines for the optimal timing of long-bone fracture stabilization in polytrauma patients: the EAST Practice Management Guidelines Work Group. *J Trauma.* 2001;50:958–967.
10. Robinson CM. Current concepts of respiratory insufficiency syndromes after fracture. *J Bone Joint Surg.* 2001;83B:781–791.
11. Scalea TM, Scott JD, Brumback RJ, et al. Early fracture fixation may be 'just fine' after head injury: no difference in central nervous system outcomes. *J Trauma.* 1999;46:839–846.
12. Johansen K, Daines M, Howey T, Helfet D, Hansen ST Jr. Objective criteria accurately predict amputation following lower extremity trauma. *J Trauma.* 1990;30:568–572.
13. Bosse MJ, MacKenzie EJ, Kellam JF, et al. A prospective evaluation of the clinical utility of the lower-extremity injury-severity scores. *J Bone Joint Surg.* 2001;83A:3–14.
14. Gregory RT, Gould RJ, Peclet M, et al. The Mangled Extremity Syndrome (MES): a severity grading system for multisystem injuries of the extremities. *J Trauma.* 1985;25:1147–1150.
15. Howe HR Jr, Poole GV Jr, Hansen KJ, et al. Salvage of lower extremities following combined orthopedic and vascular trauma: a predictive salvage index. *Am Surg.* 1987;53:205–228.

16. McNamara MG, Heckman JD, Corley FG. Severe open fractures of the lower extremity: a retrospective evaluation of the Mangled Extremity Severity Score (MESS). *J Orthop Trauma.* 1994;8:81–87.

17. Perron AD, Brady WJ, Keats TE. Orthopedic pitfalls in the ED: acute compartment syndrome. *Am J Emerg Med.* 2001;19:413–416.

18. Tiwari A, Haq AI, Myint F, Hamilton G. Acute compartment syndromes. *Br J Surg.* 2002;89:397–412.

19. Morin RJ, Swan KG, Tan V. Acute forearm compartment syndrome secondary to local arterial injury after penetrating trauma. *J Trauma.* 2009; 66:989.

20. Frink M, Hildebrand F, Krettek C, et al. Compartment syndrome of the lower leg and foot. *Clin Orthop Relat Res.* 2010;468:940.

21. Hammerberg EM, Whitesides TE Jr, Seiler JG 3rd. The reliability of measurement of tissue pressure in compartment syndrome. *J Orthop Trauma.* 2012;26:24.

22. Mubarak SJ, Owen CA. Double incision fasciotomy of the leg for decompression in compartment syndromes. *J Trauma.* 1977;59A:184–187.

23. Bondurant FJ, Cotler HB, Buckle R, Miller-Crotchett P, Browner BD. The medical and economic impact of severely injured lower extremities. *J Trauma.* 1988;28:1270–1273.

24. Georgiadis GM, Behrens FF, Joyce MJ, Earle AS, Simmons AL. Open tibial fractures with severe soft-tissue loss. Limb salvage compared with below-the-knee amputation. *J Bone Joint Surg Am.* 1993 Oct;75(10):1431–1441.

25. Scalea TM, DuBose J, Moore EE, et al. Western Trauma Association critical decisions in trauma: management of the mangled extremity. *J Trauma Acute Care Surg.* 2012;72:86.

26. Possley DR, Burns TG, Stinner DJ, et al. Temporary external fixation is safe in a combat environment. *J Trauma.* 2010;69 Suppl 1:S135.

Recommended Reading

Harris AM, Althausen PL, Kellam J, et al. Complications following limb-threatening lower extremity trauma. *J Orthop Trauma.* 2009;23:1.

Helgeson MD, Potter BK, Burns TG, et al. Risk factors for and results of late or delayed amputation following combat-related extremity injuries. *Orthopedics.* 2010; 33(9):669-76. doi:10.3928/01477447-20100722-02.

Head Trauma 11

11.1 INTRODUCTION

Traumatic brain injury (TBI) is a leading cause of death and disability worldwide, particularly in the young population. In the United States alone, TBI contributed to the deaths of more than 50 000 people in 2010. Furthermore, TBI was the main diagnosis in more than 280 000 hospital admissions and 2.2 million emergency department (ED) visits[1]. Trauma patients with co-existing TBI have higher mean length of stay in hospital, higher hospital cost and increased percentage of disability, compared with trauma victims without TBI.

The extremely high mortality and dramatic morbidity of TBI are attributed to the initial traumatic insult to which is added the secondary damage to nervous tissue from hypoxia and hypovolaemia. Hypotension and hypoxia are the consequences of almost every severe trauma. Bleeding due to trauma coexisting with TBI leaves a narrow path of resuscitation, one of the main goals of which is to optimize oxygen tissue perfusion. Early airway control (with proper immobilization of the cervical spine), provision of adequate ventilation and oxygenation and correction of hypovolemia are the key steps in protecting the brain from further damage. Prompt imaging by computed tomography (CT), whenever possible, provides additional vital information that facilitates the treating surgeon's immediate decisions.

11.2 INJURY PATTERNS AND CLASSIFICATION

Traumatic brain injuries are classified according to severity, type and mechanism of injury. Knowledge of the classification allows the trauma surgeon to grade the severity, to suspect early the presence of intracranial insult and to initiate timely appropriate diagnostic procedures and therapeutic management.

Severity is assessed clinically with the Glasgow Coma Scale (GCS), which evaluates from different parameters, collectively, the neurological status of the patient (see Appendix B). It is essential to realize that GCS is not a simple number and each of its three components has independent and substantial clinical value. Additional clinical signs and symptoms, such as focal neurological deficits, abnormal pupillary light reflexes, anisocoria and seizures contribute to the classification of TBI severity:

- *Mild TBI*: Brief loss of consciousness for a few seconds or minutes, post-traumatic amnesia (PTA) for less than an hour, normal brain imaging results, GCS score 13–15.
- *Moderate TBI*: Loss of consciousness for less than 24 hours, PTA for 1–24 hours, abnormal brain imaging findings, GCS score of 9–12.
- *Severe TBI*: Loss of consciousness or coma for more than 24 hours, PTA for more than 24 hours, abnormal brain imaging findings, GCS score of 3–8.

Type of brain injury is characterized according to the identified traumatic brain lesions:

- *Focal brain injuries:* Collision forces acting directly on the skull and the underlying brain tissue create a wide range of lesions: contusion or brain laceration, epidural or subdural haematoma, subarachnoid or intracerebral haemorrhage. Fast acquisition of brain imaging promotes early diagnosis and prompt intervention that may prove critical in determining clinical outcome. However, the majority of patients with TBI do not have a lesion suitable for neurosurgical intervention[2].
- *Diffuse brain injuries:* Sudden head movement, usually rapid deceleration often seen in motor-vehicle accidents, results in diffuse *axonal* injury and severe cerebral enema. Under extreme circumstances, the threshold of the axon's maximum elasticity may be

exceeded, affecting axonal integrity with subsequent degeneration. This devastating clinico-pathological syndrome leads to extensive damage to the brain's white matter and a variety of profound neurological deficits[3].

Both severity and type of TBI are directly associated with the *mechanism* of injury and the forces applied on cerebral parenchyma:

- *Blunt head trauma*: Comprises more than 75 per cent of head injuries and is mainly caused by motor-vehicle accidents and falls. Unless an open skull fracture is present, blunt head trauma is considered a closed injury and is of high risk for secondary brain damage. This is the main cohort of patients suffering from severe post-injury morbidity and is the main diagnostic target for a trauma surgeon. Skull fractures are often present in blunt head trauma. The significance of skull fractures should not be underestimated, as it takes considerable force to occur. A simple closed linear skull fracture identified in a skull X-ray increases chances of an intracranial haemorrhage by 400 times. All open and depressed skull fractures should be surgically treated, especially if the underlying dura is damaged.
- *Penetrating head trauma*: Patients with penetrating cerebral injury require emergency craniotomy, if there is a significant mass effect from a haematoma or the projectile trajectory. However, removal of bone or projectile fragments should not be pursued at the expense of damaging normal brain tissue. Patients presenting with a GCS score of 5 or less after resuscitation or a GCS score of 8 or less and computed tomography (CT) findings of bilateral brain injury have a particularly poor outcome and conservative treatment may be indicated.

11.3 MEASURABLE PHYSIOLOGICAL PARAMETERS OF BRAIN FUNCTION

11.3.1 Mean Arterial Pressure (MAP)

Mean arterial pressure is defined as the average arterial pressure during a single cardiac cycle and is a credible indicator of the haemodynamic status in an injured patient. It is represented mathematically by the following formula:

$$\frac{SAP + 2DAP}{3}$$

where SAP is systolic pressure, and DAP is diastolic pressure.

11.3.2 Intracranial Pressure (ICP)

Intracranial pressure (ICP) is the pressure applied on the brain inside the skull and is regulated by variations in cerebrospinal fluid volume and venous return of the brain. The normal ICP range is 7–15 mm Hg. Values over 20 mm Hg are caused by cerebral oedema or large haematomas and require surgical intervention to release the pressure on the brain.

11.3.3 Cerebral Perfusion Pressure (CPP)

The CPP is the net pressure gradient that drives cerebral blood flow to the brain. It can be calculated by the formula: CPP = MAP − ICP. The normal CPP range is 70–90 mm Hg in adults.

11.3.4 Cerebral Blood Flow (CBF)

The CBF represents the blood supply to the brain at any given time. Normal values are around 750 mL/min, which corresponds to 15 per cent of the cardiac output in the adult. It is autoregulated tightly according to the brain's metabolic demands, the blood pressure, the $PaCO_2$ and PaO_2 values and shows significant alterations in severely injured trauma patients.

11.4 PATHOPHYSIOLOGY OF TRAUMATIC BRAIN INJURY (TBI)

The initial stages of cerebral injury are characterized by two main elements: direct tissue damage and impaired regulation of CBF and metabolism. This 'ischaemia-like' pattern leads to accumulation of lactic acid due to anaerobic glycolysis, increased membrane permeability and consecutive enema formation. On a cellular level, an excessive release of neurotransmitters takes place, along with an increase of free radicals and fatty acids, occurring from membrane degradation of cellular and vascular structures. These events lead to programmed cell death (apoptosis).

11.5 INITIAL MANAGEMENT OF TBI

Only a part of the neurological damage occurs at the moment of impact. Most of the harm happens due to secondary brain injury. Therefore, a swift but meticulous approach to all patients who have suffered a TBI is essential since it is evident that *time is of essence*. The Advanced Trauma Life Support (ATLS) principles must be applied (GCS, pupils) and a cursory neurological examination can provide substantial information about the patient's neurological status. Two main pillars dictate the base of TBI patient management:

- Keep SBP >90 mm Hg (level II recommendation).
- Keep pO_2 >60 mm Hg (>8.8 kPa) (level III recommendation)[4].

These targets are critical and can provide a great challenge, especially if the patient is haemodynamically unstable due to multiple injuries. On an isolated TBI with ICP elevation autoregulation of circulation allows to compensate for the hypoperfusion, due to the cerebral oedema/haematoma, with increase of SBP. This is one of the few circumstances where a hypertensive trauma patient is identified. This 'Cushing' effect is not reproduced in a bleeding patient as the measured systolic pressure is influenced by the hypertensive TBI autoregulation and the bleeding hypotension. In such a case it is recommended to resuscitate the patient to SBP 90 mm Hg, as this would be beneficial for the cerebral perfusion and protective for the formed haemostatic thrombi on the loci of bleeding vessels.

Other systemic brain insults which have been shown to complicate the primary injured brain and must be aggressively fought are hypertension (MAP >110 mm Hg), anaemia (Hb <100 g/L), hyponatraemia (serum sodium <142 mmol/L), hyperglycaemia (blood sugar >10 mmol/L), hypoglycaemia (blood sugar <4.6 mmol/L) and fever (temperature >36.5°C)

11.6 CEREBRAL PERFUSION THRESHOLD

The main goal is to secure the provision of oxygen to the brain tissue by managing an adequate CPP. The critical CPP threshold for ischaemia is 50–60 mm Hg and values below 50 mm Hg should be avoided (level II)[4].

To maintain adequate CPP (>70 mm Hg), blood pressure must be kept high and ICP low.

Aggressive attempts to maintain blood pressure, especially with hyperosmolar volume expanders, should be avoided, because they increase the risks of adult respiratory distress syndrome (ARDS) and brain enema (level II)[4]. In recent wars a hypotensive patient with TBI was resuscitated during transportation with 250 mL of hypertonic N/S 3% infused within 20 minutes. This allowed temporal fluid shift in intravascular space and blood pressure elevation, with minimal volume infused, and is practiced in austere conditions.

11.7 INTRACRANIAL PRESSURE (ICP) THRESHOLD AND INDICATIONS FOR MONITORING

Correct and efficient CPP management in TBI patients can only be achieved by measuring ICP and blood pressure. ICP should be monitored:

- In all salvageable patients with severe TBI, with a GCS of 3–8 after resuscitation, and an abnormal brain computed tomography (CT) scan (haematoma, contusion, swelling or herniation – level III)[4].
- In all patients with severe TBI, a normal brain CT scan and at least two of the following:
  - Age over 40 years
    - Unilateral or bilateral motor posturing
  - SBP <90 mm Hg

Treatment must be initiated with ICP >20 mm Hg.

It is essential to utilize frequent CT scan as the increase in ICP results from many different injury types, each of which have different management.

11.7.1 ICP Management – Dos and Don'ts

- *Hyperventilation* can be used as a temporary measure for the reduction of elevated ICP (Level III)[4]. Hypocapnia (pCO_2: >32–35 mm Hg/>4 kPa) causes cerebral vasoconstriction, freeing space for expansion within the cranial cavity, thus lowering ICP; however, in severe hyperventilation excessive vasoconstriction leads to hypo-perfusion. Avoid excessive use of the protocol and do not hyperventilate to a pCO_2 <25 mm Hg (<3 kPa) during the first 24 hours from TBI, when cerebral blood flow (CBF) is often critically reduced (Level II)[4]. In such a case more interventional treatment is required. If hyperventilation is used, jugular venous oxygen saturation (S_jO_2 >50%)

measurements are recommended to monitor oxygen delivery.

Prophylactic hyperventilation is not recommended (level II).[4]

- *Mannitol and hypertonic saline* intravenous administration is the treatment of choice for lowering ICP. Use mannitol at a loading dose of 1 g/kg body weight over 15 minutes (level II)[4] and maintain dosing by additional equal fractions (e.g. 25 g mannitol every 6 h). Equimolar doses of hypertonic saline can also be used according to institutional protocols. Empirical mannitol use (prior to ICP measurement) is indicated in patients with signs of transtentorial herniation or progressive neurological deterioration not attributable to extracranial causes (substance abuse, hypovolemia) (level III)[4]. Mannitol is the drug of choice for improving ICP but bears a high risk of hypovolemia and arterial hypotension.

Prophylactic use of mannitol without evidence of increased ICP is not recommended.

- *High-dose barbiturate* administration is recommended to control elevated ICP, refractory to maximum standard medical and surgical treatment (level III)[4]. Barbiturate therapy must be applied on haemodynamically stable patients. Additionally, *propofol* can be used to control ICP, but high doses can produce significant morbidity (level III)[4].
- The use of steroids is *not* recommended for improving outcome or reducing ICP. In patients with moderate or severe TBI, high-dose methylprednisolone is associated with increased mortality and is contraindicated (level I)[4].

11.7.2 ICP Monitoring Devices and Application

- *Intraventricular catheter*: It is the most accurate, cost-effective and reliable ICP monitoring method. A hole is drilled through the skull and the catheter is inserted through the brain into the lateral ventricle[5]. It can be also used to drain cerebrospinal fluid (CSF) and assist to ICP reduction. When the ICP is high, catheter placement can be challenging.
- *Intraparenchymal catheter*: Parenchymal ICP monitors cannot be recalibrated during monitoring.

Parenchymal ICP monitors, using micro-strain pressure transducers, have negligible drift. The measurement drift is independent of the duration of the monitoring.

- *Subarachnoid, subdural and epidural catheters*: These less invasive techniques are lacking in accuracy and in the ability to remove excess CSF.

11.7.3 Treatment Thresholds

11.7.3.1 ICP THRESHOLDS

- Treatment should be initiated with ICP thresholds above 20 mm Hg (level II).
- A combination of ICP values and brain CT findings should be used to determine the need for treatment (level III).

11.7.3.2 CEREBRAL PERFUSION THRESHOLDS

- Aggressive attempts to maintain cerebral perfusion pressure (CPP) above 70 mm Hg with fluids and pressors should be avoided because of the risks of adult respiratory distress syndrome (ARDS) (level II).
- CPP of <50 mm Hg should be avoided (level III).
- The CPP value to target lies within the range 50–70 mm Hg. Patients with intact pressure autoregulation tolerate higher CPP values (level III).
- Ancillary minting of cerebral parameters that include blood flow, oxygenation or metabolism facilitates CPP management.

11.6.3.3 BRAIN OXYGEN MONITORING AND THRESHOLDS

- Jugular venous saturation or brain tissue oxygen monitoring measure cerebral oxygenation.
- Jugular venous saturation (<50%) or brain tissue oxygenation tension (<15 mm Hg.) are treatment thresholds.

11.8 IMAGING

- *Skull x-rays* are of limited use, unless a CT scan is not available or a penetrating injury has occurred.
- A *CT scan* is the investigation of choice for TBI. All patients with moderate or severe TBI must be submitted to a head CT scan. Deteriorating

neurological status, peritraumatic amnesia and focal neurological signs are additional criteria. The New Orleans criteria[6] propose the indication to perform CT scan in mild TBI. Patients with GCS 15 and normal neurological examination after blunt trauma are eligible for head CT if one of the following applies: headache, vomiting, age over 60 years, drug or alcohol intoxication, short-term memory deficit and seizures.

- Penetrating TBI patients should not be taken to surgery without imaging investigation.
- For haemodynamically unstable patients requiring immediate non-cranial surgery, the investigation for potential TBI is delayed.

11.9 INDICATIONS FOR SURGERY

The patient's neurological status post-TBI is the most accurate and credible indicator. Rapidly deteriorating neurological signs (requires frequent reassessment), establishment of pupillary asymmetry, haemiparesis and/or intracranial pathology amenable to surgery are absolute indications for surgical intervention.

Inability to perform head CT on a neurologically deteriorating patient, unacceptably long transfer to the nearest neurosurgical unit and a sizeable lesion that may suddenly worsen also add up to choosing the path of emergency surgical treatment.

11.9.1 Burr Holes and Emergency Craniotomy

Rapidly expanding intracranial haematomas associated with fixed dilated pupils are fatal. A prompt action in removing the compression of the brain is crucial. There are surgical interventions that can be performed by a non-neurosurgical specialist and avert progressive brain injury.

11.9.1.1 EMERGENCY 'BURR HOLE' CRANIOTOMY

Clear indications exist for performing a burr hole[7]: GCS <8 with imaging evidence of an epidural haematoma causing midline shift and unequal pupils. In the absence of a head CT, a very high clinical suspicion (e.g. a palpable fracture, with an ipsilateral fixed dilated pupil, and deteriorating neurologic status) is the only exception for performing an emergency craniotomy without imaging.

Otherwise, without imaging and/or with a GCS above 8 the craniotomy is contraindicated. Burr hole drilling sites are shown in Figure 11.1, regarding haematoma positions. The basic steps in burr hole technique are:

- Confirm the correct side and position of the haematoma.
- Shave a strip of approximately 5 cm of hair.
- Make a 3-cm incision straight down to the bone.
- Push the periosteum with a knife/swab and insert the self-retaining retractor.
- Start drilling perpendicularly to the skull and simultaneously apply saline wash.
- *Do not* stop until you feel a difference in tissue resistance or the drill stops drilling (automated clutch drills or hand drills with auto stop bits) (Figure 11.2).
- Remove bone fragments with a hook. If the haematoma is epidural, blood should come out. If it is subdural, open the dura further with a sharp knife.

Figure 11.1 Position of standard burr holes and frequent locations of epidural haematomas that are decompressed: (a) temporal (above zygoma); (b) frontal (over the coronal suture, approximately 10-cm cephalad and in line with the mid-pupillary line); (c) parietal (over the parietal eminence). (From Wilson MH, Wise D, Davies G, et al., *Scand J Trauma Resusc Emerg Med.*, 2, 20–24, 2012. With permission.)

Figure 11.2 (a) Hand-driven burr hole craniotomy drill with a set of bits. (b) The step at the tip of the bit that stops penetration to prevent inadvertent brain injury.

- If no blood comes out review location and side, *without further delaying patient transfer.*
- If fresh blood continues to ooze from the wound, *do not* try to tamponade.

The concept of emergency craniotomy is to relieve brain pressure, in order to earn time for patient transfer to a specialized neurosurgical unit. Adherence to procedure indications and technique can provide a favourable outcome in selected patients.

11.9.1.2 EMERGENCY CRANIOTOMY

This is a more complex surgical procedure that has not proven to increase survival when performed by a nonspecialist surgeon. Performance of burr hole is sufficient.

Traditional wisdom suggests that all open, depressed skull fractures should be surgically treated and that closed, depressed fractures should be elevated when the depth of the depression meets or exceeds the thickness of the adjacent skull table to alleviate compression of the underlying cortex.

The dura under the fracture must always be repaired, if damaged.

11.10 ADJUNCTS TO CARE

11.10.1 Infection Prophylaxis

- Broad-spectrum antibiotic prophylaxis is recommended for both military and civilian penetrating craniocerebral injuries, including those due to sports or recreational injuries, for all *penetrating* TBI (cephalosporin, amoxicillin/clavulanate)[8].

- Perioperative antibiotics for intubation should be administered to reduce the incidence of pneumonia (level II)[4].
- Prophylactic antibiotic use for ICP monitoring catheter placement is not recommended to reduce infection (level III)[4].

11.10.2 Antiseizure Prophylaxis

Seizure activity in the early post-traumatic period following TBI may cause secondary damage as a result of increased metabolic demands, raised intracranial pressure and excess neurotransmitter release:

- Anticonvulsants are indicated for patients who have had a seizure after TBI. The treatment regimen is also shown to decrease the incidence of early post-traumatic seizures (within 7 days of injury), continued for 6 months to 1 year. However, such seizures are not associated with a worse outcome.
- Many neurosurgeons give prophylactic anticonvulsants to all patients with significant head injury for at least the first few days after injury; however, the exact duration and role of these drugs is unclear.
- Schierhout (*Cochrane Database*)[9] recently reviewed the available evidence and concluded that while prophylactic anti-epileptics are effective in reducing early seizures, there is no evidence that treatment with prophylactic anti-epileptics reduces the occurrence of late seizures, or has any effect on death and neurological disability.
- Prophylactic use of phenytoin or valproate is *not* recommended for preventing late post-traumatic seizures (level II)[4].

11.10.3 Nutrition

Patients should be fed full caloric nutrition by day 7 post-injury (level II).

11.10.4 Deep Vein Thrombosis Prophylaxis

- Graduated or pneumatic compression stockings are recommended, until patient is ambulatory.
- Low-molecular-weight heparin should be used in combination with mechanical prophylaxis. The drawback is the increased risk of intracranial re-haemorrhage (level III).

11.10.5 Steroids

The use of steroids is not recommended for improving outcome or reducing ICP. In patients with moderate or severe traumatic brain injury (TBI), high-dose methyl-prednisolone is associated with an increased mortality and is contraindicated (level 1).

11.11 PAEDIATRIC CONSIDERATIONS

The approach for the paediatric TBI patient is similar to the one followed for the adults. Preservation of SBP >90 mm Hg is critical. Increased incidence of undrainable lesions and rapidly progressive enema in children require more intent monitoring.

11.12 PEARLS AND PITFALLS

- Always follow the ATLS principles (avoid D before completing A-B-Cs).
- Do not attribute a deterioration in level of consciousness to alcohol or drug abuse.
- Keep in mind the C-spine protection in presence of significant TBI.
- Control major bleeding from a scalp wound.
- Closely monitor TBI patients to detect early a clinical deterioration in neurological status.
- The GCS should not be used solely as a single number. It is calculated from three different parameters, each of which has its own independent significance.
- Hypotensive resuscitation applies optimally in combined TBI and systemically bleeding injury.

- The ICP elevation is caused by various intracranial injuries. Management of intracranial hypertension with conservative measures should not divert attention from identifying the specific cause of it and its etiologic management. This is feasible only via CT imaging.
- Bleeding within the cranial cavity does not kill due to volume of blood lost (the cranial cavity only has a volume of 400 cc) but due to elevation in ICP, and herniation of brainstem through tentorium that damages the cardiorespiratory centres which leads to arrest.
- Proceed to emergency craniotomy under strict and absolute indications in the absence of neurosurgical aid to avoid further harm to the patient.

11.13 SUMMARY

Traumatic brain injury is a major cause of mortality and morbidity in the trauma setting. Primary treatment in TBI focuses on prevention of secondary brain injury, mainly through preservation of normovolaemia and adequate tissue oxygenation. To the attending emergency physician, the main goal is buying time for the patient and not the definitive treatment of TBI.

REFERENCES AND RECOMMENDED READING

References

1. Centers for Disease Control and Prevention. Get the facts about TBI. http://www.cdc.gov/traumaticbraininjury/get_the_facts.html. Accessed January 2015.
2. Namjoshi DR, Good C, Cheng WH, et al. Towards clinical management of traumatic brain injury: a review of models and mechanisms from a biomechanical perspective. *Dis Model Mech.* 2013 Nov;6(6):1325–1338.
3. Andriessen TM, Jacobs B, Vos PE. Clinical characteristics and pathophysiological mechanisms of focal and diffuse traumatic brain injury. *J Cell Mol Med.* 2010;14(10):2381–2392.
4. Brain Trauma Foundation. *Guidelines for the Management of Severe Traumatic Brain Injury,* 3rd ed. http://www.tbiguidelines.org. Accessed January 2015.

5. Vender J, Waller J, Dhandapani K, et al. An evaluation and comparison of intraventricular, intraparenchymal and fluid-coupled techniques for intracranial pressure monitoring in patients with severe traumatic brain injury. *J Clin Monit Comput.* 2011;25(4):231–236.

6. Bouida W, Marghli S, Souissi S, et al. Prediction value of the Canadian CT head rule and the New Orleans criteria for positive head CT scan and acute neurosurgical procedures in minor head trauma: a multicenter external validation study. *Ann Emerg Med.* 2013;61(5):521–527.

7. Wilson MH, Wise D, Davies G, et al. Emergency burr holes: "How to do it." *Scand J Trauma Resusc Emerg Med.* 2012;2:20–24.

8. Bayston R, De Louvois J, Brown EM, et al. Use of antibiotics in penetrating craniocerebral injuries. *Lancet.* 2000;355:1813–1817.

9. Schierhout G, Roberts I. Anti-epileptic drugs for preventing seizures following acute traumatic brain injury. *Cochrane Database Syst Rev.* 2001;(4):CD000173.

Recommended Reading

Brain Trauma Foundation Guidelines. www.tbiguidelines.org.

Joseph B, Friese RS, Sadoun M, et al. The BIG (brain injury guidelines) project: defining the management of traumatic brain injury by acute care surgeons. *J Trauma Acute Care Surg.* 2014;76(4):965–969.

Maas AI, Dearden M, Teasdale GM, et al. EBIC-guidelines for management of severe head injury in adults. European Brain Injury Consortium. *Acta Neurochir (Wien).* 1997;139(4):286–294.

Burns 12

12.1 OVERVIEW

Globally, burns are a serious public health problem. There are over 300 000 deaths each year from fires alone, with more deaths from scalds, electrical burns and other forms of burns, for which global data are not available. Fire-related deaths alone rank among the 15 leading causes of death among children and young adults aged 5–29 years. Over 95 per cent of fatal fire-related burns occur in low- and middle-income countries. Southeast Asia alone accounts for just over one-half of the total number of fire-related deaths worldwide, and females in this region have the highest fire-related burn mortality rates globally. Among the various age groups, children under 5 years and the elderly over 70 years have the highest fire-related burn mortality rates. Along with those who die, millions more are left with lifelong disabilities and disfigurements, often with resulting stigma and rejection.

The suffering caused by burns is even more tragic as burns are so eminently preventable. High-income countries have made considerable progress in lowering rates of burn-related death and disability, through combinations of proven prevention strategies and improvements in the care of burn victims. Most of these advances in prevention and care have been incompletely applied in low- and middle-income countries[1].

12.2 ANATOMY

Apart from simple erythema (sunburn), all other burns constitute an open wound of greater or lesser severity. To create a dramatic analogy, a burn is similar to an evisceration with exposed bowel. In the case of the burn, it is the dermis (Figure 12.1) that is exposed to a lesser or greater extent, resulting in significant losses of fluid from the body, along with loss of the bacterial barrier,

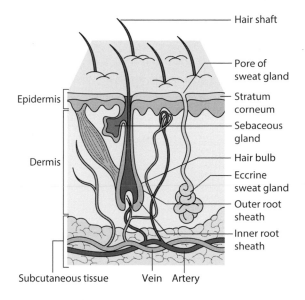

Figure 12.1 Layers and structures of the skin.

leaving the path open for infection, as well as loss of heat by convection and conduction.

In physiological terms, there is a significant loss of protein – primarily albumin – and electrolytes and haemoconcentration, along with a massive increase in energy requirements to heal the wound.

The burn wound is divided into three areas (Figure 12.2):

- Zone of coagulation.
- Zone of stasis.
- Zone of hyperaemia.

Inadequate resuscitation or the inappropriate use of ice or iced water to cool the burn may lead to deepening the burn due to vasoconstriction in the zone of stasis, extending the zone of coagulation.

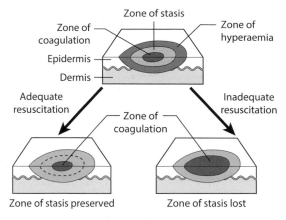

Figure 12.2 Zones of a burn.

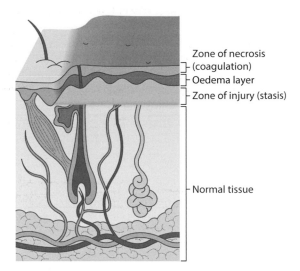

Figure 12.3 Superficial partial thickness burn.

12.3 DEPTH OF THE BURN

Burns have been traditionally divided into first, second and third degree, but the terms 'partial thickness' (superficial and deep) and 'full thickness' are more informative and will be used here. There is also a group of 'indeterminate' thickness burns, which represent a separate challenge.

12.3.1 Superficial Burn (Erythema)

'Sunburn' is painful, dry, is not blistered and will fade on its own within 7 days. It requires no debridement and is not counted in the calculation of percentage of total body surface area (TBSA). Simple oral analgesics and anti-inflammatories are all that is needed.

12.3.2 Superficial Partial Thickness

These involve the entire epidermis down to the basement membrane and no more than the upper third of the dermis. Rapid re-epithelialization occurs in 1–2 weeks. Because of the large number of remaining epidermal cells and the good blood supply, there is a very small zone of injury or stasis beneath the burn eschar (Figure 12.3).

A superficial partial thickness (SPT) burn is wet, often blistered, intensely painful and red or white (including in coloured races), blanches on pressure, and will generally heal without split-skin grafting (SSG), usually within 10–14 days. The hairs remain attached when they are pulled. The skin still feels elastic and supple. These burns are often caused by hot water and steam. They do not scar.

12.3.3 Deep Partial Thickness

Destruction of the epidermis occurs down to the basement membrane plus the middle third of the dermis. Re-epithelialization is much slower (2–4 weeks) due to fewer remaining epidermal cells and a lesser blood supply. More collagen deposition will occur, especially if the wound has not been excised and grafted within 3 weeks. The depth of the wound has a significant risk of conversion. The zone of stasis is much larger than in the SPT injury because of the lower blood flow and greater initial injury to the remaining epidermal cells (Figure 12.4).

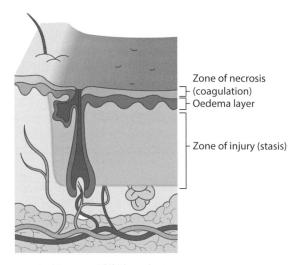

Figure 12.4 Deep partial thickness burn.

A deep partial thickness (DPT) burn is often a mixture of wet and dry. The drier it is, the deeper. Sensation is variable but is still present to touch, although often less painful. The skin texture is thicker and more rubbery. Red patches do not blanche on pressure but exhibit 'fixed skin staining' due to capillary stasis. The hairs will come out readily when pulled. If not excised, these burns take 4–6 weeks to heal and scar badly. The function of a re-epithelialized DPT burn is poor due to fragility of the epidermis and the rigidity of the scar-laden dermis.

12.3.4 'Indeterminate' Partial Thickness Burns

Indeterminate burns are usually a mixture of SPT and DPT burns, and may exhibit the clinical features of both. The history may help in deciding which is the predominant element and enable management decision making.

12.3.5 Full Thickness

Full-thickness burns involve the entire epidermis and at least two-thirds of the dermis, leaving very few dermis and epidermal cells to regenerate. Spontaneous healing is very slow, over 4 weeks. Sharp debridement is needed to remove the eschar. Scarring is usually severe if the wound is not skin grafted, and there is a high risk of infection. Induced inflammation (i.e. conversion to a full-thickness burn) is common.

Full-thickness burns are thick, dry, insensate, leathery and usually black or yellow. Thrombosis is often visible in the surface vessels. The hairs have been burned off. Escharotomies and fasciotomies may be indicated for circumferential full-thickness burns. If left, these burns will contract, become infected and scar badly. They require early excision and grafting. All electrical burns are full thickness, as are many flame and chemical burns.

12.4 TOTAL BODY SURFACE AREA (TBSA) BURNED

For the purposes of calculating the TBSA as a percentage of the entire body surface area, only SPT and DPT burns, along with full-thickness burns, are included in the calculation. Erythema – simple 'sunburn' – alone is ignored.

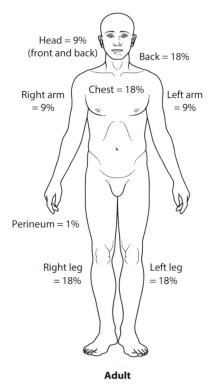

Head = 9%
(front and back)
Back = 18%
Chest = 18%
Right arm = 9%
Left arm = 9%
Perineum = 1%
Right leg = 18%
Left leg = 18%

Adult

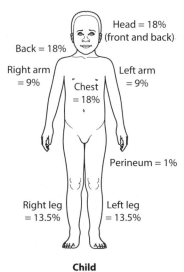

Head = 18%
(front and back)
Back = 18%
Right arm = 9%
Left arm = 9%
Chest = 18%
Perineum = 1%
Right leg = 13.5%
Left leg = 13.5%

Child

Figure 12.5 Calculation of burn size from body surface area.

All units involved in the management of burns should have a clearly established protocol, and this should include the use of a burns resuscitation chart that also shows TBSA affected, in diagrammatic form (traditionally the 'rule of nines' in the adult, and the Lund and Browder chart in the child) (Figure 12.5). The patient's palm, *including the fingers*, represents approximately 1 per cent TBSA and is useful when calculating patchy burns.

It must be emphasized that TBSA calculation is only a starting point for working out a plan of management. Subsequent management is dictated by the patient's response – not by calculated numbers.

12.5 MANAGEMENT

12.5.1 Safe Retrieval

As with all trauma, this will follow the usual Advanced Trauma Life Support (ATLS) protocols of 'Airway, Breathing, Circulation', etc. – the ABCDEs.

However, it may, in addition, include removing the casualty from the source of burning *without concomitant risk to the rescuer*. This may mean that electrical power supplies must be switched off, chemical and fuel spillages contained and fires extinguished to allow rescuers access to the casualty. Burning clothing must be removed and caustic substances washed off as much as possible, but little time should be spent at the scene.

> *Do not forget that a burned patient is still a trauma patient, and may well have suffered other major injuries in addition to the burn.*

12.5.2 First Aid

Do: Cool the burn with cold, running water. If a tap is not available, use a bucket and jug. Continue for at least 20–30 minutes and up to 2 hours from the time of injury. This will reduce the depth of the burn.

Don't: Use ice or iced water as these may extend the depth of burn. Do not use butter, egg, oil, toothpaste or any other kitchen or bathroom items. Do not let the patient get cold; removing burning clothing and leaving the patient exposed to the elements will very quickly result in hypothermia.

> *The principle is to cool the burn but warm the patient.*

Any burn produces inflammation and associated swelling and capillary leakage. The greater the TBSA affected, the greater the inflammatory response, so that any burn of over 25 per cent TBSA will produce a total body systemic reaction with resultant systemic inflammatory response syndrome (SIRS). This is unavoidable and should be anticipated.

12.5.3 Emergency Department

12.5.3.1 AIRWAY

A rapid assessment of the circumstances of the burn may well alert the medical team to the potential for an airway burn. Fires in an enclosed space (such as shack fires) with much combustible material and a prolonged extrication time will clearly represent a significant risk. Aspiration of caustic substances may produce a fierce chemical pneumonitis, and steam inhalation from boiling water may cause significant airway injury. Where obvious signs of airway injury exist (stridor, singed facial hair, soot in the nares or mouth or carbonaceous sputum), not only should supplemental oxygen be administered by 60 per cent reservoir mask, but early intubation should also be accomplished before swelling closes the upper airway.

> *It is easier to subsequently extubate a stable patient who has been intubated early, than to try a late intubation on a patient whose airway is swollen, distorted and burned.*

12.5.3.2 ANALGESIA

Partial thickness burns are intensely painful and require repeated doses of intravenous opiates, titrated against the pain. Analgesia must always be given, even if the child or adult cannot communicate with you. However, the deeper the burn gets, the fewer nerve endings survive, to the point where full-thickness burns are insensate. Nevertheless, the emotional trauma of a major burn alone requires the calming effect of opiate drugs. Providing early, adequate pain relief will reduce stress to the patient and attending medical staff alike and should be a priority in management after airway control.

Intravenous access should be accomplished and, at the same time, blood samples taken for full blood count, electrolytes, amylase, blood type and screen and glucose. In patients with a greater than 50 per cent burn, it is likely that a consumption coagulopathy may develop;

therefore, a thromboelastogram should be performed or, if this is not available, a conventional coagulation screen (international normalized ratio, activated partial thromboplastin time, platelet estimation, etc.).

If possible, arterial blood gases with an assessment of carboxyhaemoglobin should be obtained and a note made of the fraction of inspired oxygen (Fio_2) on the result so that the degree of pulmonary shunting can be calculated. This may be helpful if subsequent ventilation is required.

12.5.3.3 EMERGENCY MANAGEMENT OF THE BURN WOUND

Coverage of the burn wound in the emergency setting is best accomplished with large quantities of 'Clingfilm', which has been shown to be sterile and is available in industrial quantities. Clingfilm reduces pain by covering exposed nerve endings and contains and reduces fluid losses, while still allowing proper inspection of the burn wound. The old practice of 'mummifying' the patient in swathes of gauze and crepe bandages (with or without the addition of underlying silver creams) is unhelpful, painful for the patient, messy, time-consuming, inefficient for nursing staff and obstructive to the clinician.

12.5.3.4 FLUID RESUSCITATION

All burns over 15 per cent constitute 'major burns'. All of these will require intravenous fluid replacement, a urinary catheter to monitor output, a nasogastric tube for early feeding and at least high-care nursing. Lesser percentage burns may be treated by aggressive oral rehydration, but particularly in infants it is better to err on the side of caution, and some units still routinely resuscitate those under 12 years who have a greater than 10 per cent TBSA burn with intravenous fluids.

All fluid replacement formulae are only *guidelines* to resuscitation. Adequacy of resuscitation is based on urine output rather than slavishly following a formula such as the Parkland formula for fluid requirements. Fluid losses start at the time of burn, and fluid replacement is calculated *from the time of burn*, not from the time of admission to hospital. The Parkland formula is traditionally used to work out requirements for the first 24 hours:

TBSA% burned × 4 mL × mass in kg = requirement in first 24 hours (mL)

(If BSA >60%, use 3 mL/kg.)

The first half of the total requirement is given in the first 8 hours, and the other half over the following 16 hours; this is given as Ringer lactate. There is limited evidence that changing to a colloid solution in the next 24 hours will reduce capillary leakage. Urine output should be maintained at no more than 0.5–1 mL/kg per hour for adults and 1–2 mL/kg per hour for infants and children. If too much fluid is given, capillary leakage will increase, producing 'fluid creep' and increasing oedema as the fluid shifts into the 'third space', thus increasing the likelihood of SIRS and adult respiratory distress syndrome (ARDS)[1]. The exception would be if there were myoglobinuria, as in electrical burns, where an output over 1 mL/kg per hour would be required for an adult.

Antibiotics are not indicated for early burns within 72 hours of injury, as the burn is still essentially sterile.

12.5.3.5 ASSOCIATED INJURIES

It is easy to focus on the burn alone and miss any associated injuries. A careful history will give clues to not only the type and depth of the burn, but also the possibility of the associated injuries.

A casualty trapped in an enclosed space filled with furniture, such as in a house fire, is likely to have an airway burn and carbon monoxide poisoning, along with the possibility of toxicity from many other poisonous inhaled gases. Furthermore, if the patient had to be removed unconscious by rescuers, the length of exposure to heat and flames makes the likelihood of full-thickness burns much greater than if he or she was able to escape by him- or herself. The patient may have had to jump from a burning building to escape the flames, and have fractures or ruptured soft tissues, such as a liver or spleen.

If the patient is hypotensive on admission, it is wrong to attribute signs of shock to the burn until all other sources of shock have been ruled out. Burn shock does not usually develop in the first 24 hours post-burn. A full examination is essential once analgesia is adequate, intravenous lines (which may have to transgress a burned area of skin) are running, oxygen is being administered and the burn has been covered.

Any other injuries found during examination of the patient must be dealt with according to clinical need. Injuries that are bleeding take priority, and the normal principles of resuscitation, including damage control, apply. Most orthopaedic injuries may be deferred for definitive treatment until the resuscitation phase of the burn injury is over. This is usually within the first 48 hours. However, if the patient requires early tangential excision and SSG, it may be appropriate to attend to orthopaedic conditions at the same time, as long as the patient's physiology is not compromised.

The clinician must be alert to the possibility of deliberate abuse, especially in children, where the nature and distribution of the burn are inconsistent with the story given by the parent or caregiver. The pattern of burn and an unacceptably late presentation may be further clues to a deliberate, 'punishment' burn. Where suspicion exists, it is important to document the burn injury meticulously, with photographs if possible. Other signs of abuse should be looked for and social services contacted if appropriate.

12.5.3.6 ESCHAROTOMY AND FASCIOTOMY

In any trauma resuscitation, the purpose is to combat shock, defined as tissue hypoxia inadequate to the needs of that tissue's survival. Burns are no different, but they present with some special challenges, particularly when the airway is compromised or when circumferential full-thickness burns with a thick, unyielding eschar produce a tourniquet effect. This can occur around the chest, neck or limbs, producing a slow asphyxiation or critical limb ischaemia. Recognition of the need for escharotomy is vital and needs to be acted upon, usually within the emergency department.

An escharotomy is not necessarily a fasciotomy.

The technique is simple. Linear incisions are made deep enough to release the tension. The escharotomy wounds then gape apart, relieving the tension. The escharotomy wounds have to be extensive enough to reach normal tissue. Although a scalpel is usually adequate to achieve this, diathermy may be necessary.

Figure 12.6 shows the main incision lines for the release of eschar causing constriction. Escharotomy should be a largely painless procedure as it is only transgressing devitalized tissue, except at its limits where it may encroach upon living tissues which will be normally sensate or even hypersensate. This will not only alert the clinician to stop but ensures that constriction rings of dead eschar are not left at the limits of the escharotomy.

Despite escharotomy release, some tissues – especially in limbs – may remain ischaemic, particularly where there has been an electrical burn, which is always full thickness and frequently produces significant myonecrosis. In these cases, it may be necessary to extend the escharotomy into a fasciotomy to release the compartment syndrome. Fasciotomy is usually accompanied by profuse bleeding if the tissue within is still viable, and one should be prepared for this.

12.5.4 **Definitive Management**

12.5.4.1 'CLOSING' THE BURN WOUND

Burns are not static wounds: they are 'pathology-in-evolution'. The longer the burn remains uncovered by either the patient's own skin or an effective biological alternative, the longer it remains a significant breech of the skin's antibacterial barrier and a significant source of heat and fluid loss to the body, analogous to bowel evisceration.

From about 72 hours post-burn, surface bacteria migrate into the remaining deep dermis and below, rendering topical antiseptics and antibiotics ineffective,

Figure 12.6 Escharotomy and fasciotomy sites.

and increasing the chances of systemic septicaemia. For these reasons, there has been a move towards early excision of the wound and SSG where necessary.

Clearly, not all burns require grafting. Hot water and scalds from steam will often heal on their own within 10 days, despite their dramatic initial appearances. It is wise to wait for this time before deciding to operate. The SSG rate for these burns has been almost halved by such an approach. However, *all* burns should undergo an initial cleaning and debridement under anaesthesia as soon as possible after admission, preferably within the first 48 hours. The reasons for this are fourfold:

- This cleans the wound thoroughly and enables an appropriate choice of dressing, as Clingfilm is difficult to secure for more than 48 hours.
- It allows a proper inspection of the burn and removal of blisters, because it is not unusual for the area of the burn to be underestimated in the emergency room, and a 9 per cent burn may turn out to be 16 per cent, putting it into the 'major burn' category, with all its attendant requirements.
- It is often (wrongly) assumed that blistered burns are always SPT burns. Blistered skin should be removed, unless it is really slack, so that the clinician can be sure there is no deeper burn beneath. It is safer to excise the blister and assess the depth of the burn beneath, as it may turn out to be DPT or even full thickness.
- If it is seen that excision and SSG are required, this may be accomplished at the same visit to the operating room.

12.5.4.2 TECHNIQUE OF EXCISION AND SPLIT-SKIN GRAFTING (SSG)

Both these techniques can be accomplished by using either the Humby knife (or a modification of it) or an electric dermatome. The 'set' of the blade (depth of cut) will need to be greater for excision than for the harvesting of skin for SSG.

12.5.4.3 TUMESCENT TECHNIQUE

Blood loss can be significant in both procedures but may be minimized by using tourniquets for the limbs or the 'tumescent technique' on the torso:

1. The technique uses 2 mL 1:1000 adrenaline (epinephrine) + 40 mL 0.5 per cent plain bupivacaine added to 1 L of warm normal saline.

2. Take a 19-gauge 3.5-inch spinal needle, and attach a giving set to the bag, which is placed in a pressurized infusion device and the injection given subdermally.

3. The raised skin should feel cold (and look white in Caucasian races).

4. Once the skin has been harvested or the burn excised, adrenaline-soaked abdominal packs (5 mg in 1 L normal saline) can be applied to the wound bed, with a significant reduction in blood loss.

The SSGs are secured by skin clips, tissue glue or sutures, depending on the site, and then covered with several layers of paraffin gauze to prevent movement, followed by dry gauze and bandaging.

If infection has been a problem, activated nanocrystalline silver (e.g. Acticoat, Smith & Nephew, London, UK) may be applied and secured in place with water-soaked gauze and bandages. The dressing will remain bacterially active for up to 4 days, and may also have anti-inflammatory properties. More recently, ceramic bead compound dressings have been shown to be particularly effective in removing exudate and preventing bacterial colonization.

The choice of site for harvesting skin depends on the site that is burned (e.g. back or eyelids) and what skin is available:

- Neck skin is good for eyelids.
- Inner arm skin is good for the face.
- Wherever possible, match the colour, texture and hair growth.
- When skin substitutes are not an option, reharvesting donor sites is usually possible within 10–14 days.

It is beyond the scope of this book to discuss the many skin substitutes currently available on the market. The patient's own skin is always the best. Substitutes are often difficult to obtain, culturally unacceptable or just too expensive. The issue of substitutes only arises where the percentage TBSA is greater than the amount of harvestable skin from the patient.

12.5.4.4 ASSESSING AND MANAGING AIRWAY BURNS

12.5.4.4.1 Upper Airway

Suspicion is the watchword, with early intervention before the opportunity to protect the airway by intubation has been lost. Listening to the respiration is vital, and dyspnoea with hoarse, coarse breathing or stridor should prompt immediate action.

Upper airway burns to the larynx and trachea may be suspected by the history (e.g. a steam valve blew into the face) or by inspection of the mouth, tongue and oro-pharynx, which may be red, injected and swollen. These burns usually require intubation but generally resolve within 36 hours. It is important to remember that the burn is 'pathology-in-evolution' and that the early signs will get worse in the next 24 hours.

12.5.4.4.2 Lower Airway

The deep, 'alveolar' burn is much more difficult to detect or predict. Its rate of onset is slower, and it may only manifest itself 3–5 days after the burn. Some indication that a lower airway burn is present may come from the history of prolonged smoke exposure and raised car-boxyhaemoglobin levels. Blood gases should be taken whenever possible, and the ventilation-perfusion shunt worked out by plotting the Fio_2 against the PaO_2 (partial pressure of oxygen in arterial blood).

Although no clear guidelines exist in the literature at present, it is unusual to find a patient with a shunt of 15–20 per cent or more who has not required prolonged ventilation over a week. The alveolitis produces exces-sive lung water, and the picture is one of ARDS. It may become increasingly difficult to ventilate these patients, and nebulized heparin or acetylcysteine can be used in an attempt to reduce the stickiness of secretions. The issue of whether to perform bronchoscopy and bronchial lavage is still debated but has not been subjected to a controlled clinical trial, so no conclusions can be drawn.

12.5.4.4.3 Inhalational Toxicity

This third component of airway burns may present first as the effects of carbon monoxide poisoning are immediate.

Remember that the peak level of carbon monoxide is present at the scene and not at first measurement in the hospital.

Any carbon monoxide level of over 10 per cent is regarded as toxic, and 100 per cent oxygen should be given until the carbon monoxide level has fallen to below 5 per cent.

Pulse oximetry may be unreliable if high levels of carbon monoxide are present, as the haemoglobin is saturated with carbon monoxide and not oxygen.

Other gases such as cyanide may also have an imme-diate toxic effect, but the effects of gases like ammonia, sulphur dioxide, chlorine, hydrogen chloride, phosgene and the aldehydes may take a day or two to present. Treatment is supportive, although if cyanide is a strong possibility, sodium nitrite may be given intravenously. Methaemoglobin production is a side effect of such treatment.

12.5.4.4.4 Tracheostomy

Early tracheostomy should be considered, especially if the area of the burn includes the neck. It is quite accept-able to place a tracheostomy through the site of a burn. Once the oedema has occurred, placement of a trache-ostomy is far more difficult and hazardous. The tra-cheostomy should be well secured, as replacement may prove very difficult if it is displaced.

12.6 SPECIAL AREAS

The face, hands, perineum and feet are special areas that need special attention to obtain a good outcome.

12.6.1 Face

Biobrane is very useful for SPT burns of the face. It needs to be held in place firmly with compression for 48 hours to 'bond'. This may be accomplished by crepe bandaging, which is then removed after 2 days. Biobrane reduces pain and may be left in place until it begins to separate by itself after about 10 days, leaving new epithelium that does not need to be grafted.

12.6.2 Hands

Function is the priority for burned hands. Wrapping up in boxing glove-type dressings will rapidly result in stiff, contracted hands, so wherever possible leave the hands exposed or with minimal dressings. The prac-tice of smothering burned hands in silver sulphadi-azine cream and then placing them in plastic bags is not recommended as this macerates the remaining normal skin and just produces a pool of foul liquid in the bag in a short time. Superficial partial thickness burns can be covered with copious amounts of mupirocin ointment to combat staphylococcal and streptococcal infection, keep the burn supple and allow the occupational therapist the freedom to work without restriction.

If escharotomy is needed, it is important to try to preserve the 'pinch grip' between finger and thumb. For this reason, the incisions should be on the ulnar side of the thumb and the radial side of the fingers. It may be necessary to splint the hand at night to prevent contracture. This must be done in the 'intrinsic-plus' or 'position of function', with the wrist slightly dorsiflexed, the metacarpophalangeal joints at a right angle and the fingers in full extension (Figure 12.7).

The splint is best applied from the palmar surface and wrapped gently around the edges of the index and little fingers to stop them falling off the splint platform. It is important to place paraffin gauze between the fingers on the splint to prevent adherence to one another, with the potential for later syndactyly.

Deeper burns to the hand may be covered with a biosynthetic dressing such as Biobrane.

12.6.3 Perineum

Early catheterization is recommended, as is nursing by exposure as much as possible. Nappies/diapers coated with silver sulphadiazine cream are comfortable and practical, for both adults and children. A temporary colostomy for faecal diversion should be considered.

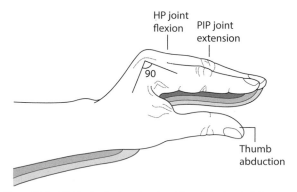

Figure 12.7 Splinting in the functional position of the hand. (MP, metacarpophalangeal; PIP, proximal interphalangeal).

12.6.4 Feet

Apart from preventing syndactyly as mentioned previously, the importance of burns to the feet is the ability to be able to weight bear, and to prevent foot-drop during the recovery period. Splints will be needed to maintain the ankle joint at a right angle.

Weight-bearing on a split-skin graft (SSG) will rapidly result in destruction of the graft. If a full thickness burn of the sole of the foot is present, it may take the skills of a reconstructive plastic surgeon to embark on lengthy cross-leg flap procedures to obtain adequate coverage that will withstand body weight. In resource-constrained countries, a below-knee amputation may seem a drastic measure but frequently returns the patient to work and his or her family quicker.

12.7 ADJUNCTS IN BURN CARE

12.7.1 Nutrition in the Burned Patient

A dietitian is an essential member of the burns team[2]. All patients with a major burn (>15 per cent TBSA) should have a nasogastric tube or fine-bore feeding tube for early enteral nutrition. This should ideally be started within 18 hours of the burn. Not only does this help in the early replacement of calories, but it also protects against gut bacterial translocation and systemic sepsis. It may in addition protect against the development of the rare Curling ulcer[3].

The aim should be, in paediatric patients at least, to provide 100 per cent of their calorie requirements down the tube, and any further food they can take orally is a bonus. Estimating the nutritional needs of burn patients is essential to the healing process. The Harris-Benedict equation is designed to calculate the calorie needs of adults, and the Galveston formula is used for children. The Curreri formula addresses the needs of both. Some studies suggest that these formulae may overestimate the calorie needs of patients by up to 150 per cent. There is no single formula that can accurately determine how many calories a patient needs, so it is important to monitor a patient's nutritional condition closely.

Protein requirements generally increase more than energy requirements, and appear to be related to the amount of lean body mass. The body loses protein through the burn, and this will be reflected in a significant drop in serum albumin level over the first week, which will take at least a month to recover despite assiduous nutritional care. However, the majority of increased protein requirements come from muscle breakdown for use in extra energy production. Providing an increased intake of protein does not stop this obligatory breakdown; it simply provides the materials needed to replace lost tissue.

Carbohydrates provide the majority of calorie intake under most conditions, including the stress of burns. Providing adequate calories from carbohydrates spares incoming protein from being used for fuel. The body breaks down carbohydrates into glucose that the body then uses for energy.

Fat is needed to meet essential fatty acid requirements and provide needed calories. Common recommendations include giving 30 per cent of calories as fat, although this can be higher if needed. Excess fat intake has been implicated in decreased immune function, and intake levels should be monitored carefully. Vitamins and trace elements are also necessary.

12.7.2 Paediatric Burn Nutrition

Providing adequate calories and nutrients is a difficult task when treating burn injuries. This task becomes even more difficult when the patient is a child. It is important to do an initial nutritional assessment early after admission as often it is children in the lower socio-economic group who get burned. This group is also more likely to be suffering from chronic malnutrition before their burn injury, giving them even less reserve with which to repair injured tissue.

12.7.3 Ulcer Prophylaxis

For more information about ulcer prophylaxis[4], see Section 14.15.

In the presence of good nutritional policies, sucralfate should be used for prophylaxis. The H_2 receptor-blockers and protein pump inhibitors should be reserved for therapy and not used for prophylaxis.

12.7.4 Venous Thromboembolism Prophylaxis

For more information about venous thromboembolism prophylaxis[5], see Section 14.15.

Patients with major burns are at high risk of venous thromboembolism. The nature of the burn is often such that mechanical devices are excluded.

Low-molecular-weight heparin should be introduced early.

12.7.5 Antibiotics

Antibiotic prophylaxis is *not* routinely used for burns. There is no substitute for good wound care, hand-washing and infection control measures. Tissue excised during tangential excision should be sent for culture, and when skin grafting, cultures (sometimes obtained by local punch biopsy) should again be sent. Sepsis should be treated topically wherever possible, and systemic antibiotics should be used only where there is evidence of systemic sepsis.

12.8 CRITERIA FOR TRANSFER

- Special areas (as above), including those involving a major joint.
- Major burns (>15 per cent TBSA, although some centres recommend >10 per cent TBSA).
- Electrical burns and lightning injury.
- All full-thickness burns of over 1 per cent in any age group.
- Chemical burns.
- Inhalation injury.
- Burn injury in patients with pre-existing medical disorders that could complicate management, prolong recovery or affect mortality.
- Any patients with burns and concomitant trauma (such as fractures) for whom the burn injury poses the greatest risk of morbidity or mortality. (In such cases, if the trauma poses the greater immediate risk, the patient's condition may be stabilized initially in a trauma centre before transfer to a burn centre. Clinical judgement and good communication will be necessary.)
- Burned children in hospitals without adequate qualified personnel or equipment.

12.9 SUMMARY

Burns are a huge problem worldwide, with the majority occurring in countries that are ill equipped to deal with them as resources are few, transport is lacking and cultural influences militate against early referral to modern facilities. Education is the cornerstone of prevention, and up to 95 per cent of burns in developing countries are preventable. Education is also, sadly, often lacking.

Nevertheless, for those who are lucky enough to reach a burns facility, modern techniques, including supportive ventilation for inhalational burns, early tangential excision and grafting, utilization of biosynthetic dressings, nanocrystalline silver technology and ceramic sphere technology, have significantly increased survival and quality of life for burn patients.

Burn care remains a 'team effort', and no amount of highly skilled grafting in the operating room will be rewarded by a happy and functional outcome if the feeding, nursing, intensive care, physiotherapy or occupational therapy is lacking.

REFERENCES AND RECOMMENDED READING

References

1. Rogers AD, Karpelowsky J, Millar AJW, Argent A, Rode H. Fluid creep in major paediatric burns. *Eur J Pediatr Surg.* 2010;20:133–138.
2. Jacobs DO, Kudsk KA, Oswanski MF, Sacks GS, Sinclair KE. Practice management guidelines for nutritional support of the trauma patient. In: *Eastern Association for the Surgery of Trauma. Practice Management Guidelines.* http://www.east.org. Accessed December 2010.
3. Muir IFK, Jones PF. Curling's ulcer: a rare condition. *Br J Surg.* 1976;63:60–66.
4. Guillamondegui OD, Gunter OL Jr, Bonadies JA, et al. Practice management guidelines for stress ulcer prophylaxis. EAST Practice Management Guidelines Workgroup. http://www.east.org. Accessed December 2014.
5. Rogers FB, Cipolle MD, Velmahos G, Rozycki G. Practice management guidelines for the management of venous thromboembolism (VTE) in trauma patients. *J Trauma.* 2002;53:142–164. Available from Eastern Association for the Surgery of Trauma, Practice Management Guidelines Workgroup. http://www.east.org. Accessed December 2014.

Recommended Reading

Greenwood JE. Development of patient pathways for the surgical management of burn injury. *Aust NZ J Surg.* 2006;76:805–811.

Herndon D, Ed. *Total Burn Care.* 3rd ed. Philadelphia, PA: Saunders Elsevier; 2007.

Websites

Brigham and Women's Hospital. Division of plastic surgery. http://www.burnsurgery.com.

Burn Survivor. Home page. http://www.burnsurvivor.com.

MetroHealth. Home page. http://www.metrohealth.org.

World Health Organization. Violence and injury prevention. Burns. http://www.who.int/violence_injury_prevention/other_injury/burns/en/index.html.

Special Patient Situations **13**

13.1 **PAEDIATRICS**

13.1.1 **Introduction**

An understanding of the different anatomy, physiology and injury patterns of the injured child is essential for a successful outcome of treatment. Many simple, familiar procedures that are taken for granted in the adult patient need to be practised in the paediatric patient before they can be safely performed in the stress of a resuscitation situation. If necessary, the need for referral should be considered as soon as the patient will tolerate safe transfer to an appropriate facility.

13.1.2 **Injury Patterns**

Certain injury patterns of paediatric trauma are becoming apparent:

- Lap belt complex:
  - Pancreatic and duodenal injury.
  - Chance fracture of the lumbar spine.
  - Horizontal contusion on the abdominal wall from the lap belt component.
- Pedestrian-vehicle crash (PVC) complex:
  - Leg and head injuries.
- Forward-facing infant complex:
  - Flexion fracture of the cervical spine.
  - Liver and spleen injury.
- Common cycle scenarios:
  - Handlebar in the epigastrium, and splenic or liver injury.
  - The fall astride with urethral or perineal injury.
- Non-accidental injury complex:
  - Injury patterns suggestive of non-accidental injury are very well known. The most vulnerable group with the highest mortality rates are infants. The presence of a severe head injury in an infant

without a clear history of a fall from a significant height or a vehicle collision should always arouse suspicion.

13.1.3 **Pre-hospital**

Prehospital interventions should be limited to basic life support with airway and ventilatory support, securing haemostasis of external bleeding and basic attempts to secure vascular access. The utility of prehospital endotracheal intubation has recently been vigorously questioned. It would appear that bag-valve and mask ventilation is at least as good as intubation in head-injured children and this should be the standard if intubation fails or if inadequate expertise exists. Extensive unsuccessful roadside resuscitative procedures are a common cause of morbidity and mortality. The younger the child and the more unstable his or her condition, the greater the tendency should be to 'scoop and run' to the nearest appropriate facility.

If a child is treated at an interim facility prior to transfer for definitive care, care should be taken to avoid unnecessary imaging, particularly computed tomography (CT) scanning, as this can cause potentially deleterious delays.

13.1.4 **Resuscitation Room**

13.1.4.1 AIRWAY

The indications for airway control are identical to those in the adult patient. The routine administration of oxygen and the stepwise system of management according to severity of airway compromise are the cardinal features of paediatric airway management. Orotracheal intubation skill without force, otherwise bothersome, or even dangerous post-extubation stridor can ensue from a traumatic intubation.

A surgical airway is seldom necessary. If it is required, a tracheostomy should be performed.

The greatest pitfalls are the danger of tube dislodgement, commonly due to failure to secure the tube adequately, or too small an endotracheal tube.

The airway of the obligate nasal breather (the neonate or infant) must not be compromised with a nasogastric tube. The clinical assessment of the cervical spine injury is less reliable in the fearful, uncooperative child, and cervical spine protection must be maintained until the neck has been passed cleared.

13.1.4.2 VENTILATION

Hypoventilation is a prominent cause of hypoxia in the injured child. Because the child depends primarily on diaphragmatic breathing, one must be particularly cautious of conditions that impair diaphragmatic movement (tension pneumothoraces, diaphragmatic rupture and severe gastric dilatation) and treat expeditiously.

Once a controlled and monitored situation has been obtained, one should avoid both barotrauma and volume trauma by providing about 6 mL/kg body weight tidal volume at the lowest pressure. Avoid lung injury from hyperventilation and barotrauma.

13.1.4.3 CIRCULATION

Frequent assessment of circulatory status is important. Children have effective compensatory mechanisms for compensating for blood loss, dependent predominantly on an adequate heart rate. Tachycardia, peripheral vasoconstriction and signs of inadequate central nervous system perfusion predominate. Hypotension is a late sign of blood loss, reflecting a class IV shock with greater than 40 per cent blood volume loss.

The practitioner must recognize and treat shock aggressively. The primary management of bleeding is surgical haemostasis. Rapid vascular access is obtained tailored to the severity of the child's shock and the practitioner's experience: central lines are reserved for the larger child and the more experienced physician. Most children respond rapidly to crystalloid resuscitation.

Do not delay the transfer of the unstable child to the operating room – establish good access and the anaesthesiologist can resuscitate while the surgeon stops the bleeding. *Never* transfer a hemodynamically unstable patient to the CT scanner. Hypothermia is critical and must be avoided. The urinary output is an invaluable aid to determine the adequacy of resuscitation.

13.1.4.4 DISABILITY

Make a quick neurological assessment including the Glasgow Coma Scale score, pupils and movements of all extremities. In general, children have a lower incidence of intracranial mass lesions requiring surgical drainage after blunt injury compared with adults. Accelerated cerebral oedema may occur in children, particularly after high-speed vehicular trauma. Signs of sudden neurologic deterioration must prompt urgent neurosurgical evaluation and consideration for placement of an intracranial pressure monitor or decompressive craniectomy. A child with signs of transtentorial herniation – a unilateral fixed, dilated pupil, ipsilateral muscle weakness and deteriorating level of consciousness – will require an urgent CT scan and prompt neurosurgical management that supersedes all other priorities except the management of the airway and the treatment of hypovolaemic shock.

13.1.4.5 CARDIAC ARREST

In children, cardiac arrest usually is not caused by ventricular fibrillation and is often heralded by bradycardia, pulseless electrical activity or asystole. The primary objective of resuscitation should be to correct the underlying cause (such as tension pneumothorax, hypovolaemia, hypothermia or hypoxia), and to provide cardiac massage and ventilatory support.

13.1.4.6 RESUSCITATIVE THORACOTOMY

Resuscitative thoracotomy is usually futile and not recommended for blunt trauma but should be considered for children with witnessed cardiac arrest and penetrating thoracic injury.

13.1.5 Specific Organ Injury

13.1.5.1 HEAD AND NECK INJURY

Most paediatric trauma deaths result from head injury. Computed tomography is the most accurate modality to evaluate paediatric patients with a suspected head injury. Diffuse intracranial lesions are more common in children than in adults. The short neck, combined with a proportionally heavy head, little muscle support and laxity of the ligaments, makes the child vulnerable to cervical injuries.

13.1.5.2 THORACIC INJURY

Young children have a more flexible thoracic cage than adults. Rib fractures in children are uncommon and indicate major injury. Pulmonary contusion is the most common injury to the chest and is commonly seen in the absence of rib fractures. Contusions are typically delayed in appearance on chest X-ray. If pathological findings (of pulmonary contusion) are visible on the admission chest X-ray, then the contusion is severe, and hypoxia should be expected to worsen over the next 1–2 days.

13.1.5.3 ABDOMINAL INJURY

Abdominal injuries must be suspected after high-energy trauma. The upper abdominal organs have little protection from the rib cage and musculature. Not surprisingly, the spleen and the liver are the most frequently injured intra-abdominal organs in children. Most children with abdominal injuries from blunt trauma can be safely treated non-operatively. For the trauma surgeon, the challenge is to identify expeditiously those patients who require surgical intervention. Patients with haemoperitoneum and haemodynamic instability not responding to resuscitation and those with clear signs of peritonitis or bowel injury as evidenced by free intraperitoneal air should be expeditiously explored. Diaphragmatic rupture and intraperitoneal bladder rupture are other early indications for surgery.

Hollow viscus injuries are relatively rare, and symptoms can be vague in the early stage after trauma. Repeated examination remains essential in the early diagnosis of these injuries. Free fluid in the absence of solid organ injury on a CT scan in a patient with an appropriate injury mechanism (e.g. lap belt injury) is highly indicative of an intestinal lesion. Recent data support the safety of serial examinations for the clinical detection of bowel injuries. Diagnosis and expeditious management of hollow visceral injuries 6–12 hours after injury does not appear to have an adverse impact on outcomes.

Pancreatic injuries are rare, and diagnosis often is delayed. Contusions can be treated non-operatively, whereas operative treatment is most often recommended in patients with transection through the distal part of the gland.

Duodenal injuries are uncommon, diagnosis often being delayed and associated with serious complications. In some countries, as many as 20 per cent of duodenal injuries in pre-school children, are related to child abuse.

13.1.5.4 GENITOURINARY INJURY

The hallmark of genitourinary tract injury is haematuria. The degree of haematuria does not correlate with injury severity, and the absence of blood in the urine does not exclude significant urological injury. The kidneys are most commonly involved. Less than 5 per cent of children with renal injuries will need operative treatment. A CT scan of the abdomen is highly sensitive and specific, although it does not reliably exclude bladder rupture unless dedicated cystography views with bladder distension are obtained.

Pelvic fracture is a rare cause for exsanguination in children, and most fractures are treated non-operatively.

13.1.6 Analgesia

A prevalent and almost irrational fear of providing children with appropriate analgesia needs to be overcome. Opiates are the primary agents recommended for both the prehospital and hospital use. Appropriate titrated doses of morphine – 0.1 mg/kg 4-hourly or when required – should be offered to the paediatric trauma patient to reduce pain and anxiety. Such an approach will facilitate resuscitation and assessment and does not mask important clinical signs, but probably enhances the interpretation by improving the patient's cooperation. However, monitoring of the patient's respiratory and haemodynamic status and level of consciousness is essential.

13.2 THE ELDERLY

13.2.1 Definition of 'Older' and Susceptibility to Trauma

Population ageing is a global phenomenon. In the United States in 1990, those over age 65 accounted for 12.5 per cent of the population, while in 2040 it is expected that this will rise to more than 20 per cent of the population. In sub-Saharan Africa, the rate of increase of those over 60 years old between 2000 and 2025 is expected to reach 145 per cent[1]. (In contrast, in Western Europe, this increase will be less than 45 per cent.) However, more older persons will mean more 'older trauma'.

What is an 'older patient'? It depends on the context. In 2000, the World Health Organization (WHO) Africa Minimum Data Set (MDS) Project collaborators agreed to use the chronological age of 60 years as a guide for the working definition of 'old'[2], although upon further deliberation in 2001, the working definition of 'older' was changed to the age of 50 years. In practical terms ageing is determined by the clinician's assessment of the patient with reference to interplay of chronology, local geographic, social, economic and biological impacts. Thus the patient may be deemed 'older' at any age between 50 and 80 years, depending on the local context. In current trauma scoring systems, the break-point for the elderly is 55 years of age. In the United States, the 12.5 per cent of the population over the age of 65 accounts for almost one-third of all deaths from injury.

Older people seem to be both more susceptible to trauma and to experience significantly higher mortality rates and complications. Contributing factors such as diminished physiological reserve and the existence of multiple medical co-morbidities present additional management challenges[3].

Certain medications such as hypnotics (e.g. zopiclone, zolpidem)[4,5] are prescribed more commonly among the older generations and have been shown to render them more susceptible to road traffic accidents and head injury. In the United States falls are the leading cause of fatalities in the U.S. construction industry: older workers have a higher rate of fatal falls than younger workers[6].

13.2.1.1 ACCESS TO TRAUMA CARE

In some settings and despite effective pre-hospital trauma triage criteria, older trauma patients are less likely to be transported to a major trauma service and have poorer outcomes than younger adult trauma patients. Older people trauma can attract greater costs and length of stay, and costs may increase with age and injury severity. Yet data show that with active, informed interventions the outcomes for older trauma patients may be substantially better than preconceptions might suggest, resulting in cost and time savings[7,8].

Awareness of these issues is essential in management of the elderly trauma patient.

13.2.2 **Physiology**

The older person's response to bodily insult, whether medical or traumatic, may often be atypical or even masked, in part due to the ageing process, and in part due to co-morbidities and attendant medications[9]. Ageing is a risk factor for microvascular dysfunction and hyperpermeability. Apart from age-related remodelling of the vascular wall, endothelial barrier integrity and function decline with age. General physiological, cellular and molecular changes occur in the vascular system as a product of ageing. Ageing leads to barrier dysfunction and vascular hyperpermeability in the periphery and the blood-brain barrier, and age-related increases occur in oxidative stress, inflammatory markers and apoptotic signalling[10]. Oxidative stress can have a negative impact in all forms of major surgery including trauma surgery; this is particularly marked in an ageing population[11].

Careful and open-minded assessment is essential in management where, as a result of the interplay of the above factors, the older trauma patient may not only present with vague and misleading signs, but also end up precipitously in extremis.

Particular consideration should be given to the following.

13.2.2.1 RESPIRATORY SYSTEM

- Decreased lung elasticity with decreased pulmonary compliance.
- Coalescence of the alveoli.
- Decrease in surface area available for gas exchange.
- Atrophy of bronchial epithelium, leading to a decrease in clearance of particulate foreign matter.
- Chronic bacterial colonization of the upper airway.

13.2.2.2 CARDIOVASCULAR SYSTEM

- Diminished pump function and lower cardiac output.
- Inability to mount an appropriate response to both intrinsic and extrinsic catecholamines and a consequent inability to augment cardiac output.
- Reduced flow to vital organs.
- Co-existing commonly prescribed medication that can blunt normal physiological responses.

13.2.2.3 NERVOUS SYSTEM

- Progressive atrophy of the brain.
- Deterioration in cerebral and cognitive functions.
- Hearing.
- Eyesight.
- Proprioception.

13.2.2.4 RENAL

- Decline in renal mass.
- Normal serum creatinine no longer implies normal renal function.
- Increased vulnerability to nephrotoxic agents (e.g. non-steroidal anti-inflammatory medication).

13.2.2.5 MUSCULOSKELETAL

- Osteoporosis causing fractures in the presence of minimal energy transfer.
- Diminution of vertebral body height.
- Decrease in muscle mass.

13.2.3 Influence of Co-morbid Conditions

In addition to the typical changes listed above, the development of disease states commonly associated with the elderly can have a significant impact on the response to injury. These can include any chronic degenerative disease, and especially the following in isolation or any combination:

- Degenerative diseases and major system dysfunction: cardiac, liver, pulmonary, renal and neurological/spinal.
- Cardiac disease including hypertension.
- Metabolic disease.
- Diabetes mellitus.
- Obesity (body mass index >30).
- Liver disease.
- Malignancy.
- Pulmonary disease.
- Renal disease.
- Neurological or spinal disease.

13.2.4 Multiple Medications – Polypharmacy

As ageing progresses, rates of drug metabolism are diminished, and accumulations readily occur with unpleasant consequences facing the unwary surgeon. All of the above must be considered within the likely context of treatments with multiple medications, which together may produce a misleading clinical picture or may even mask vital changes in clinical signs.

As ageing progresses, rates of drug metabolism are diminished, and accumulations readily occur with unpleasant consequences when the physician is unwary.

13.2.5 Analgesia

There is no reason to deny the older person adequate analgesia in any given situation. Adequate analgesia allows an improvement in physiological variables such as neuroendocrine stress responses and pulmonary function, and this in turn renders the older patient potentially suitable for major surgical procedures.

Suggested guiding principles are:

- Be mindful of the patient's physical and medication contexts, apply the most appropriate analgesic.
- Start with a low dose, not uncommonly 30 per cent of that for a healthy adult, and then titrate.
- Avoid drug combinations where possible.
- Consider a balanced analgesic regimen that includes an effective afferent block (regional analgesia), which is often appropriate.

By preventing post-operative pain and its associated neuroendocrine sequelae, major surgical procedures may be considered in patients traditionally deemed unsuitable.

13.2.6 Decision to Operate

Mortality data and expected survival curves for major abdominal surgery in the octogenarian population indicate it is safer than previously thought to operate on the elderly. These data enable the surgeon to be able to risk stratify and discuss predicted outcomes with other consultants, patients and families. If in doubt, one might have a low threshold for intervention, as otherwise the worst outcome will most likely prevail.

Although wound healing is slower than in comparable younger patients, the final result is qualitatively similar[12,13].

13.2.7 Outcome

Mortality rates are higher for comparable injuries in younger patients. The following guidelines have been recommended:

- Accept the potential for a decreased physiological reserve.
- Suspect co-morbid disease.
- Suspect multiple medications and polypharmacy.
- Suspect atypical manifestations for any given situation with masked signs.
- Look for subtle signs of organ dysfunction by aggressive monitoring.
- Assume that any alteration in mental status is associated with brain injury, and only accept age-related deterioration after exclusion of injury.
- Be aware of poorer outcomes and sudden physiological deterioration.
- Be aware of the distinction between aggressive care and futile care.

13.3 FUTILE CARE

In every environment, there are circumstances where the provision of adequate health care may not alter the outcome. In providing this care, there may be a significant drain on the resources available, and denial to others of adequate care as a result. This 'rationing' of health care may be the result of operating theatres being in use, and consequently not available, inadequate numbers of intensive care unit beds or financial restrictions.

It must be stressed, however, that all patients are entitled to an aggressive initial resuscitation and careful comprehensive diagnosis. The magnitude of their injuries should be assessed within their wider health context, and only then can the appropriateness and aggression required in their care be determined. In addition, this must all be fully discussed with the associated staff and family.

Inevitably occasions arise in the management of the older patient (as in any age group) when it is abundantly clear to the clinician that intervention is futile. The clinician must be guided by basic ethical principles, and it is essential to be humane, not to prolong life without definite and realistic therapeutic goals or without realistic expectations of a positive outcome. Opting to allow the patient a death which is comfortable and dignified may be more positive as an outcome than a futile surgical intervention.

REFERENCES AND RECOMMENDED READING

References

1. Wilson AO, Adamchak DJ, Nyanguru AC, Hampson J. A study of well-being in the elderly of Zimbabwe. *Age Ageing*. 1991;20(4):275–279.

2. Wilson AO, Nhiwatiwa R. The forgotten; the hospitalised elderly in Zimbabwe. *Cent Afr J Med*. 1991;37(4):110–114.

3. Soles GL, Tornetta P 3rd. Multiple trauma in the elderly: new management perspectives. *J Orthop Trauma*. 2011;Suppl 2:S61–S65.

4. Gustavsen I, Bramness JG, Skurtveit S, Engeland A, Neutel I, Mørland J. Road traffic accident risk related to prescriptions of the hypnotics zopiclone, zolpidem, flunitrazepam and nitrazepam. *Sleep Med*. 2008;9(8):818–822. Epub 2008 Jan 28.

5. Lai MM, Lin CC, Lin CC, Liu CS, Li TC, Kao CH. Long-term use of zolpidem increases the risk of major injury: a population-based cohort study. *Hum Factors*. 2012;54(3):303–315.

6. Dong XS, Wang X, Daw C. Fatal falls among older construction workers. *Injury*. 2014;45(9):1312–1319. Epub 2014 Feb 28.

7. Cox S, Morrison C, Cameron P, Smith K. Advancing age and trauma: triage destination compliance and mortality in Victoria, Australia. *Australas J Ageing*. 2013;Jun 17. doi:10.1111/ajag.12059.

8. Curtis K, Chan DL, Lam MK, Mitchell R, King K, Leonard L, D'Amours S, Black D. The injury profile and acute treatment costs of major trauma in older people in New South Wales. *Australas J Ageing*. 2013; Jun 17. doi:10.1111/ajag.12059.

9. Richardson J, Bresland K. The management of postsurgical pain in the elderly population. *Drugs Aging*. 1998 Jul;13(1):17–31.

10. Oakley R, Tharakan B. Vascular hyperpermeability and aging. *Aging Dis*. 2014;5(2):114–125.

11. Rosenfeldt F, Wilson M, Lee G, et al. Oxidative stress in surgery in an ageing population: pathophysiology and therapy. *Exp Gerontol*. 2013;48(1):45–54. Epub 2012 Mar 23.

12. Rubinfeld I, Thomas C, Berry S, et al. Octogenarian abdominal surgical emergencies: not so grim a problem with the acute care surgery model? *J Trauma*. 2009;67(5):983–989. doi:10.1097/TA.0b013e3181ad6690.

13. Gosain A, DiPietro LA. Aging and wound healing. *World J Surg*. 2004;28(3):321–326. Epub 2004 Feb 17.

Recommended Reading

Information Needs for Research, Policy and Action on Ageing and Older Adults: a report of the follow-up meeting to the 2000 Harare MDS Workshop: indicators for the Minimum Data Set Project on Ageing: A Critical Review in Sub-Saharan Africa June 2001, Dar Es Salaam, United Republic of Tanzania Global Programme on Evidence for Health Policy, World Health Organization.

Kauder DR. Geriatric trauma. In: *The Trauma Manual,* 3rd ed. Peitzman AB, ed. Philadelphia, PA: Wolters Kluwer Lippincott Williams & Wilkins; 2008:469–476.

Critical Care of the Trauma Patient **14**

14.1 INTRODUCTION

Most trauma mortality in the intensive care unit (ICU) occurs during the first few days of admission, primarily as a result of closed head injury, severe respiratory failure or refractory haemorrhagic shock, some of which are largely deemed as non-preventable deaths. The remainder, many of which may be preventable, occur late and are caused by multiple organ failure, infection or both.

14.2 GOALS OF TRAUMA INTENSIVE CARE UNIT (ICU) CARE

The fundamental goals of trauma intensive care unit (ICU) care are early restoration and maintenance of tissue oxygenation, diagnosis and treatment of occult injuries, and prevention and treatment of infection and multiple organ failure. Trauma ICU care is best provided by a multidisciplinary team focussed on resuscitation, monitoring and life support. In the ICU, those who take care of a patient admitted with lethal brain injury play a vital role in the support and maintenance of potential organ donors.

14.3 PHASES OF ICU CARE

14.3.1 Resuscitative Phase (First 24 Hours Post-injury)

During this phase, management is focussed on haemostatic resuscitation, and the goal of treatment is the maintenance of adequate tissue oxygenation. At the same time, occult life-threatening or limb-threatening injuries are carefully sought and should be recognized. Performing secondary and tertiary survey of all trauma patients will minimize and reduce significantly the missed injuries.

Inadequate tissue oxygenation must be recognized and treated immediately. Deficient tissue oxygen delivery in the acutely traumatized patient is usually caused by impaired perfusion or severe hypoxaemia. Although several different types of shock can be present, inadequate resuscitation from hypovolaemia and blood loss is most common.

After major trauma, some patients experience considerable delay before organ perfusion, primarily in the splanchnic circulation, is fully restored, despite apparently adequate systolic blood pressure and normal urine output. This phenomenon has been called 'occult hypoperfusion'[1]. A clear association has been identified between occult hypoperfusion or persistent hypovolemia after major trauma and increased rates of infections, length of stay, days in surgical/trauma ICU, hospital charges, multiple organ dysfunction/failure and mortality. Rapid control of bleeding and early identification and aggressive resuscitation aimed at correcting hypovolemia have been shown to improve survival and reduce complications in severely injured trauma patients, particularly with severe traumatic brain injury (TBI)[2]. However, the previously advocated practice of supranormal resuscitation to somehow drive perfusion is associated with excess lactated Ringer infusion, and an increased incidence of intra-abdominal hypertension, elevated intracranial pressure (ICP), abdominal compartment syndrome, multiple organ failure (MOF) and death[3]. An elevated fluid balance alone is an independent risk factor for adult respiratory distress syndrome (ARDS) and MOF. Currently, a more balanced approach utilizes an initial restricted or controlled volume resuscitation (SBP approximately 90 mm Hg) until surgical bleeding is controlled. A concomitant damage control resuscitation with early institution of blood components in the patient requiring more than 1–2 L of crystalloid in a 1:1:1 ratio of red blood cells (RBCs) to fresh frozen plasma (FFP) to platelets to mimic the ongoing blood losses in the severely injured, likely coagulopathic patient limits the overall amount of crystalloid infused. Simultaneously, the presence of an early trauma-associated coagulopathy (TAC) is optimally treated to minimize blood loss and reduce the recognized early mortality from coagulopathic bleeding.

14.3.1.1 'TRADITIONAL' ENDPOINTS OF RESUSCITATION

These generally include the following:

- Clinical examination: cold and clammy, blood pressure, central venous pressure, heart rate, arterial partial pressure of oxygen (PaO_2), etc., but may not identify occult hypoperfusion.
- Base deficit and lactic acidosis.
- Pulmonary artery catheter measurements, which may be used to derive measures of cardiac index and oxygen delivery.
- Gastric tonometry.
- Tissue oximetry.

14.3.1.2 POST-TRAUMATIC ACUTE LUNG INJURY

Aetiology

- Chest trauma.
- Fluid overload.
- Shock.
- Aspiration.
- Post-traumatic ARDS.
- Fat embolism syndrome.
- Pre-existing respiratory disease.

14.3.1.3 RESPIRATORY ASSESSMENT AND MONITORING

- Work of breathing.
- Respiratory rate.
- Arterial blood gases.
- Oxygen delivery and consumption.
- Bronchoscopy.

Ventilatory support should be instituted earlier rather than later; select a mode of ventilation tailored to the patient's need using appropriate volumes (frequently requires high pressures to achieve adequate ventilation in severely injured) and amounts of positive end-expiratory pressure (PEEP) (frequently greater than 10 cm/H_2O to treat progressive hypoxia).

- Non-invasive ventilation is rarely adequate in the acute setting.

- Pressure support ventilation (PSV) is poorly tolerated following severe injury.
- Lung protective ventilation (LPV) with low volume and low peak pressures is frequently not possible early in resuscitation due to severe hypoxia and low compliance – use adequate volumes despite high pressures.
- High PEEP (>10 up to 20–25 cm H_2O) for hypoxia is applied to recruit alveoli.

14.3.2 Early Life Support Phase (24–72 Hours Post-injury)

During this phase, treatment is focussed on identifiable injuries, the management of post-traumatic respiratory failure and of progressive intracranial hypertension in patients suffering from severe head injury. Usually, the diagnostic evaluation for occult injuries is now complete. Evidence of early multiple organ failure may become apparent during this time.

Major life-threatening problems that may develop at this time include intracranial hypertension, systemic inflammatory response syndrome (SIRS), early multiple organ dysfunction syndrome (MODS) and continued respiratory insufficiency. The main priorities of the early life support phase are the maintenance of tissue oxygenation, the control of ICP, an ongoing search for occult injuries, and the institution of nutritional support and withdrawal or replacement of trauma resuscitation lines or devices that may have been placed in less than ideal conditions. Further establishment of the medical history or events of the injury is also completed.

14.3.2.1 PRIORITIES

- Gas exchange and ventilatory support.
- Haemostatic resuscitation.
- Intracranial pressure (ICP) monitoring and control.
- Fluid and electrolyte balance.
- Haematological parameters.
- Occult injuries.
- Delayed intracranial haematoma formation.
  - Follow-up computed tomography (CT) scan of the head.
- Intra-abdominal injuries.
  - Follow-up CT scan or ultrasound of the abdomen.
- Cervical spine injury.
  - Completion of the radiographic survey and clinical examination if possible.

- Thoracic and lumbar spine injury.
- Extremity injury: hands and feet.
- Nerve injuries.

14.3.3 **Prolonged Life Support (>72 Hours Post-injury)**

The duration of the prolonged life support phase depends on the severity of the injury and its associated complications. Many of those who are critically injured can be successfully weaned from life support, while the more seriously injured enter a phase in which ongoing life support is necessary to prevent organ system failure. Predominant clinical concerns that arise include infectious complications that may lead to the development of late multiple organ failure or death.

The main objective of the management of patients developing MODS is to provide support for failing organ systems while attempts are made to isolate and eliminate inflammatory foci that could be perpetuating the organ system failure. In addition, prolonged immobility can cause problems with muscle wasting, joint contractures and skin compromise in pressure areas. Physiotherapy should be commenced early, with the proper use of splints, early exercise and ambulation when possible.

14.3.3.1 RESPIRATORY FAILURE

- Unexplained respiratory failure – look for occult infection or necrotic tissue.
- Tracheostomy – early.

14.3.3.2 INFECTIOUS COMPLICATIONS

The following are some infectious complications[4] that can arise:

- Nosocomial pneumonia.
  - · Gram stain of sputum and microbiological culture.
- Lung abscess and empyema.
- Surgical site infection.
  - · Superficial incisional surgical site, e.g. wound infection.
  - · Deep incisional surgical site infection.
  - · Organ/space surgical site infection, e.g. intra-abdominal abscess.
- Intravenous catheter-related sepsis.

- Bloodstream infections.
- Urinary tract infection.
- Acalculous cholecystitis.
- Sinusitis and otitis media.
- Ventriculitis and meningitis.

Antibiotic and antifungal therapy should ideally be of limited spectrum and directed toward cultures. Remember the risk of antibiotic-associated colitis, and other antibiotic-associated complications.

14.3.3.3 NON-INFECTIOUS CAUSES OF FEVER

- Drugs.
- Pulmonary embolus (PE).
- Deep venous thrombosis (DVT).

14.3.3.4 PERCUTANEOUS TRACHEOSTOMY

Percutaneous tracheostomy[5] has been shown to have fewer perioperative and postoperative complications compared with conventional tracheostomy and is now the technique of choice in critically ill patients.

Various techniques are described, with dilation by forceps or multiple or single dilators. Patient selection is important, and percutaneous tracheostomy should not be attempted if the procedure is non-elective, the landmarks are obscure in the neck or the patient has a coagulopathy. Confirmation of correct placement by fibre-optic bronchoscopy is valuable. Ultrasound scanning of the neck and routine endoscopy during the procedure appear to reduce early complications. Percutaneous tracheostomy is not suitable for children.

14.3.3.5 WEANING FROM VENTILATORY SUPPORT

During the recovery phase, the most important transition made is that from mechanical ventilation to unassisted breathing, known as weaning. Weaning begins when the causes of respiratory failure have resolved.

When signs of infection, respiratory failure or multisystem failure abate, recovery from critical illness requiring prolonged ICU care is imminent.

14.3.3.6 EXTUBATION CRITERIA ('SOA2P')

S – Secretions – minimal
O – Oxygenation – good

A – Alert
A – Airway: without injury or compromise
P – Pressures or parameters: measurements of tidal, volume, vital capacity, negative inspiratory force, etc.

14.3.4 Recovery Phase (Separation from the ICU)

During the recovery phase, the patient is weaned from full ventilatory support until he or she is breathing spontaneously and invasive monitoring devices can be removed. The patient and family are prepared for the transition from the ICU to general patient or intermediate care unit, and plans for further convalescence and rehabilitation are developed.

14.4 HYPOTHERMIA

Hypothermia is a potential complication of trauma. While hypothermia may itself cause cardiac arrest, it is also protective to the brain through a reduction in metabolic rate and thus reduced oxygen requirements. Oxygen consumption is reduced by 50 per cent at a core temperature of 30°C. The American Heart Association guidelines recommend that the hypothermic patient who appears dead should not be considered so until a near-normal body temperature is reached. However, hypothermia is on balance extremely harmful to trauma patients, especially by virtue of the way it alters oxygen delivery. Therefore, the patient must be warmed as soon as possible, and heat loss minimized at all costs, in all injured patients.

14.4.1 Re-warming

Hypothermia is common after immersion injury. Re-warming must take place with intensive monitoring. Patients who have spontaneous respiratory effort and whose hearts are beating, no matter how severe the bradycardia, should not receive unnecessary resuscitation procedures. The hypothermic heart is very irritable and fibrillates easily. Patients with a core temperature of less than 29.5°C are at high risk of ventricular arrhythmias, and should be re-warmed as rapidly as possible. Recent studies have not shown any increase in ventricular arrhythmias with rapid re-warming.

A hypothermic heart is resistant to both electrical and pharmacological cardioversion, especially if the core temperature is below 29.5°C, and cardiopulmonary resuscitation should be continued if necessary.

If the core temperature is greater than 29.5°C and fibrillation is present, one attempt at electrical cardioversion should be made. If this is ineffective, intravenous amiodarone may be helpful.

Patients with a core temperature of between 29.5°C and 32°C can generally be passively re-warmed, and if haemodynamically stable may be re-warmed more slowly. However, active core re-warming is still generally required.

Patients with a core temperature of over 32°C can generally be re-warmed using external rewarming.

Methods of re-warming include the following:

External

- Removal of wet or cold clothing and drying of the patient.
- Infrared (radiant) heat.
- Electrical heating blankets.
- Warm air heating blankets.

Note: In the presence of hypothermia, 'space blankets' are ineffective, since there is minimal intrinsic bordy heat to reflect.

Internal

- Heated, humidified respiratory gases to 42°C.
- Intravenous fluids warmed to 37°C.
- Gastric lavage with warmed fluids (usually saline at 42°C).
- Continuous bladder lavage with water at 42°C.
- Peritoneal lavage with potassium-free dialysate at 42°C (20 mL/kg every 15 minutes).
- Bilateral intrapleural lavage with warmed fluid.
- Extracorporeal rewarming via a femoral artery-femoral vein bypass.

Resuscitation should not be abandoned while the core temperature is subnormal, since it may be difficult to distinguish between cerebroprotective hypothermia and hypothermia resulting from brainstem death.

14.5 SYSTEMIC INFLAMMATORY RESPONSE SYNDROME

Two large studies have shown that 50 percent of patients with 'sepsis' are abacteraemic. It is also recognized that the aetiology in these abacteraemic patients may be burns, pancreatitis or significant destructive tissue injuries particularly when associated with shock, which all cause the release of inflammatory mediators called DAMPs. Danger activated molecular patterns (DAMPs) activate the innate and adaptive immune responses with excessive systemic inflammation and massive bystander tissue injury leading to diffuse organ injury and failure (i.e. MOF). The common theme through all of these various injuries and sepsis is that the inflammatory cascade has been initiated and runs amok. Once the inflammatory response is initiated it leads to systemic symptoms which may or may not be beneficial or harmful. The primary symptoms associated with SIRS include:

- Temperature <36°C or >38°C.
- Heart rate >90 beats per minute.
- Respiratory rate >20 breaths per minute.
- Deranged arterial gases: partial pressure of carbon dioxide ($PaCO_2$) <32 mm Hg (4.2 kPa).
- White blood count >12×10^9/L or <4×10^9/L or 0.10% immature neutrophils.

Patients who have one or more of these primary components are thought to have SIRS. A further classification of SIRS is that sepsis is SIRS plus documented infection. Severe sepsis is sepsis plus organ dysfunction, hypoperfusion abnormalities or hypotension. Finally, septic shock is defined as sepsis-induced hypotension despite fluid resuscitation. The treatment goals for septic shock include source control, early use of broad-spectrum antibiotics and circulatory support with ino-pressor agents as well as maintaining adequate organ system function.

There is no evidence for mortality reduction with the use of steroids, tight glycaemic control or use of activated protein C.

14.6 MULTISYSTEM ORGAN DYSFUNCTION SYNDROME (MODS) OR MULTIPLE ORGAN FAILURE (MOF)

Multisystem organ dysfunction syndrome is a clinical syndrome characterized by the progressive failure of multiple and interdependent organs. The 'dysfunction' identifies a phenomenon in which organ function is not capable of maintaining homeostasis, so it occurs along a continuum of progressive organ failure, rather than absolute failure. The lungs, liver and kidneys are the principal target organs; however, failure of the cardiovascular and central nervous system may be prominent

as well. The main inciting factors in trauma patients are haemorrhagic shock and infection. As life support and resuscitation techniques have improved, the incidence of MODS has increased. The early development of MODS (<3 days post-injury) is usually a consequence of shock or inadequate resuscitation, while late onset is usually a result of severe infection.

The MODS/MOF develops as a consequence of local inflammation with activation of the innate immune system and a subsequent uncontrolled or inappropriate systemic inflammatory response to inciting factors such as severe tissue injury (e.g. brain, lung or soft tissue), hypoperfusion or infection. Two basic models have emerged: the 'one-hit' model involves a single insult that initiates a SIRS, which may result in progressive MODS, whereas the 'two-hit' model involves sequential insults that may lead to MODS. The initial insult may prime the inflammatory response such that a second insult (even a modest one) results in an exaggerated inflammatory response and subsequent organ dysfunction.

Early factors that increase the risk for MODS include persistent and refractory shock with lactic acidosis and elevated base deficit, a high injury severity score (ISS) and the need for multiple blood transfusions. Advanced age or pre-existing disease may also increase a patient's risk of developing MODS because of co-morbid disease or decreased organ reserves secondary to normal ageing.

Specific therapy for MODS is currently limited, apart from providing adequate and full resuscitation, treatment of infection and general ICU supportive care. Strategies to prevent MODS include adequate fluid resuscitation to establish and maintain tissue oxygenation, debridement of devitalized tissue, early fracture fixation and stabilization, early enteral nutritional support when possible, the prevention and treatment of nosocomial infections and early mobility and resumption of exercise.

14.7 COAGULOPATHY OF MAJOR TRAUMA

Trauma patients are susceptible to the early development of coagulopathy[6], and the most severely injured patients are coagulopathic on hospital admission (see also Chapter 4). The coagulopathy is worsened by[7]:

- Haemodilution: Dilutional thrombocytopenia is the most common coagulation abnormality in trauma patients.

- Consumption of clotting factors.
- Hypothermia: Causes platelet dysfunction and a reduction in the rate of the enzymatic clotting cascade.
- Acidosis: Metabolic derangements (especially acidosis), which also interfere with the clotting mechanism.

More recently in trauma, the focus has shifted from a disseminated intravascular coagulation (DIC) type coagulopathy without microthrombi, to extensive tissue trauma in combination with reduced perfusion in which the endothelium shows an increased expression of thrombomodulin, thus binding thrombin.

With the reduced levels of thrombin there is a reduced production of fibrin. The thrombin-thrombomodulin complex activates protein C (aPC). The aPC inactivates co-factors V and VIII, causing anticoagulation. The aPC also inactivates the plasminogen activator inhibitor type 1 (PAI-1), increasing fibrinolysis. The thrombin-thrombomodulin complex also binds the thrombin activated fibrinolysis inhibitor (TAFI), reducing the inhibition of fibrinolysis. In trauma-induced coagulopathy, the shifting balance between the binding of protein C and TAFI may be the cause of the different clinical presentations. Long-standing hypotension, acidosis and ischaemia give a release of a tissue plasminogen activator. Together with a reduced liver function, consumption of coagulation factors, activated plasmin and fibrin degradation products, haemostasis is compromised. In addition, platelet survival is short and severe thrombocytopenia is common. There is also a consumptive deficiency of coagulation factors. Excess plasmin generation is reflected by reduced plasma levels of fibrin and elevated levels of fibrinogen degradation products (FDPs), with abnormal concentrations being found in 85 per cent of patients[8].

14.7.1 Management

The management of diffuse bleeding after trauma relies on haemorrhage control, active re-warming and replacement of blood products. The empirical transfusion of platelets, fresh frozen plasma and cryoprecipitate is recommended in patients with major injuries (i.e. the damage control group)[8].

Clinically, it is difficult to identify DIC as a separate entity from the coagulopathy of major trauma described above. The distinction is, however, largely academic; the key step in the management of DIC is resolution of the condition predisposing to the coagulopathy.

The condition will not resolve until the underlying cause has been corrected; while this is being achieved, component therapy is indicated. Currently, a ratio of 1:1:1 for RBC:FFP:platelets is considered most appropriate as similar to the blood being lost. In addition, tranexamic acid may have a major role in clot stabilization[9] and reversal of the coagulopathy if given early within 3 hours of injury. Despite the increased use of tranexamic acid, the gathering and validity of the data have been called into question in a major trauma centre environment. In addition, a recent study indicated that the majority of severely injured patients have a fibrinolysis shutdown, and therefore, tranexamic acid may have no effect[10].

14.8 RECOGNITION AND TREATMENT OF RAISED INTRACRANIAL PRESSURE

Early mortality in blunt trauma patients in the ICU is often caused by head injury. The primary goal in the ICU management of the patient with a severe head injury is to prevent secondary neuronal injury. One important factor that can contribute to secondary brain injury is increased ICP. Consequently, monitoring and controlling ICP and cerebral perfusion pressure is a high priority in this phase of ICU care. Other conditions that worsen brain injury include:

- Hypotension.
- Hypoxia.
- Hyperglycaemia.
- Hyperthermia.
- Hypercarbia.

14.9 RECOGNITION OF ACUTE RENAL FAILURE (ARF) AND ACUTE KIDNEY INJURY (AKI)

While the frequency of acute renal failure (ARF) is relatively low due to improved early resuscitation and restoration of perfusion, severely injured patients are still at significant risk for the development of acute kidney injury (AKI) and ARF. Several indicators of physiologic injury severity including the lowest body temperature, the highest lactate level and the need for packed red blood cells and cryoprecipitate transfusion are independently associated with a higher risk for developing ARF.

Other factors include tissue damage and necrosis, hypotension, rhabdomyolysis, the use of iodinated contrast for diagnostic tests and pre-existing conditions such as diabetes. The development of ARF complicates the ICU management of a patient, increases the length of stay[11], and is associated with an increased mortality of approximately 60 per cent. Approximately one-third of acute post-traumatic renal failure cases are caused by inadequate resuscitation, while the remainder develop as part of MODS. To prevent renal insult avoid and/or treat:

- Nephrotoxic contrast dyes and drugs.
- Hypovolaemia.
- Rhabdomyolysis.
- Abdominal compartment syndrome.
- Obstructive uropathy.

There is no indication for a 'renal protective' dopamine strategy in ARF or the initiation of dialysis in myoglobinemia. The use of treatment with diuretics in patients at risk of development of ARF cannot prevent impending ARF but can prolong the interval to dialysis for the treatment of overhydration.

14.10 EVALUATION OF METABOLIC DISTURBANCES

Disturbances in acid-base and electrolyte balance can be anticipated in patients in shock, those who have received massive transfusions and the elderly with co-morbid conditions.

Typical abnormalities may include:

- Acid-base disorders.
- Electrolyte disorders.
  · Hypokalaemia.
  · Hyperkalaemia.
  · Hypocalcaemia.
  · Hypomagnesaemia.
- Hypophosphataemia.

In acid-base disorders acidosis is most commonly due to hypoperfusion with inadequate oxygenation and anaerobic metabolism. One must identify and correct the aetiology of the disturbance, e.g. metabolic acidosis caused by hypoperfusion secondary to occult pericardial tamponade.

14.11 PAIN CONTROL/ SEDATION/DELIRIUM

A number of adverse consequences result when pain is inadequately treated. These include increased oxygen consumption, increased minute volume demands, psychic stress, sleep deprivation and impaired lung mechanics with associated pulmonary complications. Subjective pain assessment is best documented objectively and, after initiation of treatment, requires serial re-evaluation. Inadequate pain relief can be determined objectively by the failure of the patient to achieve adequate volumes on incentive spirometry, persistently small radiographic lung volumes or a reluctance to cough and cooperate with chest physiotherapy. If the patient can cooperate, visual analogue pain scores may be helpful.

Early pain control in the ICU is primarily achieved through the use of intravenous opiates. Other techniques are employed and tailored to the individual patient and injury:

- Bolus opiates.
- Morphine or fentanyl titrated intravenously.
- Patient-controlled analgesia (PCA).
- Epidural analgesia (patient-controlled epidural analgesia).
- Intrapleural anaesthesia.
- Extrapleural analgesia.
- Intercostal nerve blocks.
- Catheter techniques for peripheral nerve blocks (e.g. femoral nerve, brachial plexus, popliteal nerve and paravertebral nerve blocks).

A growing body of evidence is advocating the strategy of non-sedation to intubated patients in the ICU. A well-performed randomized control trial (RCT) has shown beneficial effects on length of stay and time in ventilator when adopting this strategy. Whether this strategy can be effectively applied to trauma patients has yet to be shown.

Delirium is a recognized complication in patients in the ICE. A breakdown of treatment strategies is beyond the scope of this chapter, but identification of causative factors, re-establishing day/night rhythm and medicamental strategies should be attempted.

14.12 FAMILY CONTACT AND SUPPORT

It is very important to establish early contact, and maintain ongoing relationships with family members in an open, honest, clear and completely transparent manner, by using simple language that is understandable when describing to explain the injuries, clinical condition and prognosis of the patient. This provides family members with essential information and establishes a relationship between the ICU care team and the family. Administrative facts, such as ICU procedures, visiting hours and available services, should also be explained. With the elderly, identifying the existence of living wills or other pre-determination documents is important. Patients and their families should be familiar with the multidisciplinary approach to patient care in the ICU as well.

14.13 ICU TERTIARY SURVEY

The tertiary survey[12] is a complete re-examination of the patient, plus a review of the history and all available results and imaging. Missed injuries are a potent cause of morbidity, and the majority will be identified by a thorough tertiary survey. A tertiary trauma survey has much to recommend it in minimizing the delay in the ultimate diagnosis of missed injury. Nevertheless, it is not a complete solution, and an ongoing analysis of errors should be undertaken at any major trauma centre.

14.13.1 Evaluation for Occult Injuries

Factors predisposing to missed injuries:

- Mechanism of injury – re-verify the events surrounding the injury.

  High-priority occult injuries:

- Brain, spinal cord and peripheral nerve injury.
- Thoracic aortic injury.
- Intra-abdominal or pelvic injury.
- Vascular injuries to the extremities.
- Cerebrovascular injuries – occult carotid/vertebral artery injury.
- Cardiac injuries.
- Aerodigestive tract injuries – ruptured bowel.

- Occult pneumothorax.
- Compartment syndrome – foreleg, thigh, buttock or arm.
- Eye injuries (remember to remove the patient's contact lenses).
- Other occult injuries – hands, feet, digits or joint dislocations.
- Vaginal tampons.

14.13.2 Assess Co-morbid Conditions

- Medical history (including drugs and alcohol).
- Contact the patient's personal physicians.
- Check pharmacy records.

14.14 NUTRITIONAL SUPPORT

14.14.1 Overview

Trauma patients are hypermetabolic and have increased nutritional needs due to the immunological response to trauma and the requirement for accelerated protein synthesis for wound healing. Early enteral feeding has been shown to reduce post-operative septic morbidity after trauma. A meta-analysis of a number of randomized trials demonstrated a twofold decrease in infectious complications in patients treated with early enteral nutrition compared to total parenteral nutrition which actually increases risk of complication compared to no supplemental enteral nutrition for up to 7 days post-injury.

Nutrition support[13,14] for critically ill and injured patients has undergone significant advances in recent decades – the direct result of scientific progress and our increased knowledge of the biology and biochemistry of key nutrient changes induced by injury, sepsis and other critical illnesses, both in adults and in children. The science of nutrition support (or, more accurately, of nutrition therapy) has become more disease based. Also called 'specialized' or 'artificial' nutrition support, nutrition therapy refers to the provision of either enteral nutrition (EN) via tube feeding or total parenteral nutrition (TPN). In contrast, 'standard therapy' refers to a patient's own volitional intake, without the provision of nutrition therapy.

Depending on the individual patient's metabolic needs, nutrition therapy helps ensure that key nutrient substrates are replenished, or added in larger amounts, to supplement specific deficiencies or to simply prevent further deterioration and clinical consequences. The benefit of early institution of either EN or TPN in the overall care of critically ill and injured patients has now been well established. After a critical illness or injury, the patient's energy and overall metabolic requirements greatly increase, in order to sustain increased metabolism and the process of wound repair.

The pre-admission nutritional status of patients is a critical factor. If patients are malnourished or have a limited nutritional reserve, their outcome is poorer. Having a low body mass index (BMI) is an independent predictor of increased mortality and of multiple organ failure. Thermal injuries, severe central nervous system (CNS) insult, sepsis and certain co-morbidities, such as cancer, chronic obstructive pulmonary disease (COPD), alcoholism and heart disease, produce added metabolic challenges and complications. Such conditions exacerbate energy expenditure and protein catabolism brought on by severe injury and critical illness, thereby evoking variation even among patients with the same disease process. It is imperative to evaluate the nutritional status of patients upon admission.

Patients with traumatic brain injury (TBI) appear to have similar outcomes whether fed enterally or parenterally. A Cochrane review has confirmed that early (either parenteral or enteral) feeding is associated with a trend toward better outcomes in terms of survival and disability compared with later feeding[16]. Patients with a TBI exhibit protein wasting and gastrointestinal dysfunction, which may be risk factors for a septic state. However, standard nutritional support may not allow restoration of the nutritional state of TBI patients[15].

To prevent malnutrition and related adverse effects, all ICU patients who are not expected to be on a full oral diet within 3 days should receive EN. Accordingly, EN is recommended as the first choice for nutrition therapy in ICU patients; however, in critically ill patients on nutrition therapy, there is a large discrepancy in the frequency of use of EN.

The American Society for Parenteral and Enteral Nutrition (ASPEN) Board of Directors and the American College of Critical Care Medicine Guidelines Committee expressed concern that continuing to provide standard therapy (that is, no nutrition therapy) beyond 7 days would lead to deterioration of the patient's nutritional status and would have an adverse effect on clinical outcome. If EN cannot be provided and if the patient has evidence of protein–calorie malnutrition (usually defined by recent weight loss of 10–15 per cent or by an actual body weight <90 per cent of the ideal body weight), then the use of TPN is mandatory. The use of TPN (versus standard therapy) in malnourished ICU patients is associated with a significantly lower rate of overall complications. Yet, the best timing for the initiation of TPN in ICU patients has not been demonstrated. On the other hand, the European Society of Parenteral and Enteral Nutrition (ESPEN) and the Canadian Society for Nutritional Sciences (CSCN) both recommend early EN initiation after ICU admission (within 24 h, per ESPEN; within 24–48 h, per CSCN). It seems reasonable to assume that all patients who are not expected to be on normal nutrition within 2–3 days after ICU admission should receive TPN, if EN is contraindicated or not tolerated. No significant differences in clinical outcome have been shown between EN versus TPN in ICU patients.

Enteral nutrition should be used when the gut is accessible and functioning[16]. Enteral nutrition is not invariably safer and better than parenteral nutrition, but a mix of the two modalities can be used safely. 'Immunonutrition' holds promise for the future[17].

Patients at risk include those with:

- Major trauma.
- Traumatic brain injury (TBI).
- Burns.
- Sepsis.

It is critical to:

- Determine energy and protein requirements.
- Determine and establish a route of administration.
- Set a time to begin nutrition support.

14.14.2 Choosing Nutritional Formula

In critically ill and injured patients, immune-modulating or immune-enhancing enteral formulations that are supplemented with agents such as arginine, glutamine, nucleic acid, omega-three fatty acids and antioxidants should be used, depending on their clinical condition. Patients with acute lung injury (ALI) or acute respiratory distress syndrome (ARDS) should be on an enteral formulation characterized by an anti-inflammatory lipid profile (that is, omega-3 fish oil, borage oil) and antioxidants[14]. Furthermore, nutritional therapy must be tailored to the individual patient's disease or disorder and unique metabolic changes. The seemingly logical strategy would be to replace deficiencies of key nutrients (such as amino acids, proteins, vitamins, minerals and trace elements) in the dose required. Early oral feeding (enteral, and/or parenteral) is most conducive to helping prevent cellular injury and clinical consequences, but, given so many complicating factors, many immune-enhancing and immune-modulating formulas have been developed for use in critically ill and injured patients.

Although it is difficult to demonstrate the precise impact of nutrition therapy, and in particular the individual effects of certain nutrients, enteral formulas fortified with immune-enhancing substrates have been associated with a significant reduction in the risk of infectious complications and a reduction in overall hospital stay. Certain nutrients can modulate inflammatory, metabolic, and immune processes. Amino acids such as arginine and glutamine improve body defenses and tumour cell metabolism, increase wound healing and reduce nitrogen loss. Also, RNA and omega-3 fatty acids modulate immune function.

14.14.3 Initiation for Enteral or Parenteral Nutrition

Enteral feeding should be started early, within the first 24–48 hours after admission if possible, but patients should be resuscitated and hemodynamically stable. Then, over the next 48–72 hours, the feedings should be advanced toward the nutrition goal for the individual patient. In the ICU patient population, the initiation of enteral feeding does not require either the presence or the absence of bowel sounds, and it does not require any evidence of passage of flatus and stool. In the setting of hemodynamic compromise (that is, when significant hemodynamic support is required to maintain cellular perfusion, including high-dose catecholamine agents, alone or in combination with large-volume fluid or blood product resuscitation), EN should be withheld until the patient is fully resuscitated and/or stable.

Either gastric or small-bowel feedings are acceptable in ICU patients. If critically ill patients are at high risk for aspiration or if they are intolerant to gastric feeding, they should be fed via an enteral access tube placed in the small bowel. The need to withhold enteral feedings because of repeated high gastric residual volumes may be a sufficient reason to switch to small-bowel feedings.

Early nutrition therapy via TPN has the potential to reduce disease severity, diminish complications and decrease the ICU length of stay, when EN is not possible, by providing ongoing requirements for calories, protein, electrolytes, vitamins, minerals, trace elements and fluids. The major indication for TPN is failure of the gastrointestinal (GI) tract. In general, TPN should be started when the GI tract cannot be used for more than 5 days in patients in a catabolic state (with or without evidence of malnutrition), or when patients cannot be fed for 3 days after major surgery. The underlying clinical conditions include short gut syndrome, severe gut dysfunction, mesenteric vascular insufficiency, bowel obstruction, GI bleeding, severe diarrhea, large volume fistulas, sepsis, severe burns and trauma associated with continuous hemodynamic instability and with severe fulminant acute and chronic pancreatitis. In many of these patient subgroups, TPN is life-saving.

14.14.4 Gut Access for Enteral Nutrition

14.14.4.1 SIMPLE

- Nasogastric tube.
- Nasoduodenal tube.
- Nasojejunal tube.

Most critically ill trauma patients should be started on early enteral nutrition. The majority do not require prolonged feeding (beyond 10–14 days), and simple nasoenteric tube feeding is then all that is required. For patients who have prolonged tube-feeding requirements, nasoenteric tubes are inconvenient, as they tend to dislodge, worsen aspiration and are uncomfortable.

14.14.4.2 MORE COMPLICATED

- *Percutaneous endoscopic gastrostomy.* This does not interfere with swallowing, is easy to nurse and has target feeding rates that are more likely to be achieved compared with nasoenteric tubes. However, it is an invasive procedure with some risk.
- *Jejunostomy.* Jejunostomy can be placed endoscopically or during laparotomy. Rates of major complications should be less than 5 per cent[18].

14.15 PREVENTIVE MEASURES IN THE ICU

14.15.1 Stress Ulceration

Stress ulceration[19] and associated upper GI bleeding has been on the decline in most ICUs for the past decade. This is, in great part, due to the improved resuscitation efforts in the prehospital environment, emergency department and operating room. Additionally, the use of acid-blocking and cytoprotective therapies has become commonplace.

Those patients at greatest risk for stress ulcer development are those with a previous history of ulcer disease, those requiring mechanical ventilation and those with a coagulopathy, regardless of whether it is intrinsic or chemically induced. Burn patients have also been labelled as high risk in historical studies.

Cytoprotective agents (e.g. sucralfate) as a preventive measure have been shown to be the most cost-effective by statistical analysis in several trials, although there are fewer cases of stress ulcer bleeding in the H_2-receptor blockade arm of these trials. However, the marked decrease in the rate of development of ventilator-associated pneumonia seen in the sucralfate population does make this therapeutic option quite attractive[14].

Intravenous H_2-receptor blockade therapy (e.g. ranitidine) to some degree blocks the production of stomach acid. Most studies demonstrating its efficacy in stress ulcer prevention do not attempt to neutralize gastric pH. Newer intravenous proton pump inhibitors may well replace H_2 blockade as the mainstay of therapy.

Perhaps the simplest and safest method of stress ulcer prevention is adequate resuscitation and early intragastric enteric nutrition. During the early resuscitative phase and while vasoactive drugs to elevate blood pressure are in use, it is not always prudent to provide nutrition enterally. It is in these circumstances that the use of acid blockade, cytoprotective agents or both is necessary.

14.15.2 **Deep Venous Thrombosis and Pulmonary Embolus**

Pulmonary embolus (PE) from DVT[20] continues to be a leading preventable cause of death in the injured patient. Recognizing the risk factors for the development of DVT and instituting an aggressive management regimen can reduce this risk from DVT in the ICU with little added morbidity. The incidence of DVT in trauma patients is 12–32 per cent and those at highest risk of fatal PE include those with spinal cord injuries, weight-bearing pelvic fracture and combined long bone fracture/TBI or long bone fracture/pelvic fracture.

A high index of suspicion in these severely injured patients should result in preventative therapy and diagnostic screening measures to be taken in the ICU. Unless haemorrhagic TBI or spinal cord epidural haematoma precludes the use of subcutaneous heparin therapy, these patients should all receive fractionated low-molecular-weight subcutaneous heparin. Unfractionated heparin does not appear to be nearly as effective in this severely injured population[21]. Similarly, unless extremity injury precludes their use, graded pneumatic compression devices should be used on all such patients. Foot pumps may also be of some benefit.

14.15.3 **Infection**

In patients with any open wounds from trauma, it is imperative that the tetanus immunization status of the patient is addressed. For those patients immunized within the previous 5 years, no additional treatment is generally needed, while booster tetanus toxoid should be administered to those who have previously received the initial tetanus series but have not been re-immunized in the preceding 5–10 years. Tetanus immune globulin should be administered to those patients who lack any history of immunization.

Patients undergoing splenectomy require immunization for *Haemophilus influenzae* type B, meningococcus and pneumococcus. Debate continues regarding the timing of administration of these vaccines in trauma patients, but it is clear that adult patients do not benefit from the antibacterial chemoprophylaxis needed in paediatric patients post-splenectomy. Due to the multiple strains of each organism, the immunizations are not foolproof in preventing overwhelming post-splenectomy infection (OPSI). Therefore, patients must be carefully counselled to seek medical attention immediately for high fevers, and healthcare providers must be aggressive in the use of empirical antibiotics in patients who may have OPSI upon presentation in the outpatient setting. Currently, booster immunization with Pneumovac is indicated every 5 years for these splenectomized patients.

Adequate wound debridement and irrigation are necessary to eliminate non-viable tissue and debris from all traumatic wounds, in order to limit infection of these wounds. Whenever possible, these wounds should be thoroughly prepared as above and closed primarily. If skin coverage is lacking, or more than 6 hours has elapsed since injury, moist dressings (to prevent tissue desiccation and further non-viable wound tissue) should be applied and changed twice per day, further wound debridement performed as indicated and skin grafts or flap coverage performed once the health of the wound can be assured. Special attention must be given to difficult wounds of the perineum (consider faecal diversion), complex fractures with soft tissue injury and contamination (osteomyelitis) and wounds on the back and occiput (as pressure may cause additional wound necrosis).

Thrombophlebitis and sepsis from intravenous cannulae are significant considerations as these intravenous lines are frequently placed under less than optimal circumstances and technique in the field and in the resuscitation areas. Removal and replacement of all such lines as early as possible, but in every instance in less than 24 hours, is paramount to avoid these infectious complications.

14.16 ANTIBIOTICS

The goal of antibiotic treatment is to improve survival; however, preventing the emergence of antibiotic resistance is also important.

There is good evidence to support the limited use of antibiotics in the critically ill trauma patient[22]. Many institutions will administer a single dose of a cephalosporin in the emergency area in all patients with open injury, irrespective of its origin. There is no evidence to support this unless surgical operation is required[23]. There is conflicting evidence regarding the need for routine antibiotics with tube thoracostomy.

For thoracoabdominal injuries requiring operation, a single dose of broad-spectrum antibiotics is indicated. Prolonged courses of antibiotics, extending beyond 24 hours, are not currently indicated in these patients.

Patients with open fractures are frequently treated with both Gram-negative and Gram-positive prophylaxis for long periods. There is no evidence for this practice or for whether the correct management should be any different from that for torso injury[24,25].

Patients in the ICU on mechanical ventilation, with or without known aspiration, have no indication for antibiotics to prevent pneumonia. In fact, this practice has hastened the onset of antibiotic resistance worldwide.

According to the Centers for Disease Control and Prevention, a diagnosis of pneumonia must meet the following criteria:

- Rales or dullness to percussion *and* any of the following:
  - New purulent sputum or a change in sputum.
  - Culture growth of an organism from blood or tracheal aspirate, bronchial brushing or biopsy.
- Radiographic evidence of new or progressive infiltrate, consolidation, cavitation or effusion,

and any of the following:

- Isolation of virus or detection of viral antigen in respiratory secretions.
- Diagnostic antibody titres for pathogen.
- Histopathological evidence of pneumonia.

For ventilator-associated pneumonia (VAP) there are new guidelines[26].

14.16.1 Ventilator-associated Pneumonia (VAP) Diagnosis

Ventilator-associated pneumonia (VAP) diagnosis interventions considered most appropriate for inclusion in the care bundle are as follows:

- Early chest X-ray with expert interpretation within 1 hour.
- Immediate reporting of respiratory secretions and Gram-stain findings, including cells.

14.16.2 VAP Treatment

VAP treatment interventions considered most appropriate for inclusion in the care bundle are as follows:

- Immediate treatment after microbiological sampling.
- Empirical therapy based on a knowledge of local pathogens and an assessment of risk factors.
- De-escalation of antibiotics in responding patients once culture results are available.
- Assessment of response to treatment within 72 hours.
- Short-therapy duration (8 days) if the patient is on an appropriate regimen and not infected by a multidrug-resistant pathogen.

Given the variations in antibiotic susceptibility profiles of VAP pathogens, both in location and with respect to changes over time, it is inappropriate to specify the use of specific antibiotic regimens.

14.17 RESPIRATORY SUPPORT

- Mechanical ventilation should be 'gentle' as high tidal volumes and pressures can damage the lungs.
- Aspiration must be prevented.
- Early tracheostomy should be undertaken.
- Pulmonary toilet and pain control should be used in patients with rib fractures.

- Lung protective ventilation (LPV) with low volume, low peak pressures and high PEEP should be used for significant or progressive hypoxia of ARDS.
- Prone ventilation may improve oxygenation in patients with ARDS or severe sepsis.
- VAP is the common hospital-acquired infection in ICU[26].
- Form early liaison with centres offering extracorporeal membrane oxygenation (ECMO).

14.18 SURVIVING SEPSIS GUIDELINES

Updated *Surviving Sepsis Campaign: International Guidelines for Management of Severe Sepsis and Septic Shock* were published in 2012[27].

A full summary of the guidelines in table form appears in Table 14.1.

Table 14.1 Summary of Surviving Sepsis Guidelines 2012

A. Initial Resuscitation – Goals

Sepsis-induced hypoperfusion is defined as hypotension persisting after initial fluid challenge or a blood lactate of ≥4 mmol/L.

1. Central venous pressure (CVP) 8–12 mm Hg
2. Mean arterial pressure (MAP) ≥65 mm Hg
3. Urine output ≥0.5 mL/Kg
4. Central venous oxygen saturation ≥70% or arterial saturation ≥90%

B. Screening for Sepsis

1. Cultures should be taken within 45 min of initial diagnosis and *before* initiation of appropriate antibiotic therapy

C. Diagnosis

1. Cultures as in B above (two samples)
   a. Through intravenous device
   b. Percutaneous
2. Identify source through imaging studies
3. Draw procalcitonin level (PCT) – preferable to CRP

D. Antimicrobial Therapy

1. Initiate empiric therapy to provide antimicrobial activity against the most likely pathogens, based on the illness, and local patterns of antibiotic surveillance.
2. Administration should occur within the first hour following recognition of sepsis, with or without septic shock.
3. Empiric therapy should not be administered for more than 3 days. Antibiotic regimen should be assessed daily, for de-escalation.
4. Duration of therapy should be 7–10 days, and antibiotics should be discontinued based on low procalcitonin, taken at days 3, 5, 7 or 10.
5. Antibiotic therapy should ideally consist of an extended spectrum beta lactam, and a fluoroquinolone (for *Pseudomonas*) or a macrolide (for *Streptococcus* or *Klebsiella*).

E. Source Control

1. A specific anatomical diagnosis for the source should be sought and intervention taken for source control within 12 h after diagnosis.
2. If intravascular devices are identified as a possible source, they should be removed as soon as possible after new access has been established.

F. Infection Prevention

1. Selective oral decontamination using oral chlorhexidine gluconate should be used throughout, to reduce the risk of ventilator-associated pneumonia.

G. Fluid Therapy

1. Crystalloid is the initial fluid of choice.
2. An initial fluid challenge of 30 mL/kg of crystalloid is suggested.
3. Fluid challenge techniques should be applied as long as there is haemodynamic improvement and there is improvement in the variables.

continued

Table 14.1 Summary of Surviving Sepsis Guidelines 2012 – *continued*

H. Vasopressors

1. Vasopressor therapy can be used to achieve a minimum MAP of 65 mm.

2. Adrenaline is to be used as the agent of first choice. (Noradrenaline is not available.)

3. Vasopressin (DDAVP) should only be used in selected circumstances.

4. Dopamine is *only* recommended in highly selected patients (e.g. patients with a low risk of tachyarrhythmias and absolute or relative bradycardia).

5. Phenylephrine is *not* recommended except in the presence of serious arrhythmias, cardiac output is known to be high and blood pressure is consistently low, and where other measures have failed.

6. Low-dose dopamine should *not* be used for renal protection.

7. All patients on vasopressors should have an arterial line placed.

I. Inotropes

1. A trial of dobutamine infusion up to 20 µgm/kg/min may be administered in the presence of:

   a. Myocardial dysfunction (elevated cardiac filling pressures and low cardiac output)

   b. Ongoing signs of hyperperfusion, despite adequate volume and MAP

2. Do *not* use a strategy to increase cardiac index to supranormal levels

J. Corticosteroids

1. Steroids should *not* be administered for the treatment of sepsis in the *absence* of shock.

2. Do *not* use intravenous hydrocortisone to treat adult septic shock patients if adequate fluid resuscitation and vasopressor therapy are able to restore haemodynamic stability.

3. If this is *not* achievable, add hydrocortisone at a dose of 200 mg/day, preferably by infusion.

4. In treated patients, hydrocortisone should be tapered when vasopressors are no longer required.

5. When cortisone is given, use continuous flow.

K. Blood Product Administration

1. Once tissue hypoperfusion has been resolved, and in the absence of extenuating circumstances (e.g. active haemorrhage, myocardial ischaemia), transfusion should *only* take place if the haemoglobin is <7 Gm/dL, to achieve a target of 7–9 Gm/dL.

2. Fresh frozen plasma (FFP) should *not* be used to correct clotting abnormalities in the absence of active bleeding or planned invasive procedures.

3. Use TEG or ROTEM goal-directed maintenance of coagulation parameters.

4. In patients with severe sepsis, administer platelets:

   a. In the absence of bleeding *only* when counts are <10 000 mm^3

   b. If risk of bleeding, administer platelets when count is >20 000 mm^3

   c. If actively bleeding, administer platelets for a minimum of >50 000 mm^3

L. Immunoglobulin Administration

1. Immunoglobulins should *not* be administered.

M. Mechanical Ventilation of Sepsis-induced ARDS (See protocol – page 87)

1. Tidal volume of 6 mL/kg based on predicted body weight.

2. Plateau pressures to be less than 30 cm H_2O.

3. PEEP should be routine, using a higher level of PEEP (8–12 cm H_2O).

4 Recruitment can be used in patients with sepsis with severe hypoxaemia.

5. Prone positioning should be used when PaO_2/FiO_2 ratio is <100.

6. Mechanical ventilation should mandate a 'head-up' position of >30°.

7. Non-invasive mask ventilation should be considered where the benefits exceed the risks.

8. A weaning protocol should be in place and mechanically ventilated patients should undergo spontaneous breathing trials regularly to evaluate weaning potential.

Table 14.1 Summary of Surviving Sepsis Guidelines 2012 – *continued*

The patient *must* satisfy the following criteria:

a. The patient must be arousable.

b. The patient must be haemodynamically stable without vasopressors.

c. There may be no new potentially serious conditions.

d. There are low ventilatory requirements.

    i. PEEP <8 cm H_2O

    ii. Pressure support <10 cm H_2O

    iii Rate <8 b.p.m.

e Low FiO_2 requirements (≤0.4) which can safely be delivered by face mask.

f. Extubate when successful and safe.

N. Sedation and Neuromuscular Blockade

1. Continuous (and even intermittent) sedation should be minimized.

2. Neuromuscular blocking agents (NMBAs) should be avoided in the septic patients *without* ARDS.

3. If required, intermittent bolus administration of NMBA should be used.

4. A *short* course only (<48 hours) of NMBA should be used with ARDS.

O. Glucose Control (See glucose protocol)

1. A protocol-based approach to blood glucose management is required.

P. Bicarbonate Therapy

1. Do *not* use sodium bicarbonate therapy for the purpose of improving haemodynamics or reducing vasopressor requirements with low pH.

Q. Deep Vein Thrombosis Prophylaxis

1. Patients should receive daily pharmacoprophylaxis against thrombo-embolism (VTE) with low-molecular-weight heparin (LMWH).

2. Patients should be treated with LMWH and intermittent compression devices.

R. Stress Ulcer Prophylaxis

1. Patients with no risk factors need no prophylaxis.

2. Trauma patients should receive sucralfate.

3. High-risk patients with bleeding risk should receive protein pump inhibitors.

S. Nutrition (See feeding protocol)

1. Administer enteral feeds within 48 h.

2. Avoid full mandatory caloric feeding during the first week or on inotropes.

3. Use nutrition with *no* immuno-modulation supplementation in severe sepsis.

14.19 ABDOMINAL COMPARTMENT SYNDROME (ACS)

14.19.1 Introduction

Raised intra-abdominal pressure (IAP) has far-reaching consequences for the physiology of the patient. There have been major developments in our understanding of IAP and intra-abdominal hypertension (IAH). The syndrome that results when organs fail as a result is known as 'abdominal compartment syndrome'. Increasingly, it is being recognized that ACS is not uncommon in trauma patients, and failure to consider its prevention, detect it in a timely fashion and treat it aggressively results in a high mortality.

14.19.2 Definition of ACS

The first World Congress on ACS was held in 2004. An internal consensus agreement relating to definitions, updated in 2013, is shown in Table 14.2. Various aspects were defined, including IAP (Definition 1), abdominal perfusion pressure (APP) (Definition 2) and IAH (Definitions 7 and 8).

Table 14.2 Consensus definitions relation to intra-abdominal pressure (IAP), intra-abdominal hypertension (IAH) and abdominal compartment syndrome (ACS) (Updated 2013 consensus)

Definition 1	Intra-abdominal pressure (IAP) is the steady state pressure concealed within the abdominal cavity
Definition 2	The reference standard for intermittent IAP measurements is via the bladder with a maximal instillation volume of 25mL of sterile saline
Definition 3	IAP should be expressed in mm Hg and measured at end-expiration in the complete supine position after ensuring that abdominal muscle contractions are absent and with the transducer zeroed at the level of the mid-axillary line
Definition 4	Normal IAP is approximately 5–7 mm Hg in critically ill adults
Definition 5	IAH is defined by a sustained or repeated pathological elevation of IAP > 12 mm Hg
Definition 6	ACS is defined as a sustained IAP ≥ 20 mm Hg (with or without an APP < 60 mm Hg) that is associated with new organ dysfunction/failure
Definition 7	IAH is graded as follows:
	Grade I: IAP 12–15 mm Hg
	Grade II: IAP 16–20 mm Hg
	Grade III: IAP 21–25 mm Hg
	Grade IV: IAP > 25 mm Hg
Definition 8	Primary IAH or ACS is a condition associated with injury or disease in the abdominopelvic region that frequently requires early surgical or interventional radiological intervention
Definition 9	Secondary IAH or ACS refers to conditions that do not originate from the abdominopelvic region
	Abdominal perfusion pressure (APP) = Mean arterial pressure (MAP) – IAP
Definition 10	Recurrent IAH or ACS refers to the condition in which ACS redevelops following previous surgical or medical treatment of primary or secondary IAH or ACS
Definition 11	Abdominal Perfusion Pressure (APP) = Mean Arterial Pressure (MAP – Intra Abdominal Pressure (IAP)
Definition 12	A polycompartment syndrome is a condition where two or more anatomical compartments have elevated compartmental pressuresv
Definition 13	Abdominal compliance is a measure of the ease of abdominal expansion, which is determined by the elasticity of the abdominal wall and diaphragm. It should be expressed as the change in intra-abdominal volume per change in IAP
Definition 14	The open abdomen is one that requires a temporary abdominal closure due to the skin and fascia not being closed after laparotomy
Definition 15	Lateralization of the abdominal wall is the phenomenon where the musculature and fascia of the abdominal wall, most exemplified by the rectus abdominus muscles and their enveloping fascia, move laterally away from the midline with time

Specifically, ACS is defined as a sustained IAP of 20 mm Hg or more (with or without an APP <60 mm Hg) that is associated with new organ dysfunction/failure (Definition 9). The ACS is also classified as follows:

- Primary ACS (Definition 10) – ACS that develops due to conditions associated with injury or illness in the abdominopelvic region. This includes conditions requiring emergency surgical or angioradiological intervention (including damage control laparotomy, bleeding pelvic fractures, massive retroperitoneal haematomas and failed non-operative management of solid organ injuries, and following disease processes such as severe acute pancreatitis.
- Secondary ACS (Definition 11) – ACS that develops from causes originating outside the abdomen, such as sepsis, capillary leak, major burns and overenthusiastic fluid resuscitation.

- Recurrent ACS (Definition 12) – ACS that develops following initially successful surgical or medical treatment of either primary or secondary ACS, or following the closure of a previously performed decompressive laparotomy.

14.19.3 Pathophysiology

The incidence of IAH in post-operative trauma patients ranges from 20 per cent to 50 per cent. It is common after many forms of emergency surgery. The causes of acutely increased IAP are usually multifactorial and are shown in Table 14.3. Raised IAP occurs commonly with overenthusiastic fluid resuscitation[28]. In addition to the direct causes shown in Table 14.3, hypothermia, acidosis and overall injury severity will further exacerbate the problem.

14.19.4 **Causes of Raised IAP**

See Table 14.3.

14.19.5 **Effect of Raised IAP on Individual Organ Function**

14.19.5.1 RENAL

In 1945, Bradley and Bradley[29], in a study of 17 volunteers, demonstrated that there was a reduction in renal plasma flow and glomerular filtration rate in association with increased IAP. In 1982, Harman et al.[30] showed that as IAP increased from 0 to 20 mm Hg in dogs, the glomerular filtration rate decreased by 25 per cent. At 40 mm Hg, the dogs were resuscitated, and their cardiac output returned to normal. However, their glomerular filtration rate and renal blood flow did not improve, indicating a local effect on renal blood flow. The situation in seriously ill patients may, however, be different, and the exact cause of renal dysfunction in the ICU is not clear owing to the complexity of critically ill patients.

The most likely direct effect of increased IAP is an increase in the renal vascular resistance, coupled with a moderate reduction in cardiac output. Pressure on the ureter has been ruled out as a cause, as investigators have placed ureteric stents with no improvement in function. Other factors that may contribute to renal dysfunction include humeral factors and intraparenchymal renal pressures.

The absolute value of IAP that is required to cause renal impairment is probably in the region of 15 mm Hg. Maintaining adequate cardiovascular filling pressures in the presence of increased IAP also seems to be important.

14.19.5.2 CARDIOVASCULAR

Increased IAP reduces cardiac output as well as increases central venous pressure, systemic vascular resistance, pulmonary artery pressure and pulmonary artery wedge pressure. Cardiac output is affected mainly by a reduction in stroke volume, secondary to a reduction in pre-load and an increase in after-load. This is further aggravated by hypovolaemia. Paradoxically, in the presence of hypovolaemia, an increase in IAP can be temporarily associated with an increase in cardiac output. It has been identified that venous stasis occurs in the legs of patients with abdominal pressures above 12 mm Hg. In addition, recent studies of patients undergoing laparoscopic cholecystectomy show up to a fourfold increase in renin and aldosterone levels.

14.19.5.3 RESPIRATORY

In association with increased IAP, there is diaphragmatic stenting, exerting a restrictive effect on the lungs, with a reduction in ventilation, decreased lung compliance, an increase in airway pressures and a reduction in tidal volumes.

In critically ill ventilated patients, the effect on the respiratory system can be significant, resulting in reduced lung volumes, impaired gas exchange and high ventilatory pressures. Hypercarbia can occur, and the resulting acidosis can be exacerbated by simultaneous cardiovascular depression as a result of raised IAP. The effects of raised IAP on the respiratory system in ICU can sometimes be life-threatening, requiring urgent abdominal decompression. Patients with true ACS undergoing abdominal decompression demonstrate a remarkable change in their intraoperative vital signs.

14.19.5.4 VISCERAL PERFUSION

Interest in visceral perfusion has increased with the popularization of gastric tonometry, and there is an association between IAP and visceral perfusion as measured by gastric pH. This has recently been confirmed in 18 patients undergoing laparoscopy in whom a reduction of between 11 per cent and 54 per cent in blood flow was seen in the duodenum and stomach, respectively, at an IAP of 15 mm Hg. Animal studies suggest that the reduction in visceral perfusion is selective, affecting intestinal blood flow before, for example, adrenal blood flow. We have demonstrated, in a study of 73 post-laparotomy patients, that IAP and pH are strongly associated, suggesting that early decreases in visceral perfusion are related to levels of IAP as low as 15 mm Hg.

Table 14.3 Causes of Raised Intra-abdominal Pressure

Massive resuscitation

Major intra-abdominal and retroperitoneal haemorrhage

Tissue oedema secondary to insults such as ischaemia and sepsis

Paralytic ileus

Ascites

14.19.5.5 INTRACRANIAL PRESSURE

Raised IAP can have a marked effect on intracranial patho-physiology and cause severe rises in intracranial pressure.

14.19.6 Measurement of IAP

The gold standard for IAP measurement involves using a urinary catheter. The patient is positioned flat on the bed. A standard Foley catheter is used, with a T-piece bladder pressure device attached between the urinary catheter and the drainage tubing. This piece is then connected to a pressure transducer online to the monitoring system. The pressure transducer is placed in the mid-axillary line and the urinary tubing is clamped. Approximately 50 mL isotonic saline is inserted into the bladder via a three-way stopcock. After zeroing, the pressure on the monitor is recorded.

Increasingly, it is recognized that IAP is not a static condition and should be measured continuously. In addition, whether IAP is measured intermittently or continuously, consideration should be given to abdominal perfusion measurement.

14.19.6.1 MEASUREMENT OF ABDOMINAL PERFUSION PRESSURE (APP)

As with the concept of cerebral perfusion pressure, calculation of the 'abdominal perfusion pressure', which is defined as mean arterial pressure minus IAP, assesses not only the severity of IAP present but also the adequacy of the patient's abdominal blood flow.

The APP has been studied as a resuscitation endpoint in four clinical trials. These demonstrated statistically significant differences in APP between survivors and non-survivors with IAH/ACS. Cheatham et al.[31], in a retrospective trial of surgical and trauma patients with IAH (mean IAP 22 ± 8 mm Hg), concluded that an APP of greater than 50 mm Hg optimized survival based upon receiver operating characteristic curve analysis. Abdominal perfusion pressure was also superior to global resuscitation endpoints such as arterial pH, base deficit, arterial lactate and hourly urinary output in its ability to predict patient outcome.

Malbrain et al.[32-34] in three subsequent trials in mixed medical-surgical patients (mean IAP 10 ± 4 mm Hg) suggested that 60 mm Hg represented an appropriate resuscitation goal. A persistence of IAH and a failure to maintain an APP of 60 mm Hg or more by day 3 following the development of IAH-induced acute renal failure was found to discriminate between survivors and non-survivors.

14.19.6.2 TIPS FOR IAP MEASUREMENT

A strict protocol and staff education on the technique and interpretation of IAP are essential.

Very high pressures (especially unexpected ones) are usually caused by a blocked urinary catheter and should be repeated.

The volume of saline instilled into the bladder is not critical but should be less than 50 mL and the same every time. A central venous pressure manometer system can be used, but it is more cumbersome than online monitoring. The size of the urinary catheter does not matter. Elevation of the catheter and measurement of the urine column provide a rough guide and are simple to perform. If the patient is not lying flat, IAP can be measured from the pubic symphysis. Real-time continuous monitoring of IAP is effective and shows trends as well as actual pressures.

14.19.7 Treatment

14.19.7.1 PREVENTION

To avoid ACS developing in the first place, in the emergency department, concepts of damage control coupled with adequate pre-hospital information will help identify patients at high risk even before they arrive in the emergency room. Avoiding excessive fluid resuscitation (damage control resuscitation) is an important factor in reducing the risk of developing subsequent ACS. In patients undergoing damage control laparotomy, it is mandatory to leave the abdomen open to prevent ACS and in anticipation of a second operation.

14.19.7.2 TREATMENT

There are a number of key principles in the management of patients with potential ACS:

- Regular appropriate monitoring of IAP in the ICU.
- Optimization of systemic perfusion, circulating volume and organ function in the patient with IAH grades I and II (i.e. ≤20 mm Hg).

- Institution of specific medical procedures to reduce IAP and the end-organ consequences of IAH/ACS, including diuretics, and removing excess ascites if present by percutaneous puncture.
- In patients with grades III to IV IAH (IAP >20 mm Hg) with evidence of new-onset organ failure not responding to non-operative management, a decompressive laparostomy performed as soon as possible.

The decompressed abdomen should be closed using a low-vacuum sandwich technique.

14.19.7.3 REVERSIBLE FACTORS

The second aspect of management is to correct any reversible cause of ACS, such as intra-abdominal bleeding. Massive retroperitoneal haemorrhage is often associated with a fractured pelvis, and consideration should be given to measures that would control haemorrhage, such as pelvic fixation or vessel embolization. In some cases, severe gaseous distension or acute colonic pseudo-obstruction can occur in ICU patients. This may respond to drugs such as neostigmine, but if it is severe, surgical decompression may be necessary. A common cause of a raised IAP in ICU is related to the ileus. There is little that can be actively done in these circumstances apart from optimizing the patient's cardiorespiratory status and serum electrolytes, and inserting a nasogastric tube.

Remember that ACS is often only a symptom of an underlying problem. In a prospective review of 88 post-laparotomy patients, Sugrue et al. found that those with an IAP of 18 mm Hg had an increased odds ratio for intra-abdominal sepsis of 3.9 (95 per cent confidence interval 0.7–22.7)[35,36]. Abdominal evaluation for sepsis is a priority, and this should obviously include a rectal examination as well as investigations such as ultrasound and computed tomography (CT) scanning. Surgery is the obvious mainstay of treatment in patients whose rise in IAP is due to post-operative bleeding.

14.19.8 Surgery for Raised IAP

As yet, there are few guidelines for exactly when surgical decompression is required in the presence of raised IAP. Some studies have stated that abdominal decompression is the only treatment and that it should be performed early in order to prevent ACS. This is an overstatement and not supported by level l evidence. The indications for abdominal decompression are related to correcting pathophysiological abnormalities as much as to achieving a precise and optimum IAP.

In general, temporary abdominal closure is superior to conventional techniques for dealing with intra-abdominal sepsis. Indications for performing temporary abdominal closure include:

- Abdominal decompression.
- When re-exploration is planned.
- To facilitate re-exploration in abdominal sepsis.
- Inability to close the abdomen.
- Prevention of ACS.

A large number of different techniques have been used to facilitate a temporary abdominal closure, including intravenous bags, Velcro, silicone and zips. Whatever technique is used, it is important that effective decompression be achieved with adequate incisions.

14.19.8.1 TIPS FOR SURGICAL DECOMPRESSION FOR RAISED IAP

- There should be early investigation and correction of the cause of raised IAP.
- Ongoing abdominal bleeding with raised IAP requires urgent operative intervention.
- Reduction in urinary output is a late sign of renal impairment. Gastric tonometry may provide earlier information on visceral perfusion.
- Abdominal decompression requires a full-length abdominal incision.
- The surgical dressing should be closed using a sandwich technique using two suction drains placed laterally to facilitate fluid removal from the wound.
- If the abdomen is very tight, pre-closure with a silo should be considered.

Unfortunately, clinical infection is common in the open abdomen, and the infection is usually polymicrobial. Particular care needs to be taken in patients undergoing post-aortic surgery as the aortic graft may become colonized. The mesh in this situation should be removed, and the abdomen left open. It is desirable to close the abdominal defect as soon as possible. This is often not possible due to persistent tissue oedema.

14.19.9 Management Algorithm

Figure 14.1 outlines an algorithm for the management of IAH and ACS.

**Intra-Abdominal Hypertension (IAH)/Abdominal
Compartment Syndrome (ACS) Management Algorithm**

Figure 14.1 Intra-abdominal hypertension (IAH) and abdominal compartment syndrome (ACS) management algorithm. (Adapted from *Intensive Care Medicine* 2006;32(11):1722–1732 and 2007;33(6):951–962. © World Society of the Abdominal Compartment Syndrome. All rights reserved.)

14.19.10 **World Society of the Abdominal Compartment Syndrome**

The concept of IAP measurement and its significance is increasingly important in the ICU and is rapidly becoming part of routine care. Patients with raised IAP require close and careful monitoring, aggressive resuscitation and a low index of suspicion for the requirement of surgical abdominal decompression.

The formation of the World Society of the Abdominal Compartment Syndrome (now WSACS – the Abdominal Compartment Society) (http://www.wsacs.org) has been a major advance, with the production of consensus definitions, the formation of a research policy, multicentre trials and the publication of the consensus guidelines on ACS.

14.20 **ORGAN DONATION**

Identification of potential organ donors from among brain-dead patients is an important role in every critical care department. It is difficult to balance the requirements of the organ transplant teams with a sympathetic and understanding approach to grieving relatives. Specific training is *vital*.

REFERENCES AND RECOMMENDED READING

References

1. Claridge JA, Crabtree TD, Pelletier SJ, Butler K, Sawyer RG, Young JS. Persistent occult hypoperfusion is associated with a significant increase in infection rate and mortality in major trauma patients. *J Trauma*. 2000;48:8–14.
2. Blow O, Magliore L, Claridge JA, Butler K, Young JS. The golden hour and the silver day: detection and correction of occult hypoperfusion within 24 hours improves outcome from major trauma. *J Trauma*. 1999;47:964–969.
3. Balogh Z, McKinley BA, Cocanour CS, et al. Supranormal trauma resuscitation causes more cases of abdominal compartment syndrome. *Arch Surg*. 2003;138:637–643.
4. Garner JS, Jarvis WR, Emori TG, Horan TC, Hughes JM. CDC definitions for nosocomial infections, 1988. *Am J Infect Control*. 1988;16:128–140.
5. Mallick A, Bodenham AR. Tracheostomy in critically ill patients. *Eur J Anaesthesiol*. 2010;27:678–682.
6. Ganter MT, Pittet JF. New insights into acute coagulopathy in trauma patients. *Best Pract Res Clin Anaesthesiol*. 2010;24:15–25.
7. Tieu BH, Holcomb JB, Schreiber MA. Coagulopathy: its pathophysiology and treatment in the injured patient. *World J Surg*. 2007;31:1055–1064.
8. Geeraedts LMG Jr, Kaasjager HAH, van Vugt AB, Frölke JPM. Exsanguination in trauma: a review of diagnostics and treatment options. *Injury*. 2009;40:11–20.
9. CRASH-2 Trial Collaborators. Effects of tranexamic acid on death, vascular occlusive events, and blood transfusion in trauma patients with significant haemorrhage (CRASH-2): a randomised, placebo-controlled trial. *Lancet*. 2010;376:27–32.
10. Moore HB, Moore EE, Gonzales E, et al. Hyprinofibrinolysis, physiologic fibrinolysis, and fibrinolysis shutdown: the spectrum of post injury fibrinolysis and relevance to antifibrinolytic therapy. *J Trauma Acute Care Surg*. 2014;77(6);811–817.
11. Bihorac A, Delano MJ, Schold JD, et al. Incidence, clinical predictors, genomics, and outcome of acute kidney injury among trauma patients. *Ann Surg*. 2010;252:158–165.
12. Janjua KJ, Sugrue M, Deane SA. Prospective evaluation of early missed injuries and the role of the tertiary trauma survey. *J Trauma*. 1998;44:1000–1006.
13. Jacobs DO, Kudsk KA, Oswanski MF, Sacks GS, Sinclair KE. Practice management guidelines for nutritional support of the trauma patient. In: Eastern Association for the Surgery of Trauma. *Practice Management Guidelines*. http://www.east.org.
14. Kreymann KG, Berger MM, Deutz NE, et al. ESPEN guidelines on enteral nutrition: intensive care. *Clin Nutr*. 2006;25:210–223.
15. Yanagawa T, Bunn F, Roberts I, Wentz R, Pierro A. Nutritional support for head-injured patients. *Cochrane Database Syst Rev*. 2000;(2):CD001530.
16. Cook AM, Peppard A, Magnuson A. Nutrition considerations in traumatic brain injury. *Nutr Clin Pract*. 2008;23:608–620.
17. Moore FA, Feliciano DV, Andrassy RJ, et al. Early enteral feeding compared with parenteral reduces postoperative septic complications: the result of a meta-analysis. *Ann Surg*. 1992;216:172–183.
18. Holmes JH 4th, Brundage SI, Yuen P, Hall RA, Maier RV, Jurkovich GJ. Complications of surgical feeding jejunostomy in trauma patients. *J Trauma*. 1999;47:1009–1012.

19. Guillamondegui OD, Gunter OL Jr, Bonadies JA, et al. Practice management guidelines for stress ulcer prophylaxis. In: Eastern Association for the Surgery of Trauma. *Practice Management Guidelines*. http://www.east.org. Accessed December 2010.

20. Rogers FB, Cipolle MD, Velmahos G, Rozycki G. Practice management guidelines for the management of venous thromboembolism (VTE) in trauma patients. *J Trauma*. 2002;53:142–164. In: Eastern Association for the Surgery of Trauma. *Practice Management Guidelines*. http://www.east.org. Accessed December 2010.

21. Boddi M, Barbani F, Abbate R, et al. Reduction in deep vein thrombosis incidence in intensive care after a clinician education program. *J Thromb Haemost*. 2010;8:121–128.

22. Hauser CJ, Adams CA Jr, Soumitra RE, Council of the Surgical Infection Society. Surgical Infection Society guidelines: prophylactic antibiotic use in open fractures: an evidence-based guideline. *Surg Infect (Larchmt)*. 2006;7:379–405.

23. Velmahos GC, Toutouzas KG, Sarkisyan G, et al. Severe trauma is not an excuse for prolonged antibiotic prophylaxis. *Arch Surg*. 2002;137:537–541.

24. Luchette FA, Bone LB, Born CT, et al. Practice management guidelines for prophylactic antibiotic use in open fractures. In: Eastern Association for the Surgery of Trauma. Practice Management Guidelines Workgroup. http://www.east.org. Accessed December 2014.

25. Hoff WS, Bonadies JA, Cachecho R, Dorlac WC. Eastern Association for the Surgery of Trauma. Practice Management Guidelines Workgroup: Update to practice management guidelines for prophylactic antibiotic use in open fractures. http://www.east.org. Accessed December 2014.

26. Rello J, Paiva JA, Baraibar J, et al. International Conference for the Development of Consensus on the Diagnosis and Treatment of Ventilator-Associated Pneumonia. *Chest*. 2001;120:955–970.

27. Dellinger RP, Levy MM, Rhodes A, et al. Surviving Sepsis Campaign: International Guidelines for Management of Severe Sepsis and Septic Shock: 2012; *Crit Care* Med. 2013;41(2):580–637.

28. Balogh Z, McKinley BA, Cocanour CS, et al. Supranormal trauma resuscitation causes more cases of abdominal compartment syndrome. *Arch Surg*. 2003;138:637–642.

29. Bradley SE, Bradley GP. The effect of increased intra-abdominal pressure on renal function in man. *J Clin Invest*. 1947;26:1010–1022.

30. Harman PK, Kron IL, McLachlan HD, Freedlender AE, Nolan SP. Elevated intra-abdominal pressure and renal function. *Ann Surg*. 1982;196:594–597.

31. Cheatham ML, White MW, Sagraves SG, Johnson JL, Block EF. Abdominal perfusion pressure: a superior parameter in the assessment of intra-abdominal hypertension. *J Trauma*. 2000;49:621–626.

32. Malbrain ML, Cheatham ML, Kirkpatrick A, et al. Results from the International Conference of Experts on Intra-abdominal Hypertension and Abdominal Compartment Syndrome. I. Definitions. *Intensive Care Med*. 2006;32:1722–1732.

33. Malbrain ML, Chiumello D, Pelosi P, et al. Prevalence of intra-abdominal hypertension in critically ill patients: a multicentre epidemiological study. *Intensive Care Med*. 2004;30:822–829.

34. Malbrain ML, Chiumello D, Pelosi P, et al. Incidence and prognosis of intraabdominal hypertension in a mixed population of critically ill patients: a multiple-centre epidemiological study. *Crit Care Med*. 2005;33:315–322.

35. Sugrue M, Buist MD, Hourihan F, Deane S, Bauman A, Hillman K. Prospective study of intra-abdominal hypertension and renal function after laparotomy. *Br J Surg*. 1995;82:235–238.

36. Sugrue M, Jones F, Deane SA, Bishop G, Bauman A, Hillman K. Intra-abdominal hypertension is an independent cause of postoperative renal impairment. *Arch Surg*. 1999;134:1082–1085.

Recommended Reading

Burch J, Moore E, Moore F, Franciose R. The abdominal compartment syndrome. *Surg Clin North Am*. 1996;76:833–842.

Cheatham ML. Abdominal compartment syndrome: pathophysiology and definitions. *Scand J Trauma Resusc Emerg Med*. 2009;17:10.

Eastern Association for the Surgery of Trauma. *Practice Management Guidelines*. http://www.east.org. Accessed December 2014.

Gaarder C, Naess PA, Frischknecht Christensen E, et al. Scandinavian Guidelines – "The massively bleeding patient". *Scand J Surg*. 2008;97:15–36.

Ivatury RR, Cheatham ML, Malbrain MLNG, Sugrue M. *Abdominal Compartment Syndrome*. Georgetown, TX: Landes Biosciences; 2006.

Ivatury RR, Porter JM, Simon RJ, Islam S, John R, Stahl WM. Intra-abdominal hypertension after life-threatening penetrating abdominal trauma: prophylaxis, incidence, and clinical relevance to gastric mucosal pH and abdominal compartment syndrome. *J Trauma*. 1998;44:1016–1021.

Schein M, Wittman DH, Aprahamian CC, Condon RE. The abdominal compartment syndrome: the physiological and clinical consequences of elevated intra-abdominal pressure. *J Am Coll Surg*. 1995;180:745–750.

Sugrue M. Intra-abdominal pressure: time for clinical practice guidelines? *Intensive Care Med*. 2002;28:389–391.

Sugrue M, Jones F, Janjua J, et al. Temporary abdominal closure. *J Trauma*. 1998;45:914–921.

Sugrue M, Bauman A, Jones F, et al. Clinical examination is an inaccurate predictor of intraabdominal pressure. *World J Surg*. 2002;26:1428–1431.

World Society for the Abdominal Compartment Syndrome. http://www.wsacs.org. Accessed December 2014.

Part 4

Diagnostic and therapeutic technology

Minimally Invasive Surgery in Trauma **15**

Minimally invasive techniques have yet to be widely adopted by trauma surgeons, unlike by their other surgical colleagues. However, selective indications for the use of these techniques are emerging rapidly in both adult and paediatric fields, especially in post-operative surveillance after non-operative management (NOM).

Physiological instability and severe head injury are contraindications to the creation of the pneumoperitoneum often used with minimally invasive techniques.

15.1 TECHNIQUE

Correct preparation and positioning of the patient for trauma laparoscopy are essential.

The patient is placed supine on a beanbag and securely strapped because abdominal organ retraction relies on dependency obtained with table rotation and tilting. Draping should allow for rapid conversion to formal laparotomy. If necessary, pneumoperitoneum should be obtained with low flow (to allow timely detection of a tension pneumothorax, leading to immediate stopping in insufflation and insertion of a thoracic drain) and maintained at low pressure (8–12 mm Hg). The first trocar should always be inserted with the open technique.

A straight or 30° scope can be used according to surgeon preferences. It has been found that 10-mm scopes are better than 5 mm as blood absorbs white light and darkens the optical field, with less intense light being transmitted by the smaller-diameter scope.

Adequate tissue handling requires 5-mm atraumatic bowel graspers inserted in ergonomically adapted ports (lateral) and skills acquired in other and regularly performed laparoscopic procedures.

15.2 THORACIC INJURY

Persistent, non-exsanguinating haemorrhage[1] can be investigated and occasionally treated by video-assisted thoracoscopic surgery (VATS)[2,3].

The VATS can be indicated in the acute setting for exploration in case of persistent bleeding of haemothorax (>300 cc within 3 hours) and to follow stab wound agents under visual control. Also, VATS can be used to exclude penetrating wounds of the heart or to perform a pericardial window in penetrating cardiac trauma potentially with appropriate release of tamponade[4].

VATS can be indicated secondarily, for evacuation of a clotted haemothorax, and for direct visualization and stapling of persistent or recurrent air leaks, with aspiration of associated haemothorax, to ligate (rare) thoracic duct injuries (when conservative medical management fails to reduce chyle leakage). It can also be indicated for extraction of foreign bodies.

15.3 DIAPHRAGMATIC INJURY

In asymptomatic patients with anterior or flank stab wounds of the lower chest or upper abdomen, the risk of an occult diaphragmatic injury is about 7 per cent. Specifically, in patients with left-sided thoracoabdominal stab wounds, the risk is 17 per cent[5].

Suspected diaphragmatic injury due to both blunt and penetrating injury can be accurately evaluated by VATS or laparoscopy.

Laparoscopy is adequate to exclude occult diaphragmatic injury after penetrating abdominal trauma or to rule out diaphragmatic injury when non-operative management of penetrating thoracoabdominal injuries is envisaged[6].

Diaphragmatic injury can be repaired laparoscopically or thoracoscopically (it is easier to work on the convex side of the muscle); however, the danger lies in that the intraperitoneal injury may be missed if thoracoscopy is used for diagnostic purposes in the acute setting.

Conversely, secondary repair of diaphragmatic injuries that have been initially missed or left untreated is an excellent indication for laparoscopic techniques, either through the thorax or via the abdomen.

All of the above assume significant laparoscopic experience on the behalf of the operator, as unfamiliarity with the anatomy and techniques required may lead to missed injury, sometimes with catastrophic results.

15.4 ABDOMINAL INJURY

15.4.1 Screening for Intra-abdominal Injury

Although initially laparoscopy appeared to be a poor screening tool after blunt trauma (16% incidence of missed intra-abdominal injuries in one series), the sensitivity and specificity of laparoscopy in detecting blunt small bowel injuries has improved considerably over the past years[7]. In abdominal stab wounds, for example, diagnostic laparoscopy can prevent an unnecessary laparotomy in one-half to more than 80 per cent of the cases, in particular by assessment of whether or not an equivocal wound has breached the peritoneal cavity.

However, sensitivity remains problematic for hollow viscus injury. Indirect signs, injection of dyes or air through gastrointestinal tubes are sometimes useful adjuncts.

In sum, laparoscopy can be used to confirm or rule out penetration into the peritoneal cavity, as well as the presence of bile or blood, while pinpointing the site of injury.

15.4.2 Splenic Injury

Successful laparoscopic splenic preservation or partial splenectomy has been reported after trauma, using fibrin glue, argon beam coagulator and by splenic-wrapping with mesh. Successful autotransfusion of haemoperitoneum aspirated from the peritoneum has also been reported. Laparoscopy is an excellent approach for secondary treatment of post-traumatic localized splenic infarcts or pseudocysts or even post-traumatic splenic artery pseudoaneurysm.

Laparoscopic management of the spleen is contraindicated in the presence of haemodynamic instability or competing injury.

15.4.3 Liver Injury

Patients failing a trial of non-operative management for hepatic injury have been managed successfully using minimally invasive surgery, including laparoscopic application of fibrin glue as a haemostatic agent[8].

Haemoperitoneum may be drained, and biliary leaks, with or without peritonitis, can be controlled via the laparoscope usually combined with endoscopic retrograde cholangiopancreatography (ERCP)[9].

Reports of successful laparoscopic treatment for intra-abdominal organs other than the liver or spleen are increasing.

15.4.4 Bowel Injury

Laparoscopic examination for penetrating injury of the bowel requires diligent and rigorous exploration in order not to miss occult or small lesions. Different techniques have been described to best run the bowel. One of these is the hand-over-hand technique, with care taken to use atraumatic graspers, to manipulate the bowel at the tip of the mesentery, and routinely explore both sides.

Laparoscopy has been used to repair small bowel injuries and to raise a colostomy to de-function the lower intestinal tract in colorectal injuries[10].

15.5 AFTER NON-OPERATIVE MANAGEMENT

After non-operative management (NOM) (especially after embolization) laparoscopy can check the abdominal cavity in case of suspicion of organ ischaemia/perforation, persistent abdominal signs in stable patients (after blunt trauma), and perform washouts in case of poor tolerance of biloperitoneum, haemobiloperitoneum or persistent occult bleeding. It can be used to treat intraperitoneal bladder rupture or release an abdominal compartment syndrome[11].

15.6 RISKS OF LAPAROSCOPY IN TRAUMA

Laparoscopy in abdominal trauma entails four specific risks:

- Missed injuries, mainly intestinal, with their attending high morbidity (and mortality).

- Gas embolism, supposedly higher when mesenteric and hepatic (venous) lesions have occurred, but apparently as rare as in any laparoscopic procedure today.
- Impeded venous return (because of raised intra-abdominal pressure).
- Increased intracranial pressure.

These last two make physiological instability and severe head injury absolute contraindications to the creation of the pneumoperitoneum, necessary for most minimally invasive techniques.

Caution is warranted as well in the presence of abdominal compartment syndrome or diaphragmatic rents[11]. While laparoscopy may rarely detect and treat the cause of the former, the risk of tension pneumothorax if there is a coexisting diaphragmatic tear requires that a large-bore needle be inserted into the thorax during the exploratory laparoscopy.

15.7 **SUMMARY**

To date, minimally invasive surgery has played only a small role in trauma surgery. Surgeons should be encouraged to incorporate laparoscopy and VATS into their protocols and gain familiarity and expertise with their use. It should, in the light of current knowledge, still be regarded as suitable only for a small group of stable patients.

REFERENCES AND RECOMMENDED READING

References

1. Lowdermilk GA, Naunheim KS. Thoracoscopic evaluation and treatment of thoracic trauma. *Surg Clin North Am.* 2000;80:1535–1542.
2. Lang-Lazdunski L, Mouroux J, Pons F, et al. Role of videothoracoscopy in chest trauma. *Ann Thorac Surg.* 1997;63:327–333.
3. Freeman RK, Al-Dossari G, Hutcheson KA, et al. Indications for using video-assisted thoracoscopic surgery to diagnose diaphragmatic injuries after penetrating chest trauma. *Ann Thorac Surg.* 2001;72:342–347.
4. Morales CH, Salinas CM, Henao CA, Patino PA, Munoz CM. Thoracoscopic pericardial window and penetrating cardiac trauma. *J Trauma.* 1997;42:273–275.
5. Leppäniemi A, Haapiainen R. Occult diaphragmatic injuries caused by stab wounds. *J Trauma.* 2003;55:646–650.
6. Friese RS, Coln E, Gentilello L. Laparoscopy is sufficient to exclude occult diaphragmatic injury after penetrating abdominal trauma. *J Trauma.* 2005;58:789–792.
7. Leppäniemi A, Haapiainen R. Diagnostic laparoscopy in abdominal stab wounds: a prospective, randomized study. *J Trauma.* 2003;55:636–645.
8. Chen RJ, Fang JF, Lin BC, Hsu YB, Kao JL, Kao YC, Chen MF. Selective application of laparoscopy and fibrin glue in the failure of nonoperative management of blunt hepatic trauma. *J Trauma.* 1998;44:691–695.
9. Griffen M, Ochoa J, Boulanger BR. A minimally invasive approach to bile peritonitis after blunt liver injury. *Am Surg.* 2000;66:309–312.
10. Mathonnet M, Peyrou P, Gainant A, Bouvier S, Cubertafond P. Role of laparoscopy in blunt perforations of the small bowel. *Surg Endosc.* 2003;17:641–645.
11. Ivatury RR, Sugerman HJ, Peitzman AB. Abdominal compartment syndrome: recognition and management. *Adv Surg.* 2001;35:251–269.

Recommended Reading

Amin PB, MagnottiLJ, Fabian TC, Croce MA. The role of laparoscopy in abdominal trauma. *Trauma.* 2011;13:137–143.

Bendinelli C, Balogh ZJ. Laparoscopy in trauma patients. In: Malik AM, ed. *Advances in Laparoscopic Surgery.* Rijecka, Croatia: InTech; 2012. http://www.intechopen.com/books/advances-in-laparoscopic-surgery/laparoscopy-in-trauma-patients. Accessed July 2015.

Brooks AJ, Boffard KD. Current technology: laparoscopic surgery in trauma. *Trauma.* 1999;1:53–60.

Carrillo EH, Reed DN Jr, Gordon L, Spain DA, Richardson JD. Delayed laparoscopy facilitates the management of biliary peritonitis in patients with complex liver injuries. *Surg Endosc.* 2001;15:319–322.

Cui H, Luckeroth P, Peralta R. Laparoscopic management of penetrating liver trauma: a safe intervention for hemostasis. *J Laparoendosc Adv Surg Tech A.* 2007;17:219–222.

Demetriades D, Hadjizacharia P, Constantinou C, et al. Selective nonoperative management of penetrating abdominal solid organ injuries. *Ann Surg.* 2006;244:620–628.

Fingerhut A, Chouillard E. Ergonomic and technical aspects of laparoscopy for trauma and non-trauma emergencies. *Eur Surg.* 2004;37(1):1–6.

Ivatury RR, Simon RJ, Stahl WM. A critical evaluation of laparoscopy in penetrating abdominal trauma. *J Trauma.* 1993;34:822–827.

Kozar RA, Moore FA, Cothren CC, et al. Risk factors for hepatic morbidity following nonoperative management multicenter study. *Arch Surg.* 2006;141:451–459.

Kozar RA, Moore, FA Moore EE, et al. Western Trauma Association critical decisions in trauma: nonoperative management of adult blunt hepatic trauma. *J Trauma.* 2009;67:1144–1149.

Letoublon C, Chen Y, Arvieux C, et al. Delayed celiotomy or laparoscopy as part of the nonoperative management of blunt hepatic trauma. *World J Surg.* 2008;32:1189–1193.

Pryor JP, Reilly PM, Dabrowski GP, Grossman MD, Schwab CW. Nonoperative management of abdominal gunshot wounds. *Ann Emerg Med.* 2004;43:345–353.

Sauerland S, Agresta F, Bergamaschi R, et al. Laparoscopy for abdominal emergencies. Evidence-based guidelines of the European Association for Endoscopic Surgery. *Surg Endosc.* 2005;20:14–29.

Uranues S, Dorr K. Laparoscopy in abdominal trauma. *Eur J Trauma Emerg Surg.* 2010;36:19–24.

Villavicencio RT, Aucar JA. Analysis of laparoscopy in trauma. *J Am Coll Surg.* 1999;189:11–20.

Radiology in Trauma **16**

16.1 **INTRODUCTION**

In a large number of patients, interventional radiology, with arterial embolization (AE), stent or stent-graft placement, has become either the first line of treatment or an important adjunct to open surgery. Clinical evaluation, however, determines the course of treatment.

Patients who are haemodynamically stable are evaluated with computed tomography (CT) for non-operative management (NOM) with or without interventional radiology. Patients who are haemodynamically unstable despite resuscitation are diagnosed with chest and pelvic X-ray, focussed abdominal sonography for trauma (FAST) and/or diagnostic peritoneal lavage, aimed at determining the most compelling bleeding source, and are then directed to the operating room for immediate operative treatment without additional imaging.

16.2 **RADIATION DOSES AND PROTECTION FROM RADIATION**

The basic dose or radiation absorbed by the tissues is the Grey (Gy) – 1 joule/Kg of tissue.

The Siewert (Sv) is used in setting radiological protection standards and contains 1000 milliSieverts (mSv):

- 1 Gy of beta or gamma radiation has 1 Sv effect.
- 1 Gy of alpha radiation has 20 Sv effect.
- 1 Gy of neutrons has 10 Sv effect.

All efforts must be made to minimize the effect of ionizing radiation on the human body.

The World Health Organization (WHO) and the International Roundtable on Community Paramedicine (IRCP) recommend a maximum annual radiation dose (Table 16.1).

- The current maximum whole-body dose is recommended not to exceed 50 mSv.

Table 16.1 Dose of Common Diagnostic Radiological Procedures

Examination	Dose (mSv)
CT – no contrast	10
CT contrast abdomen/pelvis	20
Whole-body CT	30
Chest X-ray	2
Pelvis	5
CT – no contrast	10
CT contrast abdomen/pelvis	20

Note: In the United States and Australia, 2 per cent of all malignant disease now being recorded can be attributed directly to medical radiation.

Source: ICRP publication 103: The 2007 recommendations of the International Committee for Radiation Protection. http://www.Radiologyinfo.org. Accessed January 2015.

- Note: For therapeutic oncological radiation of single-organ targets, the dose may reach 500 mSv.
- The maximum annual dose for radiation workers is 20 mSv.
- In 250 flying hours, air crew receive 50 mSv per year.

It is therefore important not to overuse the ionizing radiological diagnostic and therapeutic techniques available to us, unless benefits available exceed the risks incurred.

16.3 **PELVIC FRACTURES**

Severe pelvic fractures, particularly with disruption of the sacroiliac joints, are associated with a high risk of severe arterial and venous bleeding. The application of a sheet or external fixation may control the venous bleeding. However, arterial bleeding often requires AE, which has become the first line of treatment in patients stable enough to reach angiography. Established indications are CT evidence of ongoing bleeding, such as contrast extravasation and pelvic haematoma with bladder compression on the scan, and ongoing transfusion requirements without evidence of other extrapelvic bleeding sources.

There is also a possibility in this subgroup of patients that there may be severe venous bleeding. The patient in shock refractory to resuscitation should therefore be considered for damage control surgery with (extraperitoneal) pelvic packing (see Chapter 9) before angioembolization. Care should be taken to assess the external iliac veins as these are less amenable to packing.

Arterial embolization is carried out after performing an abdominal aortography followed by selective catheterization of the internal iliac arteries. When contrast extravasation is demonstrated, the bleeding vessels are catheterized superselectively and embolized with coils or a combination of coils and gelfoam particles. If this is not possible due to spasm or uncontrolled bleeding, a central embolization of the internal iliac arteries is performed using coils. If the patient deteriorates haemodynamically during angiography, an occlusion balloon may be placed in the infrarenal aorta to achieve haemodynamic control.

16.4 BLUNT SPLENIC INJURIES

Non-operative management of blunt splenic injuries has become the treatment of choice in haemodynamically stable patients, regardless of injury grade and grade of haemoperitoneum, in the absence of other intra-abdominal injuries requiring laparotomy. Non-operative management has been strongly motivated by the wish to preserve the spleen in order to avoid overwhelming post-splenectomy infections and laparotomy-associated morbidity. This can be achieved by using splenic AE in selected patients.

The indications for AE include CT evidence of ongoing bleeding with contrast extravasation outside or within the spleen, a drop in haemoglobin level, tachycardia and haemoperitoneum, as well as the formation of a pseudoaneurysm.

Selective catheterization of the splenic artery is performed, followed by superselective catheterization of the bleeding arteries or feeders to the pseudoaneurysm. Embolization is then performed using microcoils (which can be combined with gelfoam particles or microspheres). In this way, infarctions caused by embolization are limited to small areas.

If there are multiple bleeding arteries or selective catheterization is impossible due to spasm, central embolization of the splenic artery may be performed using microcoils. Such an embolization often contributes to decreasing the perfusion pressure, and is often enough to stop the bleeding while at the same time preserving the circulation to the spleen through collaterals existing in this area. Applying such selection criteria and technique, NOM of blunt splenic injuries may be successful in up to 85–95 per cent of patients.

16.5 LIVER INJURIES

The NOM of blunt liver injuries in haemodynamically stable or stabilized patients has become standard practice. The introduction of AE has been reported to increase the success rate of NOM to well above 80 per cent.

Operative treatment of liver injuries, even in experienced hands, still carries a high mortality and morbidity risk. Arterial embolization seems to be a valuable adjunct to operative management since most patients are haemodynamically abnormal at the end of a damage control laparotomy, and ongoing arterial bleeding is difficult to rule out clinically.

The indications for AE should include CT evidence of ongoing bleeding with contrast extravasation outside or within the liver, a drop in haemoglobin level, tachycardia and haemoperitoneum, in addition to the formation of a pseudoaneurysm. The risk of bleeding with NOM in Organ Injury Scale grades 4 and 5 liver injuries (see Appendix B, OIS Liver injuries: Table B21) is significant, and angiography in these patients should cause no controversy. In addition, angiography should be performed after damage control surgery with packing of the liver.

Angiography is performed via femoral artery puncture. Embolization is performed as peripherally as possible by the placement of microcoils alone or in combination with gelfoam particles. A completion angiogram should be performed to confirm haemostasis of the embolized vessel.

16.6 AORTIC RUPTURE AND INJURY TO MIDDLE-SIZED ARTERIES

Traumatic injuries to the aortic arch vessels are uncommon and are often a result of deceleration accidents. Physical findings are often non-specific, and diagnosis is often made on CT scanning. In haemodynamically stable patients, the use of stent-grafts has recently replaced open surgery. This includes injuries to the common carotid arteries, brachiocephalic trunk and subclavian arteries. Acute aortic traumatic transections are also well suited to the use of stent-grafts. The heparinization needed for open aortic surgery represents an additional risk factor in these patients, who often suffer from multiple associated injuries.

Currently, there are no long-term results to prove the durability of the stent-graft repair. However, due to its minimally traumatic nature, stent-graft treatment of acute aortic transections is today considered to be the first line of treatment for these patients.

RECOMMENDED READING

Asensio JA, Roldan G, Petrone P, et al. Operative management and outcomes in 103 AAST-OIS grades IV and V complex hepatic injuries: trauma surgeons still need to operate, but angioembolization helps. *J Trauma*. 2003;54:647–653.

Dent D, Alsabrook G, Erickson BA, et al. Blunt splenic injuries: high nonoperative management rate can be achieved with selective embolization. *J Trauma*. 2004;56:1063–1067.

Dondelinger RF, Trotteur G, Ghaye B, Szapiro D. Traumatic injuries: radiological hemostatic intervention at admission. *Eur Radiol*. 2002;12:979–993.

Haan JM, Biffi W, Knudson MM, et al. Western Trauma Association Multi-institutional Trials Committee. Splenic embolization revisited: a multicenter review. *J Trauma*. 2004;56:542–547.

Hagiwara A, Murata A, Matsuda T, Matsuda H, Shimazaki S. The usefulness of transcatheter arterial embolization for patients with blunt polytrauma showing transient response to fluid resuscitation. *J Trauma*. 2004;57:271–276; discussion 276–277.

Johnson JW, Gracias VH, Gupta R, et al. Hepatic angiography in patients undergoing damage control laparotomy. *J Trauma*. 2002;52:1102–1106.

Ott MC, Stewart TC, Lawlor DK, Gray DK, Forbes TL. Management of blunt thoracic aortic injuries: endovascular stents versus open repair. *J Trauma*. 2004;56:565–570.

Reed AB, Thompson JK, Crafton CJ, Delvecchio C, Giglia JS. Timing of endovascular repair of blunt traumatic thoracic aortic transections. *J Vasc Surg*. 2006;43:684–688.

Velmahos GC, Toutouzas KG, Vassiliu P, et al. A prospective study on the safety and efficacy of angiographic embolization for pelvic and visceral injuries. *J Trauma*. 2002;53:303–308.

Zealler IA, Chakraverty S. The role of interventional radiology in trauma. *Br Med J*. 2010;340:356–360.

17.1 **APPLICATIONS OF ULTRASOUND IN TRAUMA – INTRODUCTION**

After introduction of focussed assessment by sonography for trauma (FAST) in the 1990s, ultrasound (US) has rapidly become not only an available technique, but a tool coupled with clinical evaluation for the assessment and management of trauma patients.

Ultrasound could be clinically integrated in the A-B-C-D-E primary survey of any trauma patient, helping to answer to specific clinical issues. The secondary survey and the subsequent monitoring are also enhanced by US.

The use of US should never delay the definitive treatment; for this reason, any algorithm including US should start from the physiology of the patient and not from US findings.

On the other side, every US finding must be interpreted together with the mechanism of trauma, the physiology of the patient and the anatomy of the injuries.

In the perspective of a clinically integrated US, questions to be answered are simple and often require binary answers (Yes/No). For the same reasons, US in trauma is always a rapid exam, and the use by non-radiologists (surgeons, emergency physicians, intensivists) who are in charge for the patient is essential.

Appropriately trained surgeons have been demonstrated to have equal or superior accuracy than radiologists in performing clinical US.

17.2 **EXTENDED FOCUSSED ASSESSMENT BY SONOGRAPHY FOR TRAUMA (E-FAST)**

The basic application of US in trauma is E-FAST, which aims to answer the following simple questions:

- Is there free fluid (blood) in abdomen, pleural spaces and pericardium?

- Is there free air (pneumothorax) in pleural cavities?

Four areas of the abdomen are scanned for the detection of free fluid (the FAST protocol):

- Pericardial.
- Perihepatic.
- Perisplenic.
- Pelvic.

The cranial extension of the perihepatic and perisplenic views, obtained by simply sliding the probe upwards, allows a check for haemothorax.

Parasternal sagittal views on the anterior thoracic wall are used for searching the physiologic sliding of the visceral pleura (the so-called 'sliding lung'). The absence of the sliding lung and the recognition of the contact of the lung with the thoracic wall ('lung point') are US signs of pneumothorax. Lung point is not detectable in complete pneumothorax.

Sensitivity and specificity of US in the detection of haemothorax are similar to the portable chest X-rays, but the performance time for US is significantly shorter.

Sensitivity of US for the detection of pneumothorax in supine position is twice that of chest X-rays and approximates that of CT.

The E-FAST is not organ specific. That means organ injuries (liver, spleen, etc.) are not the goal and must not be included in the E-FAST protocol.

The E-FAST is non-invasive and repeatable. Whenever the physical assessment and/or the physiology of the patient require, E-FAST could be used to re-answer clinical questions.

Repeated scans have been shown to increase sensitivity for abdominal views in hemodynamically normal patients. Repetition of E-FAST is even more important where no further diagnostic investigations are available.

The amount of free fluid detected can be estimated according to some available scores in the abdomen, and at a glance in the thorax. In the abdomen, immediate and easy detection of fluid in all three views means more than 800 mL of blood is present in 85 per cent of cases.

Correlation with potential or already established injuries and with the physiological status allows the best clinical decision (observation, definitive treatment, further investigation) to rapidly be made.

- E-FAST should be performed:
  - During the primary survey in physiologically unstable patients.
  - At the end of primary survey in normal and stable patients.
  - During the secondary survey and whenever needed by changes in patient clinical status.
- E-FAST refers to B and C steps of the primary survey.

17.2.1 Indications and Results

17.2.1.1 PENETRATING ABDOMINAL TRAUMA

There is no role for US in hypotensive patients with abdominal penetrating trauma, except for those with thoracoabdominal injuries, when E-FAST could help in prioritizing the surgical approach (thorax versus abdomen first).

A positive FAST after penetrating injury in a hemodynamically normal patient is a strong predictor of significant injury (high positive predictive value). If negative, a different approach (additional diagnostic studies, clinical observation, diagnostic laparoscopy) may be required to rule out occult injury.

17.2.1.2 BLUNT ABDOMINAL TRAUMA

Even if a positive FAST exam is defined by the detection of fluid in one or more views, the meaning of positivity depends on the clinical setting, mechanism of trauma and associated lesions. The FAST significantly shortens time to definitive treatment.

A small amount of fluid in the perisplenic view in a hypotensive patient suggests other sources of shock (retroperitoneal, pelvic, thoracic, long bones bleeding; tension pneumothorax; neurogenic shock). The same small amount of free fluid in a normotensive trauma patient, with a seat belt sign, entails a high index of suspicion for hollow viscus injury.

In other words, a negative or slightly positive FAST gives information for the decision-making process which may be as useful as a grossly positive one, according to the clinical status.

17.2.1.3 PELVIC TRAUMA

Ultrasound plays a relevant role in a hypotensive patient with haemorrhagic pelvic fractures. A grossly positive exam is a marker of intraperitoneal bleeding and associated abdominal injuries and mandates surgical exploration. A negative or slightly positive FAST exam suggests pelvic bleeding is the major cause of shock. These two findings allow for the better therapeutic strategy, according to institutional resources.

17.2.1.4 BLUNT THORACIC TRAUMA

Accuracy of US in detection of haemothorax and pneumothorax is well established.

Detection of occult 'small' pneumothorax by US has similar accuracy to that of CT and can anticipate the need for drainage in mechanically ventilated patients.

17.2.1.5 PENETRATING THORACIC TRAUMA

Detection of pneumothorax and haemothorax by US cannot delay obvious indications for immediate thoracic drainage or surgery.

Ultrasound (subxiphoid or parasternal view) has replaced pericardiocentesis for the diagnosis of pericardial effusion. Penetrating precordial or transthoracic wounds suspicious for cardiac injury demonstrated accuracy in the detection of pericardial fluid of more than 97 per cent.

If it is decided that a pericardiocentesis is required (bridge to surgery or monitoring), US can help in performing a safer and easier procedure.

17.3 OTHER APPLICATIONS OF ULTRASOUND IN TRAUMA

There is an ongoing trend and evidence toward a comprehensive, clinically integrated US management of trauma, according to the clinical situation in the single patient.

In an A-B-C-D-E sequence, US could be used for assessing proper orotracheal intubation (tracheal and lung views), to speed recognition of landmarks for cricothyroidotomy or tracheostomy, for assessing presence and evolution of pulmonary contusions.

Inferior vena cava diameter and collapsibility helps in evaluation of volume status and shock management, together with the subxiphoid assessment of cardiac chambers, repletion and contractility.

Bone fractures' edges can be easily detected by US (sternum, ribs, long bones).

A more advanced application of US is contrast-enhanced US (CEUS). It could be used both for the detection of solid organ injuries in selected groups of patients (for instance, hemodynamically normal paediatric patients sustaining blunt abdominal trauma) and for the follow-up of non-operative management of parenchymatous organs (liver, spleen, kidney).

17.4 TRAINING AND PITFALLS

17.4.1 Training

Ultrasound, like any technical skill, is operator dependent. A formal training is needed for getting competence in acquisition and interpretation of US findings. Hands-on courses and proctored practice are needed.

Due to its clinical value and relatively easy learning, e-FAST training still represents the suggested first step for beginners.

Any doctor, independently of his or her own level of US skill and experience, should always match the result of his or her exam with the clinical scenario, making coherent US findings with that single patient.

17.4.2 Pitfalls

Subcutaneous emphysema makes undetectable deep structures and is a contraindication to the use of US.

Organ injuries are in general out of the scope of clinical US in trauma patients (except CEUS-FAST). Diagnosis of bowel injury, diaphragmatic rupture, retroperitoneal lesions and haematomas and solid organ injury could be considered on the basis of direct/indirect B-mode US findings, but need to be assessed with other methods when suspected.

Free abdominal fluid is not always blood. When in doubt, aspiration under US guidance can enhance the decision-making process (i.e., enteric/bile aspiration in suspected hollow viscus injury, urine in stable patient with pelvic fracture).

17.5 SUMMARY

The use of US in trauma has extended from FAST to a comprehensive US-enhanced management.

The e-FAST remains the basic diagnostic application:

- FAST is a good initial screening tool for blunt abdominal injury and shortens time to definitive treatment in hypotensive patients.
- Ultrasound is the best method for detecting haemothorax and pneumothorax in trauma patients.
- Many procedural manoeuvres could be realized under US guidance, increasing decisional process and safety.
- The clinically integrated use of US in trauma requires specific training.

RECOMMENDED READING

Blaivas M, Lyon M, Duggal S. A prospective comparison of supine chest radiography and bedside ultrasound for the diagnosis of traumatic pneumothorax. *Acad Emerg Med*. 2005;12:844–849.

Branney SW, Wolfe RE, Moore EE, et al. Quantitative sensitivity of ultrasound in detecting free intraperitoneal fluid. *J Trauma*. 1995;39:375–380.

Buzzas GR KS, Smith SR, Harrison PB, Helmer SD, Reed JA. A comparison of sonographic examinations for trauma performed by surgeons and radiologists. *J Trauma*. 1998;44:604–608.

Dulchavsky SA, Kirkpatrick AW, Billica RD, et al. Prospective evaluation of thoracic ultrasound in the detection of pneumothorax. *J Trauma*. 2001;50:201–205.

Ferrada P, Murthi S, Anand RJ, Bochicchio GV, Scalea T. Transthoracic focused rapid echocardiographic examination: real-time evaluation of fluid status in critically ill trauma patients. *J Trauma*. 2011;70:56–62.

Melniker L, Liebner E, McKenney MG, Lopez P, Briggs WM, Mancuso CA. Randomized clinical trial of point-of-care, limited ultrasonography for trauma in the emergency department: Sonography Outcomes Assessment Program (SOAP)-1 trial. *Ann Emerg Med*. 2006;48(3):227–235.

Rozycki GS, Feliciano DV, Ochsner MG, et al. The role of ultrasound in patients with possible penetrating cardiac wounds: a prospective multicentre study. *J Trauma*. 1999;46(4):543–552.

Stawicki, SP, Adkins EJ, Eiferman DS, et al. Prospective evaluation of intravascular volume status in critically ill patients: does inferior vena cava collapsibility correlate with central venous pressure? *J Trauma Acute Care Surg*. 2014;76(4):956–963.

Udobi KF, Rodriguez A, Chiu WC, Scalea TM. Role of ultrasonography in penetrating abdominal trauma: a prospective clinical study. *J Trauma*. 2001;50:475–479.

Valentino M, Serra C, Pavlica P, Barozzi L. Contrast-enhanced ultrasound for blunt abdominal trauma. *Sem Ultrasound*. 2007;28:130–140.

Williams SR, Perera P, Gharahbaghian L. The FAST and E-FAST in 2013: trauma ultrasonography. *Crit Care Clin*. 2014;30:119–150.

Zago M, ed. *Essential US for Trauma: E-FAST, Ultrasound for Acute Care Surgeons*. New York, NY: Springer-Verlag; 2014.

Part 5

Aspects of specialized care

Austere or Military Environments **18**

18.1 INTRODUCTION

Austere: severely simple, morally strict, harsh.

Harsh: unpleasantly rough or sharp, severe, cruel.

Multiple casualties: More than one patient, but can be dealt with within existing resources.

Mass casualties: Many patients with demands beyond the resources available.

Military surgery operates within the framework of a staged systematic approach to care. The role of the surgeon is not to merely operate on the individual patient, but to make every attempt at preserving the force and returning the patient back to his or her unit to fight. The team must understand their environment and contingencies. In the response to a natural disaster or a military environment, this also implies that they should not themselves become casualties.

Modern surgery and anaesthesia require infrastructure and resources, not just sutures and drugs. However, a good night's sleep and a mosquito net may be as important as the availability of an intensive care bed in providing a high standard of care. Flexibility and capability beyond one's conventional specialty are also required: surgeons do not often service generators, and anaesthetists do not often sterilize water, but they may have to.

Infrastructure requirements include shelter, power for lighting and temperature control, and water for hygiene and cooking purposes. Waste needs to be disposed of properly, medical waste disposal (particularly sharps) always being problematic. Resources include medical gases, food, drugs, fluids and other consumables such as gloves and gowns. Fluids include blood and blood products, and these in particular need a reliable and documented cold chain.

In the civilian setting, these materials and resources are provided by a series of complex supply chains that are carefully controlled and tracked, guaranteeing delivery within 24 hours anywhere in the world. To provide a similar standard of care in a deployed environment requires similar supply chains, which, in times of conflict, even the most advanced countries cannot always achieve. Following a natural disaster, or in a conflict or post-conflict environment, supply chains and systems will be disrupted and vulnerable; in a conflict, they may be deliberately targeted. No delivery can ever be guaranteed, and the team may have only what they carried off the plane.

Psychologically, some doctors do not work well out of their normal hospital or workplace, and some cannot adapt easily. In addition, the availability of a volunteer does not imply the ability or even the affability required to work in a small team. Also, individual health states need to be high: a person with diabetes, for example, is unlikely to do well without cold-chain-controlled insulin. All members of a surgical team need to understand this and have a realistic expectation of what they can – or cannot – provide in the situation in which they find themselves.

The perspective of working in an austere or military environment is quite different from the training paradigm, an academic practice with multi-tiered care or an elective private practice. Austere surgery requires a thoughtful approach to realistic surgical care within the context of the environment with which one works. In the military environment, the surgical team must alter their perspective from definitive management toward a staged approach of surgical care. Closed-loop communication to outline objectives and goals of care, especially 'up range' to the next echelon of care, is critically important.

18.1.1 Health Protection of the Deployed Surgical Team

18.1.1.1 VECTOR-BORNE DISEASE

In 2003, in Liberia, nearly 20 per cent of 225 deployed US Marines developed malaria; it was subsequently found that only 10 per cent of the population at risk had been compliant with chemoprophylaxis and none had slept under mosquito nets. Attention must be paid to the existing threats, and simple measures are effective: anti-malarial prophylaxis, long-sleeves at dawn and dusk, repellent, sleeping under nets and mosquito control measures.

18.1.1.2 ENTERIC ILLNESS

The incidence of diarrhoea among deployed military personnel from industrialized countries to lesser developed countries is typically 30 per cent per month overall, with clinical incidence between 5 and 7 per 100 person-months. The risk appears to be higher early during deployment and is associated with poor hygiene conditions and contaminated food sources. Meticulous attention to hand-washing and food source management mitigates this risk.

18.1.1.3 ROAD TRAUMA

Globally, the majority of road trauma deaths now occur in the developing world, and 50 per cent of these deaths occur among vulnerable road users, such as pedestrians, cyclists or motorcyclists. There is a risk of speeding, weak adherence to seat belt discipline and cavalier driving not only to the vehicle occupants, but also to host nation road users. A deployed westerner causing injury or death to a local child would not only be a personal tragedy for the child, the family and the driver but could also ruin a mission.

18.1.1.4 PHYSICAL, SEXUAL AND MENTAL HEALTH

Surgeons wishing to deploy need to have high health status; diabetics, for example, are unlikely to do well without their cold-chain-controlled insulin. An unfit surgeon could become a liability rather than an asset to the mission. Deployments away from home, time away from duty, availability of alcohol, interaction of deployed workers with local women prepared to undertake transactional sex and the non-use of condoms increase the risks of sexually transmitted infections.

Psychologically, some surgeons cannot adapt easily and do not work well outside of their normal hospital or workplace. Availability of a volunteer does not imply ability or the personality required to work in a small team.

18.1.2 Recent Advances in Combat Military Care

18.1.2.1 RECENT ADVANCES IN MILITARY TRAUMA CARE

Both US and UK Defence Medical Services have committed to delivering trauma care in the Joint Area of Operations aligned to the principles of the established civilian trauma systems approach, with a coherent chain of care from point of wounding through trauma hospitals to definitive specialist care and rehabilitation. This approach has borne fruit in recent conflicts in Iraq and Afghanistan, with reductions in mortality after combat injury to record levels compared to historic conflicts. Small improvements in care at every point have translated into dramatic improvements in overall performance. In one study of critically injured servicemen between 2003/4 and an injury-matched cohort in 2007/8, mortality was reduced from 47 per cent to 20 per cent. Arguably, it is this systematic approach to the care of the combat casualty that has made the difference; however, individual components are worthy of special mention:

- Personal and collective ballistic protection.
- Tourniquets.
- Haemostatic dressings.
- Medical evacuation.
- Tranexamic acid.
- Transfusion support.
- Point-of-care assessment of coagulation.
- Damage control surgery.
- Casualty evacuation (TACEVAC and STRATEVAC).
- Data capture and governance processes.

18.2 INJURY PATTERNS

In the nineteenth century, warfare was infantry based. In the twentieth century, it became mechanized and airborne, and in the twenty-first century, combat is asymmetric, with possibly only one side in uniform. To quote General Sir Rupert Smith, author of *The Utility of Force*[1], the modern battlefield is 'amongst the people'. Injuries sustained in contemporary combat operations are inflicted on combatant and non-combatant alike: in a recent review of activity at a coalition hospital in Afghanistan, 60 per cent of casualties were local nationals, including women and children.

Similarly, in an urban setting of Somalia[2], casualty distribution in military personnel was similar to that of the Vietnam War[3]: 11 per cent died on the battlefield, 3 per cent died after reaching a medical facility, 47 per cent were evacuated and 39 per cent returned to duty. Over the past decade of conflict in Iraq and Afghanistan, US and coalition military casualties exceeded 5300 hostile deaths[4], 1472 non-hostile deaths (due to disease, non-battle injury, and other causes) and over 52 000 troops wounded in action. Casualty rates in Iraq and Afghanistan have been considerably lower than during the Vietnam conflict, and a greater proportion of troops wounded have survived their wounds (<2 per cent mortality). The leading causes of injury among casualties in Afghanistan and the Iraq war were explosive devices and gunshot wounds. Death is instantaneous in over 35 per cent of those killed in action, and the most common cause of death is exsanguinating haemorrhage (>90 per cent).

Wounding patterns are modified by the presence or absence of modern ballistic protection (armour). In a review of coalition combat deaths up to the end of 2009, there had been >6000 allied military deaths in Iraq and Afghanistan. The leading cause of death was blast mechanisms followed by gunshot wounds. Chest or abdominal injury (40 per cent) and traumatic brain injury (35 per cent) were the main causes of death for soldiers killed in action.

The defining injury pattern in recent counter-insurgency operations is that caused by improvised explosive devices (IEDs): the combination of bilateral lower limb amputation with pelvic fracture and perineal injury[1,2] has been described as the 'signature injury' of the conflict in Afghanistan.

Chest or abdominal injuries (40 per cent) and brain injuries (35 per cent) were the main causes of death for soldiers killed in action. The case fatality rate in Iraq was approximately half as high as in the Vietnam War. In contrast, the amputation rate was twice as high. Approximately 8–15 per cent of the deaths appeared to be preventable.

In the UK Role 3 hospital in Afghanistan the overall survival rate was 93.2 per cent (Table 18.1). The survival rate was influenced by the nationality of the patient (Table 18.1) with the reduced rate among the Afghan population attributed to the lower use of personal protective equipment (PPE) and increased co-morbidities.

Wounding patterns are modified by the presence or absence of modern ballistic protection (armour) and the pre-hospital timeline. Many fatal penetrating injuries

Table 18.1 Activity at a Coalition Hospital in Afghanistan

	Survivors	Deaths	Recovery Rate (%)
UK military	1906	58	97
Coalition military and entitled civilians	1206	42	97
Afghan	3250	367	90
Totals	6362	467	93.2

are likely to be caused by missiles entering through areas not protected by body armour, such as the face and junctional areas in the neck, face, groin and buttocks. Injuries can be sustained by gunshot or the effect of conventional explosive munitions (air-delivered bombs, artillery shells, rocket-propelled grenades or hand grenades). The proportion of penetrating injuries due to bullets or fragments will depend on the nature of the battle, with blunt injury and burns likely to comprise a significant component of the injuries in conventional manoeuvre warfare. However, the defining injury pattern in recent counter-insurgency operations is that caused by IEDs, which cause a combination of blast and missile wounds.

One of the characteristics of military wounding is early lethality, with a high proportion of deaths occurring soon after injury. Of those who survive to reach hospital, the majority will have injury to the extremities. Protocols for casualty assessment, tourniquet application, the use of haemostatic wound dressings, and the direct transfer of casualties from ambulance to operating theatre are designed to recognize that exsanguination remains the main cause of preventable battlefield death. In a recent review of deaths of servicemen after combat injury, although 85 per cent of deaths were considered non-preventable, half of those that were considered to be potentially survivable were the result of intracavity haemorrhage[5].

Military medical practitioners have been described as 'working at the interface of two dynamic technologies, warfare and trauma management'. In addition to the problems of dispersed battlefields, highly mobile front lines, extended lines of logistics and a delay in evacuation, the modern military surgeon is likely to be called upon to treat civilians, including females (especially obstetric care) and children, as well as service personnel, with a requirement to offer immediate care well away from their speciality; problems in ophthalmology, maxillofacial surgery, ear, nose and throat medicine, paediatrics, gynaecology, tropical medicine or even public health will fall under the remit of the military surgeon. These challenges are magnified by the nature of modern surgical training, with its accent on early training in sub-specialties, combined with the decline in the popularity of trauma surgery and surgical intensive care. Military surgeons therefore have to be trained in a variety of specialties and undergo multiple course training (including team training) – before they deploy.

When it comes to providing care outside of one's specialty, a rational approach in the context of one's environment should prevail. To quote Albert Einstein, 'everything should be as simple as possible...but not simpler'.

Modern all-arms battle presents a vast array of potential wounding agents, from high-velocity military rifles, shrapnel from mortars or mines, blast from any explosive, and chemical, biological and nuclear exposure (depleted uranium in shells) to motor vehicle crashes. The latter is often the most common cause of injury. It is imperative that military medical personnel become familiar with the medical consequences of toxin exposure, the illnesses caused by these agents and the measures required to protect military healthcare providers.

18.3 EMERGENCY MEDICAL SERVICES SYSTEMS

The patient presenting to the surgical team in a civilian hospital has already been part of a 'supply chain'. Consider the victim of a road traffic collision. Summoning help requires the existence of an intact telephone or radio system, appropriately trained individuals arriving in suitably equipped vehicles and an unimpeded journey, delivering an appropriately 'packaged' patient, to the hospital. In the deployed environment, this pre-hospital chain is particularly vulnerable. Patients may experience delays of hours or days getting to care, which will in turn influence how they present to the surgical team. During such dynamic care, detailed pre-hospital protocols are critically important to optimize outcome.

Deployed military medical systems usually consist of a crescendo series of levels (echelons or roles) of care in military medical treatment units, traditionally called roles 1–4:

Role 1: Close to the point of injury, a casualty either applies self-aid or receives 'buddy aid' (such as field dressing or tourniquet application). The next stage is care by a military paramedical provider, then by a doctor or nurse at an aid post (role 1 facility).

Role 2: This echelon of medical treatment facility is designed for the evacuation from role/echelon 1 facilities, triage and resuscitation, treatment and holding of patients until they can be returned to duty or evacuated. Surgery may be possible at this level (role 2[+]).

Role 3: Role 3 facilities include specialist diagnostic resources (such as CT scanning), specialist surgical and medical capabilities, preventive medicine, food inspection, dentistry and operational stress management teams. The archetypal recent role 3 hospital was the Joint Force Hospital in Camp Bastion, Afghanistan.

Role 4: Role 4 medical support provides definitive care of patients for whom the treatment required is longer than the theatre evacuation policy or for whom the capabilities usually found at role 3 are inadequate. This would normally include specialist surgical and medical procedures, reconstruction, rehabilitation and convalescence. This level of care is usually highly specialized, time consuming and normally provided in the country of origin. Under unusual circumstances, this level of care may be established in a theatre of operations.

The situation becomes complicated when casualties move between systems (e.g. military to host nation, or non-governmental organization to military), having received surgery in the first system. Because standards of care can vary enormously between systems, these casualties need a thorough examination and re-evaluation. Soldiers have been trained and issued their equipment *before* the disaster or injury occurs, in order to perform immediate aid on themselves or each other; civilians, however, have not. It is critically important that full documentation accompanies the patient in order to prevent overtreatment.

18.3.1 Incident Management and Multiple Casualties

At incidents in which bombs are involved or secondary devices are suspected, the '4 Cs' must be adopted, as presented in Table 18.2.

Table 18.2 Four Cs of Incident Management

- Confirm
- Clear
- Cordon
- Control

Confirm: Incident commanders must be clear about what is happening and about the risk and position of further hazards. Factors that must be considered are clearance priorities, cordon locations, safe areas, access and egress routes and rendezvous points.

Clear: The scene should be cleared to a safe distance. This distance will vary depending on the terrain. The method and urgency of clearance will depend on the incident.

Cordon: Cordons establish the area in which the rescue effort is taking place and define safe zones and tiers of command. An outer cordon should be established as a physical barrier preventing accidental or unauthorized access to the site. An inner cordon may be set up around wreckage, especially if hazards still exist.

Control: Once cordons are set up, the control of the cordons and scene is maintained by clear rendezvous and access points.

Once the '4 Cs' have been established, medical management and support can begin (Table 18.3).

Table 18.3 Medical Management and Support

* Command and Control
* Safety
* Communication
* Assessment
* Triage
* Treatment
* Transport

Command and control: This is the paramount principle. If good command and control are not established, the initial chaos will continue, and the injured will suffer regardless of how well some individual casualties are treated. Command usually overrides control. Command implies the overall responsibility for the mission, whereas control implies the authority to modify procedures or actions by services.

Safety: Healthcare workers must remember that their own safety is paramount and that they must not become casualties themselves. This may include infectious agents that may occur coincidently during a natural disaster.

Communication: Communication is the transmission between a sender and a receiver, preferably such

that the receiver is in no doubt about the intent and need of the sender. Every major incident inquiry has identified failings in communications. Without good communication, command and control is impossible. When a formal medical record system may not exist, simply writing instructions over wound bandages may suffice.

Assessment: This is a constant process. Commanders should always consider the current situation, what resources are required and where these can be obtained.

Triage: In any situation when there is more than one casualty, a system of triage must be used (see Section 18.4). There are many different systems in use (Table 18.4).

Treatment: At the scene of any ballistic incident, treatment teams may be faced with casualties with multiple serious injuries. Treatment must follow the <C>A-B-C paradigm (see below).

Transport: Not every patient needs to travel in an ambulance. Buses or other multipassenger vehicles should be used to move the walking wounded. The judicious use of other resources, including armoured vehicles and aircraft, is essential.

Table 18.4 Triage Categories

Priority	Label Colour	Description
T1	Red	Immediate
T2	Yellow	Urgent
T3	Green	Delayed
Dead	White or black	Dead
T4	Blue (not standard)	Expectant

18.4 TRIAGE

Effective triage is crucial in an efficient military healthcare system. It was first described by Napoleon's surgeon, Dominique Jean Larrey, who introduced a system of sorting casualties as they presented to field dressing stations. His priority, and the aim of the system, was to identify those soldiers who had minor wounds, and therefore could with minor treatment return to the battle. Although we might now call this reverse triage, he had introduced a formal system of prioritizing casualties. Triage remains a fundamental principle in modern military medicine. It is dynamic and should be applied at all levels of medical care, from the point of wounding to definitive surgical care.

The system for 'surgical triage' may be slightly different from the triage system used in resuscitation, but the same principles apply. Those requiring life-saving surgical intervention take priority over patients requiring limb-saving surgery in the forward locations, and taking into account all the other factors, the key question will be 'Do they need to go on the table at all?' Overtriage is a feature of all mass casualty situations; however, a rate of overtriage is acceptable to avoid missing patients who really did require an intervention. In a series of 1350 laparotomies from the Vietnam War, based on the clinical assessment of wounded soldiers, the rate of negative laparotomy was 19.2 per cent. In a modern military setting, an accurate screening tool (perhaps using computed tomography [CT] or focussed abdominal sonography for trauma [FAST]) can be very useful.

Effective triage is crucial in an efficient military healthcare system. It is dynamic, and must be applied at all levels of medical care, from the point of wounding to definitive surgical care. Triage must be repeated at every point of care, or at any point of deterioration. Patients compensate, change condition and deteriorate without prior warning. In civilian practice, 'expectant' patients are rarely categorized because resources are typically unlimited. In the military environment, care is often 'rationed'. The needs of the dying, who will require 50 per cent of the resources of a surgical team to save them, need to be balanced against the needs of the next 10 patients who arrive.

The following are patterns of injury for non-survivors in a military or austere environment:

- Long bone amputations.
- Open skull fracture.
- Full thickness burns >30 per cent.
- Head injury with GCS <8.
- Arrival in cardiac arrest.

Triage depends on resources (see Table 18.5).

Table 18.5 Factors Affecting Triage

- Patient load and severity
- Medical capability and supply
- Local situation and safety
- Available evacuation assets and flight times
- Theatre medical assets

Transfer time will also dictate who requires life-saving interventions at that point and who can wait until they reach the next echelon of medical care. Equipment will always be in limited supply in these forward locations and must be used appropriately as re-supply will take time. The flow of casualties in a fast-moving battle will also influence how many and what type of casualties should be operated on. The prospect of incoming serious casualties will change triage decisions for the wounded already at the medical facility. If there is only one surgical table available forward, 'Who goes on first?' and 'Do they need to go on at all?' may be simple questions to ask, but the answers are anything but straightforward.

The need for effective triage poses difficult questions. A patient with extensive multiple injuries, who would get maximum effort and resources in a civilian trauma centre, may need to be labelled 'expectant' if several other patients face a better chance of survival given early access to the limited equipment and expertise available. Thus, an awareness of the overall tactical picture on the part of the senior surgeon is paramount. It may be wise to remember that triage, including surgical triage, means doing the 'best for the most', and expectant treatment for some may eventually benefit the 'most'.

18.4.1 Forward Surgical Teams and Triage

Many military healthcare teams around the globe are now incorporating far-forward resuscitative surgery capabilities into doctrine and mission planning. Although these forward surgical teams provide only a limited trauma surgical capability, they aim to provide life- and limb-saving surgery to the select group of potentially salvageable patients who would otherwise die or suffer permanent disability due to delays in evacuation from the fast-moving modern battlefield. However, such a surgical team will necessarily have a very limited scope of activity and requires the commitment of other military assets in order to protect the medical workforce.

These teams should be capable of providing life-saving thoracoabdominal haemorrhage control, control of contamination within body cavities, temporary limb revascularization, stabilization of fractures and evacuation of major intracranial haematomas. Each nation has a slightly different balance and skill mix within this forward surgical capability, but most will normally provide the three main tenets of forward care: a resuscitation capability, one or more surgical tables and a critical care capability.

Most nations 'mission-tailor' their teams to the specific operational environment, and sizes range from as few as six members to larger teams of more than 30. As part of the casualty estimate, military planners need to decide on the number of surgical tables required and the speed at which they can safely transfer patients to the next echelon of care ('emptying the back door'). The size and sophistication of the attached critical care element will be determined by the capability of tactical aeromedical evacuation. If there is no such facility, either in- or out-country, the first few patients may fill a facility and render it completely ineffective.

Forward surgical teams must be light, mobile and rapidly deployable to allow them to respond in an uncertain battlefield. Restrictions and constraints within these teams are many and include limitations of space and equipment, poor lighting and the need to achieve some degree of climate control for the human resources and, particularly, for blood and other products. Some re-sterilization of surgical tools may be possible, but disposable equipment, water and especially oxygen will all be limited.

Human factors of physical and emotional fatigue will also affect how long the surgical team can endure the challenges of operating in austere and dangerous environments without reinforcement or resupply. The teams will often have to function independently but may also deploy as augmentation of an existing medical facility during a casualty surge. Even in wartime, the best surgical teams could not operate for more than 18 hours at a time over a sustained period without breaking after 3 days.

There is a difference between a well-equipped relatively static 'field' (or combat support) hospital and a 'forward surgical team'. The *raison d'être* of the team is delivery of the life- and limb-saving surgery as far forward as possible to a select group of potentially salvageable patients who would otherwise suffer due to delays in evacuation from the battlefield. Without patient selection (by security perimeter or guard-force) a small team will not function.

Triage is challenging, it requires difficult decisions to be made, but it remains crucial to the effective use and efficiency of the forward surgical teams.

18.5 MASS CASUALTIES

One of the fundamental planning parameters for medical support is an estimate of the numbers and types of casualty expected. An estimate of the numbers and types of casualty, the resources required to deal with them per phase of battle and their evacuation is the cornerstone of operational medical planning. Casualty estimates are major resource-drivers and will determine what capabilities are required and at what level. The medical support for a specific operation will therefore be planned in light of the perceived threat.

Mass casualties, however, may occur for many reasons, and the cause of the major incident may not have been identified as one of the known 'threats'. The term 'mass casualty' is of course, relative, and for a small team, this number may be as low as three casualties. Multiple motor vehicle crashes, downed helicopters, floods and even earthquakes have recently produced mass casualty situations or major incidents for military forces around the world. All these incidents have produced an unexpected surge in casualties, far greater than the casualty estimate that each operation had declared. The key in all these events was that the medical facilities were overwhelmed, and available resources could not meet the required demand.

When major incidents produce mass casualties in civilian situations, for example from rail crashes or as a result of urban terrorism events, there are often a number of receiving hospitals to choose from to spread the load of casualties. This luxury is rarely available in the military environment. In some situations, other nations' medical facilities may be available, but often the only available 'receiving hospital' will be the forward surgical team. Triage remains the key to effective medical management of a mass casualty event, especially when large numbers of wounded arrive at the location in a short space of time. Equipment, manpower and transport will be in short supply, so sound training and adherence to the principles of triage should ensure effective use of the limited resources available.

In civilian practice, advanced triage tools have been developed to predict workload capacity in mass casualties. Critically injured casualties exceeding more than one per hour may rapidly exceed the capability of competent trauma teams. A good estimate to reliably predict patient volume after a mass casualty event is shown in Figure 18.1. Typically, 50 per cent of total patient volume will occur within one hour of an incident. More than 75 per cent of casualties will have arrived by the second hour. Therefore, total patient volume and requisite staffing may be somewhat predictable in an isolated mass casualty event.

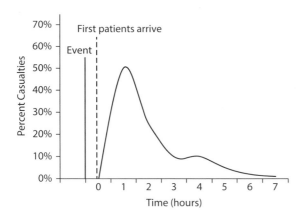

Figure 18.1 Per cent casualties arriving to casualty reception.

After triage and treatment, transport remains the third key element of medical support in a mass casualty event. Unlike in a civilian environment, where there will be many options for both ground and air transport, transport is likely to be very limited in the military mass casualty situation. Regular and effective triage will determine who is transported first, and by what means, to ensure that the right patient arrives at the right time at the next level of medical care.

18.6 **EVACUATION**

It is recognized that speed of evacuation[4,5] from point of wounding to first surgical intervention is a critical determinant of outcome. The Korean War saw the introduction of helicopter evacuation of the wounded from the front line to mobile army surgical hospitals (MASH), with onward transport by fixed-wing aircraft to base hospitals. During the Vietnam conflict, the average pre-hospital time for combat casualties treated at a US Navy hospital was 80 minutes. Limited provision of aircraft in a combat setting has meant that medical evacuation has used assets earmarked for other purposes; for example, during Operations Desert Shield/Desert Storm in 1991, many patients were successfully airlifted using converted cargo aircraft. This concept of using cargo aircraft was originally validated in World War II and is still in vogue today. Dedicated aeromedical capability in the military now exists with two distinct models: the UK Medical Emergency Response Team (MERT) and the US Air Force helicopter rescue fleet known as PEDROS (named after the call sign of the first US Air

Force HH-43 rescue helicopters in the Vietnam conflict). A landmark study documented prohibitively long pre-hospital times. Since the introduction of a dedicated air asset, pre-hospital times from wounding to point of care have fallen to approximately 45 minutes.

In Afghanistan a successful international system of evacuation assets provides cover to the whole theatre of operations. The different evacuations provide different levels of care ranging from a flight medic to complex ICU capability. A recent study of more than 900 patients evacuated to a role 4 facility demonstrated a <0.02 per cent mortality with significantly injured soldiers (mean injury severity score of 23)[6].

18.6.1 **Forward Surgical Teams**

Many military healthcare teams around the globe are now incorporating far-forward resuscitative surgery capabilities into doctrine and mission planning. Although these forward surgical teams can provide trauma surgical capability for only a limited number of patients, they aim to provide life- and limb-saving surgery to the select group of potentially salvageable patients who would otherwise die or suffer permanent disability due to delays in evacuation. However, such a surgical team will necessarily have a very limited scope of activity and require commitment of other military assets in order to protect the medical workforce.

These teams are designed to be capable of providing life-saving thoraco-abdominal haemorrhage control, control of contamination within body cavities, temporary limb or carotid revascularization, stabilization of fractures and evacuation of major intracranial haematomas. Each nation has a slightly different balance and skill-mix within their forward surgical capability, but most will normally provide the three main tenets of forward care: a resuscitation capability, one or more surgical tables and a critical care capability. Most nations 'mission-tailor' their teams to the specific operational environment, and sizes range from as little as 6 members to larger teams of 30 plus. As part of the casualty estimate, military planners need to decide on the number of surgical tables required and the speed at which they can safely transfer patients to the next echelon of care ('emptying the back door'). The size and sophistication of the attached critical care element will be determined by the capability of tactical aeromedical evacuation (TACEVAC). If there is no such facility, either in- or out-country, then the first few patients will fill a facility and render it completely ineffective.

Strategic evacuation (STRATEVAC) is the evacuation of casualties from the Joint Operational Area to the home nation, another North Atlantic Treaty Organization (NATO) country or other safe area. The Royal Air Force utilizes critical care air support teams (CCASTs) and the United States uses critical care air transport teams (CCATTs). These teams are led by senior doctors and can continue virtually all intensive care interventions throughout the transfer period (such as mechanical ventilation, provision of vasoactive drugs and even extra-corporeal membrane oxygenation), thus providing an intensive care air bridge between deployed and home nation facilities.

Forward surgical teams must be light, mobile and rapidly deployable to allow them to respond in an uncertain battle space. Restrictions and constraints within these teams include limitations of space and equipment, poor lighting and the need to achieve some degree of climate control for the human resources and, particularly, for blood products. Some re-sterilization of surgical tools may be possible, but consumable equipment, including water and oxygen will be limited. Human factors of physical and emotional fatigue will also affect how long the surgical team can remain effective in austere and dangerous environments without reinforcement or re-supply.

There is a difference between a well-equipped relatively static 'field' (or combat support) hospital and a 'forward surgical team'. The *raison d'être* of the team is delivery of the life and limb-saving surgery as far forward as possible to a select group of potentially salvageable patients who would otherwise suffer due to delays in evacuation from the battlefield. Without patient selection (by security perimeter or guard-force) a small team will not function.

18.7 RESUSCITATION

18.7.1 Overview

The treatment and resuscitation available will alter with each echelon of care; resources and complexity of care generally increase as the casualty moves away from the battlefield. Exsanguinating haemorrhage remains the most common cause of death among those killed in action during military conflicts. Although the principles remain the same, resuscitation of wounded combatants remains a formidable challenge on the battlefield and there are some crucial differences to consider in this environment. Unlike in the urban setting, the military must consider weight and therefore quantity of supplies that can be transported into austere locations. Large volumes of fluids at any stage in the resuscitation process are therefore not a feasible option. More importantly, recent conflicts have demonstrated improved mortality with a balanced haemostatic resuscitation. Replacing crystalloid with early utilization of blood products, to include fresh whole blood, has even made its way to the far forward treatment station[7]. For patients with uncontrolled haemorrhagic shock in whom surgical intervention is not immediately available, the goal of maintaining a systolic arterial pressure of 70 to 80 mm Hg (palpable radial pulse) is now generally accepted (Table 18.6).

18.7.2 **Damage Control Resuscitation**

Approximately 90 per cent of casualties are in a stable condition on arrival at hospital; however, 7–10 per cent of combat casualties will require massive transfusion and it is in these maximally injured that major improvements in care have been achieved recently.

Arguably the most important change in military trauma care in recent years has been the introduction of the concept of damage control resuscitation[9,10]. Damage control resuscitation can begin in the pre-hospital MERT phase; however, it more typically begins after rapid initial assessment in the emergency department (ED) and progresses through the operating room (OR) into the intensive care unit (ICU). In the severely injured casualty, damage control resuscitation consists of two parts: first, pre-surgical fluid therapy is limited to keep blood pressure at approximately 90 mm Hg, preventing renewed bleeding from recently clotted vessels (in practice this means limiting crystalloid fluid infusion and using the casualty's conscious level and/or presence of a radial pulse as a guide). Second, intravascular volume restoration is accomplished by using thawed plasma as a primary resuscitation fluid in at least a 1:1 or 1:2 ratio with packed red cells and empiric transfusion with platelets.

Difficulty in obtaining vascular access can be experienced in austere conditions, when hypotension, low ambient temperature and tactical considerations, such as the presence of mass casualties or operating light restriction, can conspire to frustrate attempts at vascular access; intraosseous access is an attractive option in these scenarios[8].

Table 18.6 Clinical Considerations in Penetrating Injury

Catastrophic Haemorrhage

- Penetrating wounds to the groins, axilla and neck. Consider haemostatic agents.
- Penetrating wounds to major limb vessels/traumatic amputations. Consider early use of tourniquet.

Airway and C spine

Simple first: Jaw thrust, oral airway.

Airway at risk from:

- Burn injury
- Disruption from fragments
- Compression from penetrating vascular injury in the neck

Consider early anaesthesia and intubation (aided by fibre-optic scopes and use of small-diameter endotracheal tubes) or early surgical airway

Cervical Collars: limited role in pure penetrating injury and may conceal developing haematoma in the neck; are needed in mixed injury as occurs in bombings.

Use of cervical collars is a balance of risk: protection of C spine versus concealing injury.

Breathing

- Needle decompression for tension pneumothorax.
- Manage sucking chest wounds with Asherman seals and then consider chest drainage.

Circulation

- Catastrophic bleeding should have been controlled early. Smaller external bleeds can be managed with simple first aid measures of compression and elevation. Ongoing internal bleeding from penetrating cavity injury needs to be suspected or recognized from history and clinical findings.
- Difficulty in obtaining vascular access can be experienced in austere conditions, when hypotension, low ambient temperature and tactical considerations, such as the presence of mass casualties or operating light restriction, can conspire to frustrate attempts at vascular access; intraosseous access is an attractive option in these scenarios.

Deficit

The majority of casualties who sustain a high-energy penetrating brain injury do not survive to medical care. Casualties who survive to care from penetrating injury are generally a preselected group and in the absence of obvious devastating injury should be resuscitated as above to minimize secondary injury. There is an obvious conflict between hypotensive resuscitation for cavity bleeding and the need to maintain cerebral perfusion, and this becomes a judgement call at the time.

Environment

Hypothermia needs to be treated managed with warm air blankets and environmental control. The temperature of any fluid given to trauma patients, particularly in a military or austere environment, is crucial. Any fluid used in resuscitation must be warmed to avoid further cooling of a haemorrhagic casualty. The actual process of warming the fluids remains a considerable challenge and in most cases requires improvization on behalf of the provider.

Blood is the gold standard fluid of choice in such casualties, particularly those in profound shock, and is now carried by many military resuscitation teams forward of the first surgical teams; however, in many military healthcare systems, blood will not be available and other fluids need to be carried. Options available to resuscitation teams include isotonic crystalloids, colloids, hypertonic saline and hypertonic saline plus colloid. The choice of fluid remains unresolved and may in fact be less important than the quantity and rate of fluid infused in patients with uncontrolled haemorrhage.

Difficulty in obtaining vascular access can be experienced in austere conditions, when hypotension, low ambient temperature and tactical considerations, such as the presence of mass casualties or operating light restriction, can conspire to frustrate attempts at vascular access; intraosseous access is an attractive option in these scenarios[8].

The temperature of any fluid given to trauma patients, particularly in a military or austere environment, is crucial. Any fluid used in resuscitation must be warmed to avoid further cooling of a haemorrhagic casualty. The actual process of warming the fluids remains a considerable challenge and in most cases requires improvisation on behalf of the provider. Locally available re-warming/protective devices, such as plastic bags, use of hot car engines, etc., may suffice.

The concept of damage control resuscitation[9,10] implies that rather than treat haemorrhage per se, efforts are primarily directed at stopping any bleeding, using local methods such as pressure, topical agents such as zeolite (QuikClot) and chitosan (HemCon), and regional haemostasis with the use of tourniquets.

This is followed by rapid evacuation to a surgical facility where damage control surgery can take place. Resuscitation fluids are minimized where possible, and the early transfusion of blood and blood products where available is encouraged. An example of this is the UK Damage Control Resuscitation protocol (Table 18.7).

Table 18.7 UK Damage Control Resuscitation Protocol

1	For the first hour after injury, resuscitate to a palpable radial pulse, and after this (if not in surgery) resuscitate to a 'normal' blood pressure (an approach known as novel hybrid resuscitation and taught on the UK Battlefield Advanced Life Support course [BATLS]).
2	For severely injured casualties, recognize they are likely to be coagulopathic early – and resuscitate with blood, thawed plasma and platelets (blood and plasma initially in a 1:1 ratio).
3	Balance the need for volume replacement against the risk of overtransfusion – reassess constantly.
4	Use tranexamic acid early.
5	Monitor blood gases, lactate, calcium and potassium – with active management of falling calcium or rising potassium.
6	With blast casualties anticipate lung injury and ventilate using adult respiratory distress syndrome protocols.
7	Ensure that the anaesthesia team and surgical team work closely together to ensure the correct sequencing of damage control procedures.

18.7.3 Damage Control Surgery in the Military Setting

The typical civilian damage control patient is likely to require the direct attention of at least two surgeons and one nurse during the first 6 hours, full invasive monitoring, multiple operations, massive transfusion of blood and products, and prolonged ICU stay, with a high mortality. The utility of this philosophy was even recently labelled as 'impractical for common use in a forward military unit during times of war'. However, experience in the current counter-insurgency conflicts has led to a widespread adoption of the philosophy of damage control surgery in the military context as 'minimally acceptable care' with rapid procedures and pragmatic objectives. Current military surgical efforts are framed within a 'damage control' mindset, with temporary

revascularization of limbs and damage control laparotomy providing good control.

In the far-forward, highly mobile, austere military environment, it is quite likely that the surgeon will not have the luxury of being able to perform definitive surgery on every casualty. Short, focussed operative interventions can be used on peripheral vascular injuries, extensive bone and soft tissue injuries and thoracoabdominal penetrations in patients with favourable physiology, instead of *definitive* surgery being provided for every injured soldier. This may conserve precious resources such as time, operating table space and blood. Instead of applying these temporary abbreviated surgical control (TASC) manoeuvres to patients about to exhaust their physiological reserve, as in classic damage control, TASC is applied when the limitations of reserve exist outside the patient.

This philosophy relies heavily on the military medical system, with post-operative care and evacuation to the 'resource-replete environment' a priority. In the military, the key would seem to be triage (i.e. patient selection). The philosophy for the military surgeon exposed to numbers of casualties in the setting of limited resources remains to do the best for the most, rather than expend resources on limited numbers of critically wounded.

18.8 **BLAST INJURY**

Blast injury is the physiological and anatomical insult to the human body caused by the physical properties of an explosion. The shock wave that results from the explosion is referred to as the blast wave; its leading edge is the blast front and the rush of air caused by the blast wave is the blast wind.

In open air, the force of a blast rapidly dissipates, but within confined spaces the blast wave is actually magnified by its reflection off walls, floors and ceilings, increasing its destructive potential. Because water is less compressible than air, an underwater blast wave propagates at high speeds and loses energy less quickly over long distances, being approximately three times greater in strength than that which is detonated in the air.

Blast injury has been classified into four specific and distinct categories that reflect the mechanism of tissue injury and physical tissue damage that occur as a result of blast phenomena: primary, secondary, tertiary and quaternary blast injury:

- *Primary blast injury*: This refers to the effects of direct pressure (barotrauma) due to either underpressurization or overpressurization relative to atmospheric pressure. Gas-enclosing organs, such as the lung, tympanic membrane (the most common injury) and bowel, are the most vulnerable.

- *Secondary blast injury*: These are penetrating injuries caused by blast projectiles and debris. They are the leading cause of death and injury in both military and civilian terrorist attacks, except in cases of major building collapse.
- *Tertiary blast injury*: Displacement injuries result from persons or objects falling or being thrown because of the blast wave. Structural collapse or large airborne fragments lead to crush injury and extensive blunt trauma.
- *Quaternary blast injury*: This includes asphyxia, burns and inhalation injuries.
- *Quinary blast injury*: This is an early hyperinflammatory state, thought to be due to exposure to 'unconventional' materials used in the manufacture of the explosive.

18.8.1 Diagnosis and Management of Primary Blast Injuries

18.8.1.1 BLAST LUNG INJURY (BLI)

This may be immediately lethal or present a pattern similar to blunt trauma, with pulmonary contusion, often without rib fractures or chest wall injury. The earliest sign of blast lung injury is systemic arterial oxygen desaturation, often in the absence of other symptoms.

Radiological features can range from a typical 'butterfly pattern' bihilar shadowing on the chest X-ray to a 'white-out'. Management is principally supportive. Mechanical ventilation and effective chest drainage form the mainstay of treatment. High-peak inspiratory pressures should be avoided to decrease the chance of iatrogenic pulmonary barotraumas.

18.8.1.2 RUPTURE OF THE TYMPANIC MEMBRANE

All explosion victims should be evaluated with an otoscopic examination. Small perforations typically heal within a few weeks, and treatment should be expectant, with topical antibiotics if the ear canal is full of debris. Some authors suggest that early operative intervention be considered in patients with large perforations that are unlikely to heal. Some studies have reported a high (30 per cent) incidence of permanent high-frequency hearing loss 1 year after injury.

18.8.1.3 INTRA-ABDOMINAL INJURIES

Primary blast injury to the gastrointestinal tract is rare. The characteristic bowel lesion is a mural haematoma, ranging in severity from a minor submucosal haemorrhage to full-thickness disruption and perforation. The ileocaecal junction and colon are the most commonly affected sites, and delayed perforation can occur. Pneumoperitoneum alone may be a non-specific sign only associated with bowel perforation in less than 50 per cent of the patients.

Rupture of solid organs has been observed in the absence of other mechanisms of injury. Management should be in accordance with the principles of damage control. Diagnostic peritoneal lavage can be difficult to interpret because of the high incidence of retroperitoneal and mesenteric haematoma. Patients can also develop haematemesis or melena without obvious intraperitoneal involvement due to mucosal and submucosal haemorrhage. Colonoscopy is not recommended because of the risk of perforation.

18.8.1.4 OTHER INJURIES

- Transfer of kinetic energy from the blast wave to the eye can result in rupture of the globe, serous retinitis and hyphaema. Ophthalmology consultation should be obtained.
- The most common blast-induced arrhythmias, in addition to bradycardia, are premature ventricular contractions and asystole. The treating physician should be aware that haemorrhaging, explosion-injured patients may not have the expected compensatory tachycardia and may become hypotensive without rapid resuscitation.
- Traumatic amputations from primary blast injury are uncommon and controversial as to whether the blast wave alone is the cause.
- Primary blast injury can also result in cranial fractures around air-filled sinuses and focal neurological deficits as a result of air embolism. There are data supporting the concept of blast-induced brain injury, with psychological as well as physical symptoms.

18.9 BATTLEFIELD ANALGESIA

Relief of pain is an important consideration for both the wounded person and the military caregiver[14,15]. Provision of effective analgesia is humane but also attenuates the adverse pathophysiological responses to pain, and is likely to aid evacuation from the battlefield and maintain morale. Analgesia may be given at self- and buddy-aid levels; protocols to guide medical and paramedical staff in the provision of safe and effective analgesia are available.

Analgesia methods used in recent conflicts include

- Simple non-pharmacological.
  - Reassurance.
  - Splinting of fractures.
  - Cooling of burns.
- Oral analgesics.
  - Non-steroidal anti-inflammatory drugs.
  - Paracetamol.
- Nerve blocks and infiltration of local anaesthesia.
- Intramuscular and intravenous opiates.
- Fentanyl 'lollipops'.

Methods under development include intranasal ketamine, fentanyl and inhalational analgesics, such as methoxyflurane inhalation.

18.10 BATTLEFIELD ANAESTHESIA

Battlefield anaesthesia presents many challenges, including the need to maintain airway control, hypothermia of the casualty, restricted drug availability, lack of supplementary oxygen and the possible requirement for prolonged post-operative mechanical ventilation. Mass casualty situations are also a constant possibility in the military arena.

Surgery requires both adequate analgesia and anaesthesia. No single agent can provide both an appropriate level of anaesthesia and analgesia, hence a combination of drugs and techniques is required. The choices of anaesthetic are narrowed in austere conditions, being limited to general anaesthesia (either intravenous or inhalational), regional anaesthesia or none at all. For surgical exploration of body cavities, general anaesthesia is most frequently chosen, while a regional aesthetic may be more appropriate for injuries of the extremities or perineum.

In the field, rapid sequence induction (RSI) is the norm, using fast-acting hypnotic and neuromuscular blocking agents to facilitate rapid airway control. In the absence or limitation of supplemental oxygen supplies, RSI becomes even more crucial as pre-oxygenation of the patient's lungs is often not possible. There are several RSI cocktails used in the pre-hospital setting, most using a combination of an induction agent, a paralyzing agent and analgesia. Sedation, amnesia and analgesia can then be maintained with intravenous agents such as ketamine, benzodiazepines and opiates.

For long procedures or surgical sites involving the abdomen or thorax, a combination anaesthetic that includes an inhalational agent such as isoflurane may be used. British surgical teams use a portable 'triservice apparatus' that does not require a compressed gas source, and they have gained much experience with this technique of field anaesthesia. his 'draw-over' type of vaporizer is currently also in use by US forces in austere settings.

Regional anaesthesia remains an important option in battlefield anaesthesia, as it provides both patient comfort and surgical analgesia, while maintaining patient consciousness and spontaneous ventilation. With the relatively large number of extremity wounds in modern conflicts, and certainly in the mass casualty setting with a limited anaesthesia capability, regional aesthetic techniques should not be overlooked. Continuous infusion nerve blocks provide excellent analgesia for post-operative casualties during evacuation.

The pragmatic approach is to build systems around managing the severely injured patient and then adapt them to other situations when necessary.

18.10.1 Induction of Anaesthesia

Rapid sequence induction of anaesthesia (RSI) is the accepted standard for the trauma casualty. Indications for RSI in the emergency department include

- Casualties requiring immediate airway protection or mechanical ventilation.
- Uncontrollable agitation or Glasgow Coma Score (GCS) <8.
- Severe uncontrollable pain.

In cases of non-compressible haemorrhage such as intra-abdominal bleeding, RSI is usually more appropriately performed on the operating table with the casualty prepared for immediate surgery.

Prior to RSI, equipment and team preparation is paramount. A trained anaesthetic assistant should be available and ideally a second clinician whose role is to administer drugs and to monitor vital signs. A team member should be designated to perform thoracostomy should a tension pneumothorax become evident. In the event of cervical spine control being necessary, any cervical collar should be opened or removed and replaced with manual in-line stabilization by another team member. All equipment should be checked daily and again prior to casualty arrival. Minimum equipment immediately available includes

- Self-inflating bag and correctly sized face mask.
- Two sizes of laryngoscope (MAC 3 and 4 for adults).
- Appropriately sized endotracheal tubes.
- Failed/difficult intubation equipment.
- Bougie.
- Oropharyngeal and nasopharyngeal airways.
- Laryngeal mask airway (ideally second generation, e.g. ProSeal, iGel).
- Alternative laryngoscope (e.g. AirTraq, Glidescope if available).
- Surgical airway equipment.
- Working suction.
- Monitoring including end-tidal CO_2, ECG, NIBP and SpO_2.

Choice of induction agent(s) is not prescriptive. The aim is to preserve cardiac output as far as possible. For this reason most military anaesthetists favour ketamine (1–2 mg/kg) in major trauma. In the most severely injured a lower dose than that suggested may be required. The choice of muscle relaxant in RSI has long been suxamethonium (1.5 mg/kg), by virtue of its rapid onset and offset. An alternative to this is rocuronium (1.2 mg/kg), which provides good intubating conditions within 60 seconds. The much longer time to offset neuromuscular blockade is argued as advantageous should the need for a surgical airway arise. Rocuronium is also the drug of choice for RSI in cases of hyperkalaemia, burns older than 24 hours and spinal cord injuries older than 10 days. Immediate reversal is with sugammadex 16 mg/kg. This may not be available in the deployed environment.

Extreme care should be taken with RSI in hypovolaemic casualties. If possible severe hypovolaemia should be corrected prior to induction to avoid the risk of pulseless electrical activity (PEA) cardiac arrest. The aim of resuscitation should be to achieve a normal blood pressure in controlled haemorrhage and a palpable radial pulse in uncontrolled haemorrhage. If immediate RSI is required, the dose of induction agent should be reduced accordingly. Ventilation should be established minimizing the respiratory rate (e.g. 6 bpm) and airway pressures (avoid positive end-expiratory pressure [PEEP]).

18.10.2 Maintenance of Anaesthesia

Anaesthesia can be maintained initially by use of IV agents. This is particularly useful if induction has taken place in the emergency department and further imaging is needed or if there is a delay prior to transfer to the operating theatre.

Fentanyl (1–2 µg/kg initially) is used as an adjunct to blood product resuscitation by virtue of its effect as a sympatholytic countering the extreme vasoconstriction seen in extreme hypovolaemia. This permits further volume resuscitation and avoids rebound hypertension. Further doses are titrated during DCR/DCS up to 15 µg/kg.

Midazolam (0.02–0.05 mg/kg initially) can be used to maintain anaesthesia immediately following RSI in addition to fentanyl. Further boluses of 0.02 mg/kg can be titrated to anaesthetic effect. Anaesthesia for surgery is usually maintained with a volatile agent. In ongoing hypovolaemia, volatile use should be carefully titrated along with fentanyl according to physiological parameters. The Tri-Service Anaesthetic Apparatus (TSAA) (UK Defence Medical Services) can be used to administer a volatile anaesthetic without a supply of compressed gas. It can be used in conjunction with an oxygen concentrator that preserves supplies of cylinder oxygen. The US Defence Medical Services have 'drawover' anaesthesia apparatus similar to the TSAA. An alternative to volatile anaesthesia is total intravenous anaesthesia (TIVA). In its simplest form, this could be bolus administration of ketamine for short cases. Syringe drivers are now in common use and allow for a variety of TIVA drugs to be used.

Epidural anaesthesia is usually not undertaken in the most austere environments. This is due to difficulty in ensuring a consistently sterile environment for safe catheter placement, as well as the requirement for specialist equipment and the need for trained staff to escort in evacuation. In the mature deployment with a robust logistical and evacuation chain, epidural placement may be considered.

Spinal anaesthesia is a common technique in developing countries where there may be a lack of trained anaesthesia practitioners; the risk of airway complications associated with general anaesthesia can thus be avoided. Placement of a spinal block in the shocked casualty leads to catastrophic hypotension from loss of sympathetic tone. Spinal anaesthesia should be avoided in this situation. In patients where spinal anaesthesia may be appropriate, the risks of infection from placement in the field may outweigh any benefits.

18.10.3 Damage Control Anaesthesia in the Military Setting

Anaesthesia for 'damage control' procedures and major cavity injury is really a fusion of continuing resuscitation and critical care (see also Chapter 19). This requires optimization of haemodynamic status, re-warming of the casualty and pain relief. One of the biggest challenges will be reversing the hypothermia that is almost universal in haemorrhagic patients in these conditions. As well as warming all intravenous fluids and ventilator circuits, an active re-warming device will be required. If a return to the operating theatre for more definitive surgery is not planned in the forward location, critical care must be maintained throughout the aeromedical evacuation.

18.11 CRITICAL CARE

If damage control is going to be the norm for the far-forward surgeon, a critical care capability must be a part of the forward surgical team structure. The priorities will be therefore be optimization of haemodynamic status, re-warming of the patient, control of coagulopathy, pain relief and preparation for return to theatre or evacuation depending on the situation. The healthcare providers looking after the critical care of a patient in these surroundings face many of the problems already identified for the anaesthetic provider. As stated above, one of the biggest challenges will be reversing the hypothermia that is almost universal in haemorrhagic patients in these conditions. Therefore an active re-warming device will be required, as well as warming all intravenous fluids and ventilator circuits. If a return to the operating theatre for more definitive surgery is not planned in the forward location, critical care must be maintained throughout the aeromedical evacuation.

18.12 TRANSLATING MILITARY EXPERIENCE TO CIVILIAN TRAUMA CARE

Six aspects of military trauma care have been identified as contributing to recent good outcomes for patients wounded in combat[16-18].

18.12.1 Leadership

Current military trauma care systems are delivered by consultants.

18.12.2 Front-end Processes

The treatment of patients wounded by military weapons is fundamentally geared toward the concept of damage control. Correction of a patient's deranged physiology is recognized as a greater priority than definitive anatomical repair. In addition, the key hospital infrastructure (emergency department, operating room, CT scanner and ICU) is planned around the needs of the time-critical patient, ensuring that all key components are close to one another.

18.12.3 Common Training

It is considered that the common military training model (from first aid to multidisciplinary field hospital simulation) facilitates effective team working and delivery of appropriate human and other resources at the right time for wounded patients.

18.12.4 Governance

Military trauma systems operate a robust and diligent framework that, through a vigorous review of injury data, clinical processes and patients' outcomes, provides feedback to improve the system's performance.

18.12.5 Rehabilitation Services

Formal, dedicated rehabilitation specialists and facilities are recognized as being fundamental to favourable long-term outcomes.

18.12.6 Translational Research

Integrated basic and clinical research streams feed rapid improvements in all aspects of care to clinicians, which can then be introduced into clinical care.

18.13 SUMMARY

These are exciting times in which to be a military medical practitioner. Dramatic changes in the global world order have shifted the priorities for military planners, and surgical doctrines also have to adapt to the likely scenarios of future conflict. Low-density dispersed battlefields, highly mobile operations, extended lines of evacuation and logistic supply, civilian wounded and the possibility of chemical, biological and nuclear attack all mean that military doctors will have to demonstrate their adaptability and resourcefulness, as well as their surgical skills. Whether labelled 'TASC' or 'damage control', limited initial surgery is likely to be part of the surgeon's armamentarium.

In summary, in the operational or deployed humanitarian setting, resources are more limited, and the word 'finite' achieves a new meaning. Professional flexibility is paramount. Triage and intervention may be modified by an open or closed back door, or by open skies. Environmental protection is minimal when compared with civilian structures. Surgery has to be tailored taking into consideration operational realities. Procedures such as simple burr holes, evacuation of a retro-orbital haematoma (compressing the optic nerve), damage control thoracotomy and laparotomy, shunting of vascular injuries, fasciotomies and, above all, the extent of debridement required are new skills to be learnt.

Experience of war advances trauma care; the concentration of the severely wounded in the hands of well-resourced, motivated clinicians provides the impetus for advances in the surgical care of the wounded. This recent period of conflict has certainly provided opportunities for advancement on many levels. Each mission will bring a new set of technical and personal challenges. But, as Hippocrates [c. 460 BC–c. 377 BC] said: 'He who wishes to be a surgeon, must first go to war'.

REFERENCES AND RECOMMENDED READING

References

1. Smith R. *The Utility of Force: The Art of War in the Modern World.* 2012; Allen Lane (Penguin Books UK): London.
2. Mabry RL, Holcomb JB, Baker AM, et al. United States Army Rangers in Somalia: an analysis of combat casualties on an urban battlefield. *J Trauma.* 2000;49(3):515–528.
3. Hardaway RM III. Vietnam wound analysis. *J Trauma.* 1978;18:635–642.
4. iCasualties.org. Casualty Reports, 2014. http://icasualties.org. Accessed September 29, 2014.
5. Eastridge BJ, Mabry RL, Seguin P, et al. Death on the battlefield (2001–2011): implications for the future of combat casualty care. *J Trauma Acute Care Surg.* 2012;73(6 Suppl 5):S431–S437.
6. Ingalls N, Zonies D, Bailey JA, et al. A review of the first 10 years of critical care aeromedical transport during Operation Iraqi Freedom and Operation Enduring Freedom: the importance of evacuation timing. *JAMA Surg.* 2014;149(8):807–813.
7. Cordova CB, Capp AP, Spinella PC. Fresh whole blood transfusion for a combat casualty in austere combat environment. *J Spec Oper Med.* 2014;14(1):9–12.
8. Cooper BR, Mahoney PF, Hodgetts TJ, Mellor A. Intraosseous access (EZ-IO) for resuscitation: UK military combat experience. *J R Army Med Corps.* 2007;153(4):314–316.
9. Holcomb JB. Damage control resuscitation. *J Trauma.* Jun 2007;62(6 Suppl):S36–S37.
10. Rappold JF, Pusateri AE. Tranexamic acid in remote damage control resuscitation. *Transfusion.* Jan 2013;53 Suppl 1:96S–99S.
11. Holcomb JB, Helling TS, Hirshberg A. Military, civilian, and rural application of the damage control philosophy. *Mil Med.* 2001;166(6):490–493.
12. Rotondo MF, Zonies DH. The damage control sequence and underlying logic. *Surg Clin North Am.* 1997;77(4):761–777.
13. Granchi TS, Liscum KR. The logistics of damage control. *Surg Clin North Am.* 1997;77(4):921–928.
14. Fisher AD, Rippee B, Shehan H, Conklin C, Mabry RL. Prehospital analgesia with ketamine for combat wounds: a case series. *J Spec Op Med.* Winter 2014;14(4):11–17.
15. Clifford JL, Fowler M, Hansen JJ, et al. State of the science review: Advances in pain management in wounded service members over a decade at war. *J Trauma Acute Care Surg.* Sep 2014;77(3 Suppl 2):S228–S236.
16. Beekley AC, Starnes BW, Sebesta JA. Lessons learned from modern military surgery. *Surg Clin North Am.* Feb 2007;87(1):157–184, vii.
17. Caterson EJ, Carty MJ, Weaver MJ, Holt EF. Boston bombings: a surgical view of lessons learned from combat casualty care and the applicability to Boston's terrorist attack. *J Craniofac Surg.* Jul 2013;24(4):1061–1067.
18. Dubose J, Rodriguez C, Martin M, et al. Preparing the surgeon for war: present practices of US, UK, and Canadian militaries and future directions for the US military. *J Trauma Acute Care Surg.* 2012;73(6 Suppl 5):S423–S430.

Recommended Reading

BALLISTICS: HISTORY, MECHANISMS, BALLISTIC PROTECTION AND CASUALTY MANAGEMENT

Mahoney PF, Ryan JM, Brooks AJ, Schwab CW. *Ballistic Trauma: A Practical Guide*, 2nd ed. London, UK: Springer Verlag; 2005.

Miller FP, Vandome AF, McBrewster J, eds. *Ballistic Trauma: Physical Trauma, Weapon, Ammunition, Small Arms, Semiautomatic Pistol, Machine Gun, Submachine Gun, Assault Rifle, Public Health, Firearm, War*. Beau Bassin, Mauritius: World Health Organization/Alphascript Publishing; 2009. http://www.alphascript-publishing.com/.

Ryan J. *Ballistic Trauma: Clinical Relevance in Peace and War*. London, UK: Arnold; 1997.

Volgas DA, Stannard JP, Alonso JE. Ballistics: a primer for the surgeon. *Injury* 2005;36:373–379.

BLAST INJURY

Bala M, Rivkind AI, Zamir G, et al. Abdominal trauma after terrorist bombing attacks exhibits a unique pattern of injury. *Ann Surg.* 2008;248:303–309.

Champion HR, Holcomb JB. Injuries from explosions: physics, biophysics, pathology, and required research focus. *J Trauma.* 2009;66:1468–1477.

Ciraulo DL, Frykberg ER. The surgeon and acts of civilian terrorism: blast injuries. *J Am Coll Surg.* 2006;203:942–950.

DePalma RG, Burris DG, Champion HR, Hodgson MJ. Blast injuries. *N Engl J Med.* 2005;352:1335–1342.

Neuhaus SJ, Sharwood PF, Rosenfeld JV. Terrorism and blast explosions: lessons for the Australian surgical community. *A NZ J Surg.* 2006;76:637–644.

Ritenour AE, Baskin TW. Primary blast injury: update on diagnosis and treatment. *Crit Care Med.* 2008;36(Suppl.):S311–S317.

WAR SURGERY

Advanced Life Support Group. *Major Incident Medical Management and Support*, 2nd ed. London, UK: BMJ Books; 2002.

Buckenmaier C, Bleckner L. The Military Advanced Regional Anesthesia and Analgesia Handbook. 2010 Borden Institute Washington DC.

Butler FK Jr, Hagmann JH, Richards DT. Tactical management of urban warfare casualties in special operations. *Mil Med.* 2000;165(4 Suppl):1–48.

Calderbank P, Woolley T, Mercer S, et al. Doctor on board? What is the optimal skill-mix in military pre-hospital care? *Emerg Med J.* 2010;Sep 15 [Epub ahead of print].

Coupland RM. *War Wounds of Limbs: Surgical Management.* Oxford, UK: Butterworth Heinemann; 2000.

Coupland R, Molde A, Navein J. *Care in the Field for Victims of Weapons of War.* Geneva, Switzerland: International Committee of the Red Cross; 2001.

Department of the Army. *War Surgery in Afghanistan and Iraq: A Series of Cases, 2003–2007.* Textbooks of Military Medicine. Washington, DC: Department of the Army; 2008.

Dufour D, Kromann Jensen S, Owen-Smith M, et al. *Surgery for Victims of War*, 3rd ed. Geneva, Switzerland: International Committee of the Red Cross; 1998.

Giannou C, Baldan M. *War Surgery: Working with Limited Resources in Armed Conflict and Other Situations of Violence.* War Surgery Vol. 1. ICRC Publication 2009 ref. 0973. Geneva, Switzerland: International Committee of the Red Cross.

Greaves I, Porter KM, Revell MP. Fluid resuscitation in pre-hospital trauma care: a consensus view. *J R Coll Surg Edin.* 2002;47:451–457.

Greenfield RA, Brown BR, Hutchins JB, et al. Microbiological, biological, and chemical weapons of warfare and terrorism. *Am J Med Sci.* 2002;323:326–340.

Hodgetts TJ, Mahoney PF, Evans G, Brooks A, eds. Battlefield Advanced Trauma Life Support. *J R Army Med Corps.* 2006; 152(2 Suppl): 5–72.

Holcomb J. Causes of death in US Special Operations Forces in the global war on terrorism: 2001–2004. *US Army Med Dep J.* 2007(Jan–Mar):24–37.

Husum H, Ang SC, Fosse E. *War Surgery Field Manual.* Penang, Malaysia: Third World Network; 1995.

Husum H, Gilbert M, Wisborg T. *Save Lives, Save Limbs: Life Support for Victims of Mines, Wars and Accidents.* Penang, Malaysia: Third World Network; 2000.

International Committee of the Red Cross. *First Aid in Armed Conflict and Other Situations of Violence.* Geneva, Switzerland: ICRC; 2006.

Journal of the Royal Army Medical Corps. Wounds of Conflict (Vol. 147, No. 1, February 2001), Combat Casualty Care (Vol. 153, No. 4, December 2007), Wounds of Conflict II (Vol. 155, No. 4, December 2009). http://www.ramcjournal.com. Accessed December 2010.

Lounsbury DE, Brengman M, Bellamy RF, eds. *Emergency War Surgery.* Third United States Revision. Washington, DC: Borden Institute; 2004.

North Atlantic Treaty Organization. *Emergency War Surgery NSATO Handbook 2010*. Washington, DC: Borden Institute. http://www.bordeninstitute.army.mil/other_pub/ews/EWS.ZIP. Accessed December 2014.

Roberts P, ed. *The British Military Surgery Pocket Book*. AC No. 12552. London, UK: HMSO; 2004.

Santry HP, Alam HB. Fluid resuscitation: past, present, and the future. *Shock*. 2010;33:229–241.

Willy C, Voelker HU, Steinmann R, Engelhardt M. Patterns of injury in a combat environment. 2007 update. *Chirurg*. 2008;79:66–76.

Trauma Anaesthesia 19

19.1 INTRODUCTION

Trauma anaesthetists are an essential part of the trauma team working in close collaboration with the surgeon. Trauma anaesthesia is involved in the entire chain of trauma care, from pre-hospital, to emergency room, often multiple operating room episodes, intensive care and pain management.

Trauma anaesthesia as a subspecialty of anaesthesiology requires broad experience in all modes of anaesthesia and a flexible approach to applying this knowledge. Strategies that work in elective cases may not be appropriate for trauma patients. The trauma anaesthetist participates in and contributes to the decision-making process during the initial resuscitation and provides resuscitation and anaesthesia in the perioperative setting.

Because of this comprehensive involvement and the frequent multiple surgeries for some severely injured, trauma anaesthetists may be a consistent asset throughout the entire treatment process.

19.2 PREPARATION FOR DAMAGE CONTROL

Damage control surgery (DCS) describes the strategy of limiting surgical intervention in haemodynamically compromised trauma patients by restricting procedures to early control of haemorrhage and contamination, and postponing the definitive anatomical repair until the patient is more stable.

19.2.1 Introduction

In this chapter we will cover the aspects of trauma anaesthesia related to damage control in trauma. Anaesthetic involvement in specific situations, such as head trauma, is dealt with in the other relevant chapters. Special skills are also described in those chapters.

19.2.2 Planning and Communicating

When the trauma patient enters the emergency room the trauma anaesthetist should take charge of the airway, optimize oxygenation and resuscitation, taking account in particular the patient's neurologic condition and temperature.

The trauma team should then decide the optimal process of care for that individual. Interventions in the emergency room (ER) should be limited to those that are essential for survival. Ensuring adequate venous access and perhaps an extra-large-bore IV cannula may make an important difference; an arterial line may not be worth the time. Together with the surgeon, the anaesthetist has an important role in initiation of diagnostics or surgery depending on the clinical condition.

The anaesthetist has a crucial role in optimizing the physiology to match the surgical strategies. Assessment of ongoing dynamic changes and reaction to treatment is an essential contribution to the decision-making process.

The planned strategy for resuscitation and surgery should be communicated closely between the surgeon, the anaesthetist and the team, coordinated by the trauma team leader.

19.3 DAMAGE CONTROL RESUSCITATION (DCR)

With the development of the concepts of DCS in the early 1990s, it became clear that anaesthetic strategies needed to adapt to special needs aiming at a comprehensive and multidisciplinary resuscitation approach. The non-surgical management needs to be maximally time efficient and supportive in order to provide the best possible conditions for early surgical haemostasis[1]. The DCS and damage control anaesthesia combine together in the concept of 'damage control resuscitation' aiming to rapidly stop bleeding, restore blood volume, aggressively preventing and correcting coagulopathy, hypothermia and acidosis[2].

The five principal pillars of DCR are:

- Limit or omit fluid administration, early use of blood product.
- Monitor permissive hypotension.
- Target coagulopathy.
- Prevent and treat hypothermia.
- Facilitate early use of tranexamic acid where indicated.

The DCR aims to treat and prevent conditions which exacerbate haemorrhagic shock and the ensuing systemic inflammatory response. The DCR addresses the pathophysiologic consequences of tissue trauma and blood loss and reduces the risks of overly aggressive fluid resuscitation, while targeting correction of metabolic derangements and coagulopathy. The concept of limiting operative stress by delaying definitive repair until after control of haemorrhage and after the patients improves his or her physiology is supported by DCR. The importance of an early transfer to an intensive care unit (ICU) for subsequent normalization of microcirculation, correction of coagulopathy and re-warming are stressed. Therefore, patients in the damage control pathway can be expected to arrive in ICU in a critical and under-resuscitated state. Early and optimal flow of information about the situation and specific needs between the surgical, anaesthetic and ICU teams is key for optimal management. Therefore, trauma resuscitation requires prolonged multidisciplinary collaboration, starting in the pre-hospital setting and continuing through emergency departments and operating theatres to the ICU.

In most civilian trauma centres of the developed world, less than 10 per cent of the trauma workload qualifies for damage control strategy. Precise and early identification of these patients is of the essence as the overuse of this approach may lead to significant morbidity and hospital resource use. With early haemorrhage control and optimal resuscitation, some patients may rapidly improve their hemodynamic state. Therefore, even if initially considered for the DCR pathway, they might now be suitable for definitive care. Constant re-assessment is crucial and the role of the anaesthetist in providing continued information about the patient's hemodynamic and organ perfusion is key for joint decision making.

In this chapter we describe the strategy and the pathophysiology behind the three non-surgical pillars of DCR.

19.3.1 Limited Fluid Administration

Aggressive fluid resuscitation to restore normal circulatory function has long been the mainstay of the initial approach for haemorrhagic shock. In 2004, Moore et al. coined the term 'bloody vicious cycle', showing that crystalloid administration leads to a transient rise in blood pressure, followed by increased haemorrhage, which requires further fluid administration, leading to the sequence of hypotension, fluid bolus, re-bleeding and deeper hypotension. It is currently accepted that administration of high volumes of fluid before achieving definitive haemostasis increases the rate of bleeding by raising cardiac output, with increased blood pressure counteracting local vasoconstriction and reopening spontaneously clotted vessels. In addition to dilutional coagulopathy, large volumes of crystalloid fluids have deleterious effects on organ function, the endothelium and immunological and inflammatory mediators. All of these are associated with poor outcome. Recent studies have shown that high volumes of crystalloids increase reperfusion injury and leukocyte adhesion, resulting in an increased incidence of infectious complications and multiple organ failure (Table 19.1)[3].

During ongoing surgical bleeding, clear fluids should be limited to minimal amounts or even omitted until definitive control of haemorrhage has been achieved. Early use of blood and blood products in this critically bleeding group of trauma patients reduces crystalloid administration and is the mainstay of resuscitation in damage control. Some even recommend to limit the use of crystalloids in trauma-related haemorrhagic shock to a function of carrier of drugs and to keep lines open between blood product administrations. Preferred types of crystalloids are balanced solutions such as Ringer lactate solution or Plasmalyte 0.9%. Sodium chloride solution ('normal saline') can contribute to hyperchloraemic acidosis which may have an adverse effect on renal function. Synthetic colloids containing starches have shown to interfere with fibrin polymerization, coating of platelets, blocking of fibrinogen receptor (GPIIb-IIIa) and von-Willebrand type 1-like syndrome and cause coagulopathy (colloid-induced coagulopathy), increased bleeding and transfusion requirements. Starch solutions have also been associated with an increased risk of renal failure and increased mortality in the critically ill[5], although the discussion is still ongoing.

Table 19.1 Consequences of Aggressive Crystalloid Resuscitation[3]

Respiratory	Capillary permeability
	Pulmonary oedema, which also results in acute lung injury (ALI)/acute respiratory distress syndrome (ARDS)
Gut	Intestinal permeability
	Bacterial translocation
	Paralytic ileus
	Abdominal compartment syndrome (ACS)
	Anastomotic dehiscence
Heart	Myocyte action potential
	Ventricular dysfunction
	Arrhythmia
	Membrane polarization
	Disruption of phosphorylation
	Cellular oedema
	Apoptysis
Blood	Dilution of coagulation factors
	Increased blood loss
	Counteracting vasoconstriction
	Oncotic pressure
Vessels	Catecholamine release
	Vascular resistance to catecholamines
Inflammatory Pathways	Activation of inflammation (TNFα, interleukins, SIRS)
	Early vasoplegia
Endothelium	Damage to endothelial integrity
	Capillary leak

Source: Adapted from Cotton BA, Guy JS, Morris JA, Jr., Abumrad NN, *Shock*, 26(2), 115–121, 2006; and Kozar RA, Peng Z, Zhang R, et al., *Anesth Analg.*, 112(6), 1289–1295, 2011. With permission.

Limiting fluid administration raises the question of how to maintain blood pressure. The use of vasopressors for hemodynamic support during resuscitation after injury is controversial. While arginine vasopressin and phenylephrine have shown to provide some beneficial effects in patients with traumatic brain injury, lung contusion or in animal models with haemorrhagic shock[6], a prospective multicentre study on blunt trauma patients has shown an increased mortality in patients with early vasopressors use[7]. Therefore, hypovolemic shock should be treated primarily by volume replacement, but low doses of vasopressors might be useful to counteract the sympatholytic and cardiovascular depressant effect of anaesthetic agents.

In regard to the question around maintaining blood pressure, what blood pressure goal should be aimed for during the acute resuscitation of bleeding trauma patients?

19.3.2 Permissive Hypotension

Permissive hypotension is a strategy to reduce blood loss by limiting systolic pressure to the minimum necessary to maintain perfusion of vital organs. In massively bleeding patients, raising blood pressure to normal levels before achieving surgical haemostasis has been shown to enhance bleeding by displacing clot[5] formed during the body's attempt at primary haemostasis ('popping the clot'). The strategy is not new, and was reported during World War I, when Cannon stated that 'Haemorrhage in the case of shock may not have occurred to a marked degree because blood pressure has been too low, and flow too scant to overcome the obstacle offered by the clot. If the pressure is raised before the surgeon is ready to check any bleeding that may take place, blood that is sorely needed may be lost'[4]. Although safe limits of blood pressure in terms of preservation of organ perfusion are unknown, systolic blood pressure of 80 mm Hg, and in the case of concomitant severe brain trauma, mean arterial pressure (MAP) of over 80 mm Hg are recommended. While there is no hard evidence for these limits, it is very clear that such low pressures should be maintained for the shortest possible time in order to limit vital organ ischaemia. The importance of early surgical haemostasis and the need for the DCR concept being applied as a whole has to be emphasized.

19.3.3 Targeting Coagulopathy

Early and aggressive administration of blood and blood products has shown to improve survival after trauma-related haemorrhagic shock[8]. Lost blood volume should be replaced by blood products aiming at near equal ratios of packed red blood cells (PRBC): fresh frozen plasma (FFP): platelets[9,10]. Such regimens have demonstrated improved outcome. Data suggest that plasma-based resuscitation when compared to crystalloids is better at preserving endothelial integrity. Administration of FFP after haemorrhagic shock has anti-inflammatory properties and a potential glycocalyx-restoring capacity[11].

Up to 30 per cent of injured patients present with impaired coagulation on arrival at the care facility. The presence of trauma-related coagulopathy is a surrogate marker of the extent and severity of tissue trauma and shock and correlates with mortality. Coagulation abnormalities related to severe trauma have several causal factors including consumption of clotting factors and platelets, dilution after administration of fluids and, fibrinolysis as well as hypothermia and acidosis. Early identification of patients with acute traumatic coagulopathy (ATC) is crucial for timely initiation of haemostatic resuscitation[12,13]. Early blood gases are a quick and helpful tool to identify patients in shock. Base deficit or lactate has shown to provide a reliable correlation with the need for massive transfusion and risk of death. A base deficit of >2 mmol/L correlates with class 2, and BD >6 mmol/L with class 3 shock according to the ATLS definition[14]. In the absence of timely laboratory assessment, in patients with evidence of impaired end-organ perfusion and extensive tissue trauma, initiation of haemostatic resuscitation may be indicated even before biologic or viscoelastic confirmation of ATC. Early administration of blood products raises logistic challenges. The implementation of a massive transfusion protocol (MTP) is recommended, which will allow the ready availability of blood products. Availability of a MTP has shown to be associated with a reduction of organ failure and improved 30-day survival after severe trauma[15]. The putative mechanism is potentially related to earlier transfusion of plasma and platelets.

While the optimal ratio of pRBC:FFP:platelets is unclear, haemostatic resuscitation is generally recommended initiated with a fixed ratio close to 1:1:1[16] followed by a switch, as early as possible, to goal-directed resuscitation guided by viscoelastic haemostatic assays[17] (VHAs) (see also Chapter 4).

Fibrinolysis is a key feature of the ATC. The CRASH-2 trial[18] showed a 30 per cent mortality reduction after the administration of tranexamic acid in trauma patients at risk of significant haemorrhage. A bolus of 1 g of tranexamic acid, followed by an infusion of 1 g over 8 hours, has become used within many MTPs. It should be given as early as possible to bleeding trauma patients; if treatment is not given until 3 hours or later after injury, it is less effective and could even be harmful. In major haemorrhage, fibrinogen reaches critically low values earlier than other coagulation factors or platelets. Replacement is generally necessary to maintain a plasma concentration of 150–200 mg/dL and its early use (in the form of cryoprecipitate or fibrinogen concentrate) has been integrated in many MTPs even though strong evidence supporting this is lacking. Further data are needed.

Despite the increased use of tranexamic acid, the gathering and validity of the data has been called into question in a major trauma centre environment. In addition, a recent study indicated that the majority of severely injured patients have a fibrinolysis shutdown, and therefore, tranexamic acid may have no effect[19].

Tranexamic acid is not widely used routinely outside of Europe, and its greatest use may be where increased clot lysis is shown to be present (e.g. using thrombo-elastography).

19.3.4 **Prevent and Treat Hypothermia**

Hypothermia below 35°C had a profound impact on surgical site infection rates after trauma laparotomy. Hypothermia also adversely affects coagulation as well as cardiac output and function in most bodily organs. Hypothermia and acidosis compromise thrombin generation kinetics via different mechanisms. Hypothermia primarily inhibits the initiation phase, whereas acidosis severely inhibits the propagation phase of thrombin generation. Similarly, hypothermia and acidosis affect fibrinogen metabolism differently. Hypothermia inhibits fibrinogen synthesis, whereas acidosis accelerates fibrinogen degradation, leading to a potential deficit in fibrinogen availability. Thus, the specific steps related to hypothermia prevention and treatment are:

- Keep the operating room (OR) temperature warm (25°C or higher). Maintaining a warm OR on patient arrival helps keep patients warm.
- Have additional warming devices available, including a forced air device system, fluid warmers on the IV line, warm IV solutions, and warm blankets.
- Have a system to warm all solutions that are to be used in the surgical field.

19.3.5 **Key Messages**

- Assess arterial blood gases on every trauma patient to aid decision making.
- Before surgical control of haemorrhage:
  - · Limit crystalloid fluid resuscitation.
  - · Do not use synthetic colloids.
  - · Commence blood products and goal-directed haemostatic resuscitation early.
  - · Allow blood pressure to be below normal during early haemorrhage control.
- Arrange early transfer to ICU and effective multidisciplinary communication.

19.4 DAMAGE CONTROL SURGERY

19.4.1 Anaesthetic Procedures

Being able to predict situations is a key skill for the trauma anaesthetist and is derived from extensive experience. The anaesthetist should be able to predict how the patient physiology will evolve over a short period of time, and his or her response to treatment. The anaesthetist should anticipate the treatment the patient will receive and the route the patient will need to take to get to a stable state.

19.4.1.1 AIRWAY

In order to be able to correct hypoxia, manage CO_2, protect the airway and facilitate interventions most severe trauma patients will require intubation. Anaesthetists who deal with airway management on a daily basis are probably the best group to perform this task, but if other groups are to perform this they should be trained to perform it to the same standards and quality. Intubation in patients with possible neck trauma is a recognized difficult airway management situation. There are difficult airway algorithms available to assist decision making for situations. An oral tube may be impossible, a laryngeal mask not suitable and a surgical airway the only and fastest option. This decision needs to be made before the patient decompensates, and skill and experience are required to make the decision in a timely manner. The anaesthetist may need to rely on his or her own skills rather than wait for another individual. The skill of establishing a surgical airway needs to be taught and practised to be retained.

19.4.1.2 BREATHING

Mechanical ventilation is a life-saving treatment but also has increased dangers for trauma patients. Trauma patients are at increased risk of volume and barotrauma and acute respiratory distress syndrome (ARDS) from mechanical ventilation, referred to as ventilator induced lung injury (VILI). The injured lung is more susceptible to maldistribution of pressure between healthy and injured parts, leading to collapse in some areas with overdistension in others even at lower tidal volumes. The anaesthetist needs to apply judicious amounts of positive end-expiratory pressure (PEEP) and a ventilation strategy aimed at minimizing overdistension of the lung.

Damage to the thoracic wall and to the lung increase the risks of pneumothorax, air embolism and VILI adding to the original acute lung injury. During ventilation the anaesthetist needs to be aware of these potential complications and the options for treatment.

While ventilating the patient the anaesthetist also needs to take into account associated injuries and the influence of ventilation on injury. For example PEEP, $PaCO_2$ and PaO_2 are important in traumatic brain injury treatment strategies. The PEEP may reduce blood pressure, especially in the presence of hypovolaemia. Furthermore, PEEP at high levels (>12 mm Hg) may increase intracranial pressure (ICP). Nevertheless, it has also been demonstrated that in brain-injured patients during mechanical ventilation, the application of moderate levels of PEEP (up to 8 cm H_2O) provided protection against the occurrence of lung injury, probably by restoring lung volume and reducing lung heterogeneity – that is atelectasis, airway closure and tidal expiratory flow limitation. Mean arterial pressure (MAP) and ICP monitoring and prevention of hypoxia are essential for prevention of secondary brain injury. $PaCO_2$ also affects ICP, and the aim is to achieve normocarbia ($PaCO_2$ 35–45 mm Hg). Hypocarbia increases cerebral vasoconstriction, leading to decreased cerebral blood flow (CBF), which may decrease ICP but also cause ischaemia. Decreasing $PaCO_2$ (by hyperventilating the patient) is a treatment strategy that should be limited to short duration management of critically raised ICP (e.g. en route to an intervention for reducing the ICP, e.g. surgery). Hypercarbia increases CBF by vasodilatation and increases ICP in severe brain injury with the risk of decreasing cerebral perfusion pressure and causing or worsening secondary brain injury.

19.4.1.3 CIRCULATION

Control of exsanguinating bleeding has taken priority over the airway breathing circulation changing the ABC mnemonic to C (control of catastrophic bleeding)-A-B-C, certainly in the pre-hospital and military settings.

19.4.1.4 VASCULAR ACCESS

Vascular access is required for the administration of resuscitation drugs and blood transfusion. The ATLS approach calls for two large-bore intravenous (i.v.) cannulas. The rationale is not to put twice as much volume in (permissive hypotension) but to have redundancy and availability when required. With a second i.v. you can have a separate access for medication that cannot be mixed and as backup if you have a dysfunctional line.

If one of the i.v.s is a small-calibre one there is the option to change it to a larger one using a wire Seldinger technique that will allow exchange for a rapid infusion catheter. Another way to gain better i.v. access is to apply a tourniquet above the small catheter, infuse 60 mL of i.v. fluid and insert a larger-bore i.v. catheter above the small catheter in the now distended vein.

If the need for a rapid infusor system is foreseen, a 14-gauge (at least) catheter will be needed to allow high flow (500–800 mL/min). The i.v. lines used for the rapid infusor should not have one-way valves such as in use in the ICU and only high-flow three-way stopcocks if you really need them. Medication should have a separate line from the high-flow system. A central venous line allows multiple ports, central venous pressure measurement and high flow fluid administration as well as venous blood gas measurements. A central venous line allows early intravenous feeding.

The larger the bore of the i.v. cannula, the greater the flow (Figure 19.1).

19.4.2 **Monitoring**

Besides the standard anaesthesia monitoring, a five-leads electrocardiogram (ECG) in case of thoracic injury is advisable. Blunt cardiac injury can be detected by changes in ECG and treated with supportive therapy. Ventilation should be monitored with pulse oximetry for adequate oxygenation and end-tidal (ET) CO_2 for assuring adequate respiratory minute volume. The $ETCO_2$ further informs us about cardiac output decreasing in the case of circulatory collapse.

An arterial line provides the opportunity for beat-to-beat blood pressure monitoring, blood sampling and

Figure 19.1 Time in seconds to infuse 1 L of clear fluids versus catheter gauge.

physiological status, but should not delay time to surgery or intervention. Arterial line insertion is first attempted peripherally (radial or brachial or dorsal foot arteries), secondarily moving proximally (femoral or axillary arteria) in difficult situations with massive bleeding.

In the OR, in due time and according to the clinical condition, hemodynamic status can be evaluated by accessing cardiac output. The purpose is to evaluate the status of the blood volume and cardiac function in order to secure normovolaemia and perfusion, meanwhile avoiding hypo- as well as hypervolaemia. In the early dramatic phase of damage control resuscitation (DCR) using pulse, BP, pulse oximetry and $ETCO_2$ can be the only possibilities, but when more control is achieved hemodynamic monitoring can be intensified according to the clinical condition.

Haemodynamic monitoring is a means of checking cardiac output and performing volume estimation:

- Pulse and BP.
- Central venous pressure or central venous saturation ($S_{cv}O_2$) accessed via a central line.
- Transthoracic or transoesophageal echocardiogram – focus assessed transthoracic echocardiography (FATE).
- Mixed venous oxygen saturation via pulmonary artery catheter (rarely indicated in damage control).
- Minimally invasive cardiac output estimation via arterial line.

Monitoring of a bispectral index (BIS) may prevent awareness during trauma anaesthesia, although BIS responses to ketamine administration are atypical and can be paradoxical.

Monitoring urine output may give some indication of the volume status. Due consideration should be given to insertion of a urine catheter in the case of suspected urethra injury.

Temperature monitoring is essential in trauma management. Intraoperative normothermia is an important quality performance measure for patients undergoing surgery as it should be in trauma management.

19.5 **ANAESTHESIA INDUCTION IN HYPOVOLAEMIC SHOCK**

19.5.1 **Introduction**

Anaesthetizing a severely injured patient requires a thorough knowledge of the medications used and their altered pharmacokinetics and pharmacodynamics in the hypovolemic, acidotic and hypothermia trauma patient. The principal goal of anaesthesia for trauma patients is to provide analgesia, unconsciousness and amnesia and eventually muscle relaxation without further deteriorating the deranged physiology and hemodynamic situation. In traumatic brain injury, systolic blood pressure <90 mm Hg and PaO_2 <60 mm Hg are independently associated with increased morbidity and mortality.

The pharmacokinetics (absorption, distribution, metabolism and elimination) change significantly with hypovolemic shock. The severely injured patient is in a condition of increased sympathetic tone in attempts to redistribute the circulation to brain and heart. In shock, the body becomes the equivalent of a single compartment model, a blood-brain circuit, at the expense of the perfusion of gut, liver, kidneys and muscles. Intravenous drugs will be almost instantaneously distributed to heart and brain, resulting in more rapid-onset, higher brain concentrations and more profound effects. Further, many anaesthesia induction agents show a high protein binding. Hence, in hypovolemic shock and especially after fluid resuscitation, reduced plasma protein binding leads to increased availability of free drug

with higher effect site concentration and concomitantly increased adverse haemodynamic effects.

Anaerobic metabolism and metabolic acidosis will alter the distribution of ionizable drugs, leading to enhanced brain concentration. Furthermore, in shock, hepatic and renal blood flow is markedly decreased, impairing the intrinsic metabolic capacity leading ultimately to an increase in the free fraction of drugs and prolonged action. Drugs with a high hepatic extraction rate, such as propofol, ketamine, and morphine and synthetic opioids, will show a prolonged duration of action.

19.5.2 **Drugs for Anaesthesia Induction**

The effect site equilibration constant, cited as t½Keo, represents the time necessary for the administered drug to reach an appropriate anaesthetic concentration in the brain. The longer the t½Keo of a drug, the higher the initial plasma concentration needed to achieve a rapid anaesthetic concentration. Hence, intravenous anaesthetic agents with the shortest t½Keo are generally best suited for a rapid induction in the severely injured, hypovolaemic patient (Table 19.2).

Table 19.2 Effects of Anaesthetic Induction Agents

Induction Agent	Effector Site Equilibration (t½Keo)	Haemodynamic Effects	Comments
Propofol	≤20 min	↑ HR unchanged (1) Cardiac output Blood pressure Laryngeal reflexes Vagotonic	Poorly suited for rapid induction in haemodynamic compromise Potential increase in intracranial pressure outweighed maintenance of haemodynamics
Ketamine	±2 min	Heart rate Cardiac output Blood pressure Sympathomimetic	Minimal dose adjustment needed in hypovolaemic shock
Etomidate	±2.5 min	Cardiac output Blood pressure Steroid synthesis Heart rate Inotropy Laryngeal reflexes	Possible adrenocortical suppression
Thiopental	±1.5 min	Vasodilatation	Dose reduction required, ideally <3 mg/kg
Benzodiazepines	±9 min	Cardiac output SVR Sympathetic tone|	Time to reach effector site is slow

Commonly used anaesthetic drugs have a direct depressant effect on the cardiovascular system, inhibit compensatory mechanisms and carry a high risk to further deteriorate the haemodynamic status of trauma patients. Subsequent positive pressure ventilation will impair venous return and contribute to further haemodynamic impairment. Recognition of masked hypovolemia and an accurate estimation of its extent are crucial in the choice of type and dose of anaesthetic drugs.

For induction of general anaesthesia, the most commonly used drugs include ketamine, thiopental, etomidate, midazolam and propofol. For the choice of the most suited induction agent, the patient's physiology, comorbidities and the anaesthetist's experience should be taken into consideration. All anaesthetic induction agents can be vasodepressors and have potential to cause hypotension. The skill and experience of the anaesthetist are the most important determinants for a good outcome. Short-term use of a vasopressor can reverse vasodepressor effects but it must be emphasized that continued need for vasopressors in the trauma patient population is associated with poor outcomes.

19.5.2.1 PROPOFOL

Propofol has a long t1/2Keo of up to 20 minutes, indicating that for rapid induction a higher initial dose is required. However, in shocked patients, propofol shows an increased end-organ sensitivity (e.g. lower C50) and a slower intercompartmental clearance. Haemorrhagic shock has shown shift of the concentration/effect relationship to the left, demonstrating a 2.7-fold decrease in the effect site concentration required to achieve 50 per cent of the maximal effect in the BIS scale. In shock, potency of propofol is increased, and the dose required to reach effect site concentration is 5.4-fold reduced. Therefore, rapid induction can be performed with propofol, but a high dose is required in patients exhibiting increased organ sensitivity. This, in view of the important concomitant negative effects on haemodynamics, makes propofol a poor choice for the trauma setting, but if used, dose reduction to approximately one-third is highly recommended.

19.5.2.2 KETAMINE

Ketamine is a highly lipid-soluble drug. At a physiologic pH, almost 50 per cent is dissociated and only 12 per cent is bound to plasma proteins. This ensures a rapid blood-brain equilibration and fast clinical onset.

Ketamine is the least likely agent to cause cardiovascular depressant effects. Its direct negative inotrope effect is counteracted by a stimulatory effect on the cardiovascular system, probably by a centrally mediated sympathetic response and inhibition of noradrenaline re-uptake. In the severely shocked patient with a state of catecholamine exhaustion or resistance to further catecholamine effect, the direct effects of ketamine on myocardial depression may outweigh the indirect sympathetic effects and haemodynamic collapse may still occur. A reduction of the induction dose to 0.25 to 0.5 mg/kg i.v. may be indicated. Ketamine has further shown to provide anti-inflammatory proprieties; however its clinical impact in trauma patients remains to be determined. Ketamine has reportedly both raised and lowered intracranial pressure. In traumatic brain injury, the cerebral autoregulation is impaired and the CBF is directly depending on the cerebral perfusion pressure. Maintenance of hemodynamic stability may therefore outweigh potential risks. Further, ketamine reduces cerebral oxygen consumption' and the cerebral vasodilatation as observed in spontaneously breathing patients may be reduced by controlled ventilation.

19.5.2.3 ETOMIDATE

Haemorrhagic shock produces minimal changes in the pharmacokinetics and pharmacodynamics of etomidate. Etomidate preserves the pressor response to intubation, and shock affects only minimally its ability to reach the effector site rapidly. Its central and peripheral volumes are only lightly decreased in acute hypovolemia, increasing its blood levels by about 20 per cent. Therefore, unlike as with other hypnotics, only minimal adjustments in induction dose are required to achieve the same drug effect in haemorrhagic shock. As compared to propofol, no increased drug sensitivity had been demonstrated for etomidate. These points provide etomidate with a good safety profile as an induction agent in trauma patients.

However, in many countries etomidate was withdrawn after the CORTICUS study, which showed that in septic patients even a single dose may suppress the corticoadrenal axis for up to 67 hours. In the non-septic trauma patients, suppression of steroid synthesis does not seem to be associated with worse outcome as increased on mortality or prolonged length of stay.

19.5.2.4 THIOPENTAL

Thiopental exhibits several desirable properties in the shocked patient as a short t1/2 Keo (1.5 min) and a tendency to preserve autonomic responsiveness as a reflex tachycardia or the pressor response to laryngoscopy. However, its usefulness in the setting of hypovolemic shock is compromised by the important negative inotropy and arteriolar vasodilation, leading to severe hypotension in shocked patients. Doses must therefore be carefully adapted to values if possible below a range of 3 mg/kg.

19.5.2.5 MIDAZOLAM

Midazolam in induction dose has shown to significantly decrease plasma norepinephrine concentration and alters baroreflex control of the heart rate. It also causes reduction of systemic vascular resistance and left ventricular stroke work index. Hence, in hypovolemic patients, it may further decrease blood pressure and prevent compensatory tachycardia. Additionally, midazolam is highly protein bound, inhibiting a rapid entry into the brain effector site. The half-life for closure of its imidazol-ring, which enhances lipid solubility and brain entry, is long (10 min), making this agent of little value for rapid sequence induction (RSI).

There is no hard outcome evidence supporting one agent over the other, but whatever agent is chosen, induction doses must be adapted to the patient's physiology, and most often reduced. Many use a combination of induction drugs combining their different effects. Normalization of haemodynamic parameters with aggressive fluid resuscitation prior to induction has not proven to completely reverse the increase in induction drug potency.

Maintenance of anaesthesia during damage control procedures in the haemodynamically compromised patient requires a careful choice and titration of drugs. Perioperative awareness is well recognized during emergency anaesthesia, often as a consequence of dose reduction. A comparison of patients treated by ketamine induction and maintenance with volatiles versus no maintenance drug showed a perioperative awareness rate of 11 per cent versus 43 per cent. The choice of the optimal maintenance drug is influenced by the patient's physiology and his or her injury profile. For traumatic brain injury and trauma to the spinal cord, intravenous anaesthesia as with propofol is recommended, while as in other settings inhalational anaesthesia might be more suited. A BIS measure might be a valuable help in preventing awareness in the severely shocked patient with altered dose requirements.

19.6 BATTLEFIELD ANAESTHESIA

Battlefield anaesthesia is both an anaesthetic as well as an operational problem (see also Chapter 18). It is not an exclusive medical problem. It occurs in an environment that both provides the platform from which you treat and influences the decision making.

Battlefield anaesthesia presents many challenges, including the need to maintain airway control, hypothermia of the casualty, restricted drug availability, lack of supplementary oxygen and the possible requirement for prolonged post-operative mechanical ventilation. Mass casualty situations are also a constant possibility in the military arena. Surgery requires both adequate analgesia and anaesthesia. No single agent can provide both an appropriate level of anaesthesia and analgesia, hence a combination of drugs and techniques is required. The choices of anaesthetic are narrowed in austere conditions; these are limited to general anaesthesia (either intravenous or inhalational), regional anaesthesia or none at all. For surgical exploration of body cavities, general anaesthesia is most frequently chosen, while a regional anaesthetic may be more appropriate for injuries of the extremities or perineum. In the field, RSI is the norm, using fast-acting hypnotic and neuromuscular blocking agents to facilitate rapid airway control. In the absence or limitation of supplemental oxygen supplies, RSI becomes even more crucial as pre-oxygenation of the patient's lungs is often not possible. There are several RSI cocktails used in the pre-hospital setting, most using a combination of induction agent paralyzing agent and analgesia. Sedation, amnesia and analgesia can then be maintained with intravenous agents such as ketamine, benzodiazepines and opiates.

For long procedures or surgical sites involving the abdomen or thorax, a combinaetion anaesthetic that includes an inhalation agent such as isoflurane may be used. British surgical teams use a portable 'tri-service apparatus' that does not require a compressed gas source, and they have gained much experience with this technique of field anaesthesia. This 'draw-over' type of vaporizer is currently also in use by several other countries in austere settings. The draw-over configuration places the ventilator distal to the vaporizer, entraining ambient air and vapour across the vaporizer in the same manner as the spontaneously breathing patient.

Regional anaesthesia remains an important option in battlefield anaesthesia, as it provides both patient comfort and surgical analgesia, while maintaining patient consciousness and spontaneous ventilation. With the relatively large number of extremity wounds in modern conflicts, and certainly in the mass casualty setting with a limited anaesthesia capability, regional aesthetic techniques should not be overlooked. Continuous infusion nerve blocks provide excellent analgesia for post-operative casualties during evacuation.

19.6.1 Damage Control Anaesthesia in the Military Setting

Anaesthesia for 'damage control' procedures and major cavity injury is really a fusion of continuing resuscitation and critical care. This requires optimization of haemodynamic status, re-warming of the casualty and pain relief. One of the biggest challenges will be reversing the hypothermia that is almost universal in haemorrhagic patients in these conditions. As well as warming all intravenous fluids and ventilator circuits, an active re-warming device will be required. If a return to the operating theatre for more definitive surgery is not planned in the forward location, critical care must be maintained throughout the aeromedical evacuation.

19.6.2 Battlefield Analgesia

Relief of pain is an important consideration for both the wounded and the military caregiver. Provision of effective analgesia is humane but also attenuates the adverse pathophysiological responses to pain, and is likely to aid evacuation from the battlefield and maintain morale. Analgesia may be given at self- and buddy-aid levels; protocols to guide medical and paramedical staff in the provision of safe and effective analgesia are available.

Analgesia methods used in recent conflicts include:

- Simple non-pharmacological.
- Reassurance.
- Splinting of fractures.
- Cooling of burns.
- Oral analgesics.
  - · Non-steroidal anti-inflammatory drugs.
  - · Paracetamol.
- Nerve blocks and infiltration of local anaesthesia.
- Intramuscular and intravenous opiates.

- Fentanyl lollipops.
- Methods under development – intranasal, ketamine, fentanyl and inhalation analgesics (e.g. methoxyflurane inhalation).

REFERENCES

1. Moore FA, McKinley BA, Moore EE: The next generation in shock resuscitation. *Lancet*. 2004;363(9425):1988–1996.
2. Holcomb JB, Jenkins D, Rhee P, et al. Damage control resuscitation: directly addressing the early coagulopathy of trauma. *J Trauma*. 2007;62(2):307–310.
3. Kasotakis G, Sideris A, Yang Y, et al. Inflammation, host response to injury. I: Aggressive early crystalloid resuscitation adversely affects outcomes in adult blunt trauma patients: an analysis of the Glue Grant database. *J Trauma Acute Care Surg*. 2013;74(5):1215–1221; discussion 1221–1222.
4. Cannon WB. The preventive treatment of wound shock. *J Am Med Assoc* 1918; 70: 618–21.
5. Zarychanski R, Abou-Setta AM, Turgeon AF, et al. Association of hydroxyethyl starch administration with mortality and acute kidney injury in critically ill patients requiring volume resuscitation: a systematic review and meta-analysis. *JAMA*. 2013;309(7):678–688.
6. Stadlbauer KH, Wagner-Berger HG, Raedler C, et al. Vasopressin, but not fluid resuscitation, enhances survival in a liver trauma model with uncontrolled and otherwise lethal hemorrhagic shock in pigs. *Anesthesiology*. 2003;98(3):699–704.
7. Sperry JL, Minei JP, Frankel HL, et al. Early use of vasopressors after injury: caution before constriction. *J Trauma*. 2008;64(1):9–14.
8. Spahn DR, Bouillon B, Cerny V, et al. Management of bleeding and coagulopathy following major trauma: an updated European guideline. *Crit Care*. 2013;17(2):R76.
9. Gunter OL, Jr., Au BK, Isbell JM, Mowery NT, Young PP, Cotton BA. Optimising outcomes in damage control resuscitation: identifying blood product ratios associated with improved survival. *J Trauma*. 2007;65(3):527–534.
10. Holcomb JB, Wade CE, Michalek JE, et al. Increased plasma and platelet to red blood cell ratios improves outcome in 466 massively transfused civilian trauma patients. *Ann Surg*. 2008;248(3):447–458.
11. Kozar RA, Peng Z, Zhang R, et al. Plasma restoration of endothelial glycocalyx in a rodent model of hemorrhagic shock. *Anesth Analg*. 2011;112(6):1289–1295.

12. Brohi K, Singh J, Heron M, Coats T. Acute traumatic coagulopathy. *J Trauma*. 2003;54(6):1127–1130.

13. Brohi K, Cohen MJ, Ganter MT, et al. Acute traumatic coagulopathy: initiated by hypoperfusion: modulated through the protein C pathway? *Ann Surg*. 2007;245(5):812–818.

14. Mutschler M, Nienaber U, Brockamp T, et al. Renaissance of base deficit for the initial assessment of trauma patients: a base deficit-based classification for hypovolemic shock developed on data from 16,305 patients derived from the TraumaRegister DGU®. *Crit Care*. 2013;17(2):R42.

15. Cotton BA, Au BK, Nunez TC, Gunter OL, Robertson AM, Young PP. Predefined massive transfusion protocols are associated with a reduction in organ failure and postinjury complications. *J Trauma*. 2009;66(1):41–48; discussion 48–49.

16. Hess JR, Holcomb JB, Hoyt DB. Damage control resuscitation: the need for specific blood products to treat the coagulopathy of trauma. *Transfusion*. 2006;46(5):685–6.

17. Stensballe J, Ostrowski ST, Johansson P. Viscoelastic guide to resuscitation. *Curr Opin Anesthesiol*. 2014;27:212–218.

18. Shakur H, Roberts I, Bautista R, et al. Effects of tranexamic acid on death, vascular occlusive events, and blood transfusion in trauma patients with significant haemorrhage (CRASH-2): a randomised, placebo-controlled trial. *Lancet*. 2010;376(9734):23–32.

19. Moore HB, Moore EE, Gonzales E, et al. Hyprinofibrinolysis, physiologic fibrinolysis, and fibrinolysis shutdown: the spectrum of post injury fibrinolysis and relevance to antifibrinolytic therapy. *J Trauma Acute Care Surg*. 2014;77(6):811–817.

Appendices

Appendix A
Trauma Systems

A.1 INTRODUCTION

Care of the injured patient has been fundamental to the practice of medicine since recorded history. The word 'trauma' derives from the Greek meaning 'bodily injury'. The first trauma centres were used to care for wounded soldiers in Napoleon's armies, and the first modern trauma centre was the Birmingham Accident Hospital in the United Kingdom, opened in 1944 in what was then the Queen's Hospital.

The lessons learned in successive military conflicts have advanced our knowledge of care of the injured patient. The Korean conflict and the Vietnam War established the concept of minimizing the time from injury to definitive care. The extension of this concept to the management of civilian trauma led to the evolution from the 1970s onwards of today's trauma systems. The Middle East and Afghan conflicts in the last decade resulted in massive progress in the sphere of military trauma care, with significant enhancement in civilian care as well. For the first time, prospective high-quality research has taken place in the conflict situation.

A.2 INCLUSIVE TRAUMA SYSTEM

In principle, a hospital that provides acute care for the severely injured patient (a trauma centre) should be a key component of a system that encompasses all aspects and phases of care, from prevention and education to pre-hospital care, to acute care, and through to rehabilitation (Figure A.1). The initial trauma systems did not consider the non-trauma centre hospitals, even though they cared for the majority of patients, those who were

Figure A.1 The inclusive trauma system.

less severely injured. Instead, these trauma systems were driven by the major or severely injured trauma patient who required immediate treatment, optimally at a trauma centre.

A system must be fully integrated into the emergency medical services (EMS) system and must meet the needs of all the patients requiring acute care for injury, regardless of severity of injury, geographical location and population density. The trauma centre remains an essential component, but the system recognizes the necessity for other healthcare facilities. The goal of the most cost-effective trauma care is to match the facility's resources with the needs of the patient.

The goal of the system is to match the regional needs and facilities with the resources and patient care loads required.

A.3 COMPONENTS OF AN INCLUSIVE TRAUMA SYSTEM

The structure of a trauma care system involves a number of components and providers, each of which must be adapted to a specific environment. These components and providers, graphically represented in Figure A.2, are:

- Administrative components.
  · Leadership.
  · System development.
  · Legislation.
  · Finances.
- Operational and clinical components.
- Injury prevention and control.
- Human resources – workforce resources.
- Education.
- Pre-hospital care – EMS system.
- Ambulance and non-transporting guidelines.
  · Communications systems.
  · Emergency disaster preparedness plan.
- Definitive care facilities.
  · Trauma care facilities.
  · Interfacility transfer.
  · Medical rehabilitation.
- Information systems.
- Evaluation.
- Research.

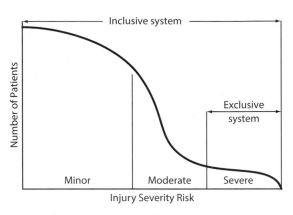

Figure A.2 The components of an inclusive trauma system.

A.3.1 Administration

The system requires administrative leadership, authority, planning and development, legislation and finances. Together, these components form an outer sphere of stability that is vital for the continuation of activities directly related to patient care. The diversity of the population, as defined by the environment (urban or rural) or by special segments of the population (the young or the elderly), must be addressed by the system.

A.3.2 Prevention

Prevention reduces the actual incidence of injury and is cost-efficient for the system and for society. Injury prevention is achieved through public education, legislation and environmental modification.

A.3.3 Public Education

Public education leads to a change in behaviour and thus minimizes injury exposure. Education includes the proper recognition of injury and efficient access to the EMS system. These components stimulate the necessary political and legislative activity to establish legal authority, leadership and system changes.

The development of a system is a major challenge for any community. The concept of centralizing trauma care creates potential political and economic problems, since the normal flow of patients might be altered by trauma triage protocols. Trauma systems, by their nature, will direct the care of the most critically injured patients to a limited number of designated 'trauma centres'. The trauma system will only succeed if all parties are involved in the initial planning, development and implementation.

It is crucial that doctors, and especially surgeons, are involved in the system-planning process. They should help to establish standards of care for all clinical components and participate in planning, verification, performance improvement and system evaluation.

A.4 MANAGEMENT OF THE INJURED PATIENT WITHIN A SYSTEM

Once the injury has been identified, the system must ensure easy access and an appropriate response at the scene of injury. The system must assign responsibility and authority for care and triage decisions made prior to trauma centre access. Triage guidelines must be accepted by all providers and used to determine which patients require access to trauma centre care. This coordination requires direct communication between pre-hospital care providers, medical direction and the trauma facility.

The trauma centre, which serves as the definitive specialized care facility, is a key component of the system, and is different from other hospitals within the system in that it guarantees immediate availability of *all* the specialities necessary for the assessment and management of the patient with multiple injuries. These centres need to be integrated into the other components of the system to allow the best match of resources with the patients' needs. The system coordinates care between all levels of the facility, so that prompt and efficient integration of hospital and resources can take place according to patient need.

Access to rehabilitation services, first in the acute care hospital and then in more specialized rehabilitation facilities, is an integral part of the total management of the patient. It is important that the patients be returned to their communities when appropriate.

A.5 STEPS IN ORGANIZING A SYSTEM

A.5.1 Public Support

Public support is necessary for the enabling and necessary legislation to take place. The process takes place as follows:

- Identification of the need.
- Establishment of a patient database to assist with need and resource assessment.

- Analysis to determine the resources available.
- Resource assessment, formulated to identify the current capabilities of the system.
- Highlighting of deficiencies and formulation of solutions.

A.5.2 Legal Authority

This is established once the need for a system has been demonstrated. Legislation will be required to establish a lead agency with a strong oversight or an advisory body composed of healthcare, public and medical representatives. This agency will develop the criteria for the system, regulate and direct pre-hospital care, establish pre-hospital triage, ensure medical direction, designate the proper facilities to render care, establish a trauma registry and establish performance improvement programmes.

A.5.3 Establish Criteria for Optimal Care

These must be established by the lead authority in conjunction with health and medical professionals. The adoption of system-wide standards is integral to the success of any system.

A.5.4 Designation of Trauma Centres

This takes place through a public process directed by the lead agency. Consideration must be given to the role of all acute care facilities within the particular region. Representatives from all these facilities must be involved in the planning process.

The number of trauma centres should be limited to the number required (based on the established need) for the patient population at risk of major injury. Having too many trauma centres may weaken the system by diluting the workload, thus reducing the experience for training, and will unnecessarily consume resources that are not fully utilized.

Development of a system requires that all the principal players be involved from the beginning. There must be agreement about the minimal data that will be contributed by *all* acute care facilities. Without the data from the hospitals managing the less severely injured, the data will be incomplete, and skewed toward major injury.

A.5.5 **System Evaluation**

Trauma systems are complex organizational structures with evolving methods and standards of care. It is necessary to have a mechanism for ongoing evaluation, based on:

- Self-monitoring.
- External evaluation.

A.6 **RESULTS AND STUDIES**

The Skamania conference was held in July 1998, with the purpose of evaluating the evidence regarding the efficacy of trauma systems. During the conference, the evidence was divided into three categories: that resulting from panel studies, registry comparisons and population-based research.

A.6.1 **Panel Review**

An overview of panel studies was presented at the Skamania conference. The critique of panel reviews is that they vary widely, and interrater reliability has been very low in some studies. Furthermore, autopsy results alone are inadequate, and panel studies vary regarding the process of review and the rules used to come to a final judgement. In general, all panel studies were classified as weak class III evidence. Nevertheless, MacKenzie came to the conclusion that when all panel studies are considered collectively, they do provide some face validity and support of the hypothesis that treatment at a trauma center versus a non-trauma center is associated with fewer inappropriate deaths and possibly disabilities.

A.6.2 **Registry Study**

Jurkovich and Mock reported on the evidence provided by trauma registries in assessing overall effectiveness. They concluded fairly emphatically that this was not class I evidence, but that it was probably better than a panel study. Their critique of trauma registries included the following six items: data are often missing, miscodings occur, there may be interrater reliability factors, the national norms are not population based, there is less detail about the causes of death and they do not take into account prehospital deaths. A consensus of the participants at the Skamania conference concluded that registry studies were better than panel studies but not as good as population studies.

A.6.3 **Population-based Studies**

Populated-based studies probably also fall into class II evidence. They are not prospective randomized trials, but, because of nature of the population-based evidence, they cover all aspects of trauma care, including pre-hospital, hospital and rehabilitative. A critique of the population-based studies pointed out that there are a limited number of clinical variables, and it is difficult to adjust for severity of injury and physiological dysfunction. There are other problems, although these probably apply to all studies, including secular trends, observational issues and problems with longitudinal population mortality studies.

A.7 **SUMMARY**

Although there are difficulties with all three types of study, each may also offer advantages to various communities and regions. All three types may also influence health policy, and all can be used pre- and post-trauma system start-up. There was consensus at the Skamania conference that the evaluation of trauma systems should be extended to include an economic evaluation and assessment of quality-adjusted life-years.

RECOMMENDED READING

American College of Surgeons. Regional trauma system: optimal elements, integration, and assessment. In: Committee on Trauma. *Resources for Optimal Care of the Injured Patient 2015 (Orange Book),* 6th ed. Chicago, IL: American College of Surgeons; 2015. http://www.facs.org. Accessed December 2014.

Coimbra R, Hoyt DB, Bansal V. Trauma systems, triage, and transport. In: Mattox KL, Moore EE, Feliciano DV, eds. *Trauma,* 7th ed. New York, NY: McGraw-Hill; 2013:54–76.

Jurkovich GJ, Mock C. Systematic review of trauma system effectiveness based on registry comparisons. *J Trauma.* 1999;47(Suppl.):S46–S55.

MacKenzie EJ, Rivara FP, Jurkovich GJ. A national evaluation of the effect of trauma-center care on mortality. *N Engl J Med.* 2006;354(4):366–378.

MacKenzie EJ, Weir S, Rivara FP, et al. The value of trauma center care. *J Trauma.* 2010;69(1):1–10.

Peterson TD, Mello MJ, Broderick KB, et al. Trauma care systems 2003 (updated February 10, 2007). *American College of Emergency Physicians: Guidelines for Trauma Care Systems.* http://www.acep.org. Accessed December 2014.

Pruitt BA. Trauma systems: Evidence, research, action. The Skamania symposium 1998. *J Trauma.* 1999. Supplement 47 no 3.

Appendix B
Trauma Scores and Scoring Systems

B.1 INTRODUCTION

Estimates of the severity of injury or illness are fundamental to the practice of medicine. The earliest known medical text, the Smith Papyrus, classified injuries into three grades: treatable, contentious and untreatable.

Modern trauma scoring methodology uses a combination of an assessment of the severity of anatomical injury with a quantification of the degree of physiological derangement to arrive at scores that correlate with clinical outcomes.

Trauma scoring systems are designed to facilitate pre-hospital triage, identify trauma patients suitable for quality assurance audit, allow an accurate comparison of different trauma populations and organize and improve trauma systems.

In principle, scoring systems can be divided into:

- Physiological scoring systems, based on the body's response to injury.
- Anatomical scoring systems, based on the physical injury that has occurred.
- Scoring systems based on both anatomical injury description and physiological response.
- Outcome analysis systems, based on the result after recovery.

B.2 PHYSIOLOGICAL SCORING SYSTEMS

B.2.1 Glasgow Coma Scale (GCS)

The Glasgow Coma Scale (GCS)[1], devised in 1974, was one of the first numerical scoring systems (Table B.1). The GCS has been incorporated into many later scoring systems, emphasizing the importance of head injury as a triage and prognostic indicator.

Table B.1 Glasgow Coma Scale

Parameter	Response	Score
Eye opening	Nil	1
	To pain	2
	To speech	3
	Spontaneously	4
Motor response	Nil	1
	Extensor	2
	Flexor	3
	Withdrawal	4
	Localizing	5
	Obeys command	6
Verbal response	Nil	1
	Groans	2
	Words	3
	Confused	4
	Orientated	5

B.2.2 Paediatric Trauma Score (PTS)

The Paediatric Trauma Score (PTS)[2] (Table B.2) has been designed to facilitate triage of children. The PTS is the sum of six scores, and values range from –6 to 12, with a PTS of 8 or less being recommended as the trigger to send the child to a trauma centre. The PTS has been shown to accurately predict risk for severe injury or mortality but is not significantly more accurate than the RTS and is a great deal more difficult to measure.

B.2.3 Revised Trauma Score (RTS)

Introduced by Champion et al., the Revised Trauma Score (RTS)[3] evaluates blood pressure, the GCS and the

Table B.2 Paediatric Trauma Score (PTS)

Clinical Parameter	Category	Score
Size (kg)	>20	2
	10–20	1
	<10	−1
Airway	Normal	2
	Maintainable	1
	Unmaintainable	−1
Systolic blood pressure (mm Hg)	>90	2
	50–90	1
	<50	−1
Central nervous system	Awake	2
	Obtunded/decreased LOC	1
	Coma/decerebrate	−1
Open wound	None	2
	Minor	1
	Major/penetrating	
Skeletal	None	2
	Closed fracture	1
	Open/multiple fractures	−1

Note: The values for the six parameters are summed to give the overall PTS. LOC, level of consciousness.

Table B.3 Revised Trauma Score (RTS)

Clinical Parameter	Category	Score	× Weight
Respiratory rate (breaths per minute)	10–29	4	0.2908
	>29	3	
	6–9	2	
	1–5	1	
	0	0	
Systolic blood pressure	>89	4	0.7326
	76–89	3	
	50–75	2	
	1–49	1	
	0	0	
Glasgow Coma Scale score	13–15	4	0.9368
	9–12	3	
	6–8	2	
	4–5	1	
	3	0	

Note: The values for the three parameters are summed to give the triage-RTS. Weighted values are summed for the RTS.

respiratory rate to provide a scored physiological assessment of the patient.

The RTS can be used for field triage, and enables prehospital and emergency care personnel to decide which patients should receive the specialized care of a trauma unit. An RTS score of 11 or less is suggested as the triage point for patients requiring at least level 2 trauma centre status (surgical facilities, 24-hour X-ray, etc.). An RTS of 10 or less carries a mortality of up to 30 per cent, and these patients should be moved to a level 1 institution.

The difference between RTS on arrival and best RTS after resuscitation will give a reasonably clear picture of the prognosis. By convention, the RTS on admission is the one documented.

The RTS (non-triage) is designed for retrospective outcome analysis. Weighted coefficients are used, which are derived from trauma patient populations, and provide a more accurate outcome prediction than the raw RTS (Table B.3). Since a severe head injury carries a poorer prognosis than a severe respiratory injury, the weighting is therefore heavier. The RTS thus varies from 0 (worst) to 7.8408 (best). The RTS is the most widely used physiological scoring system in the trauma literature.

B.2.4 Acute Physiologic and Chronic Health Evaluation II: APACHE II

The APACHE II score[4] is used to evaluate mortality, and prognosis in ICU patients.

Calculation is based on a number of physiological and clinical comorbidity parameters, as well as age[5]. Each parameter can score 0 points, considered as normal physiology, to a maximum of 4 points (Table B.4).

Mortality interpretation is based on overall score (Table B.5).

B.3 ANATOMICAL SCORING SYSTEMS

B.3.1 Abbreviated Injury Scale (AIS)

The Abbreviated Injury Scale (AIS)[6] is an anatomically based, consensus-derived, global severity-based scoring system that classifies each injury by body region according to its relative importance on a six-point ordinal scale.

The AIS was developed in 1971 as a system to describe the severity of injury throughout the body. The AIS has been periodically upgraded, and AIS-2005 (update 2008) is currently in use.

Table B.4 APACHE II Scoring

Input	Measured	Measured	Points
Temperature (°C)	36–38°		0
	34.0–35.9°	38–38.5°	1
	32–33.9°	38.5–39°	2
	30–31.9°	39–40.9°	3
	≤29.9°	≥41°	4
Heart rate	70–109		0
	—	—	1
	55–69	110–139	2
	40–54	140–179	3
	<40	≥180	4
Mean arterial pressure (mm Hg)	70–109		0
			1
	50–69	110–129	2
		130–159	3
	≤49	≥159	4
Respiratory rate (b.p.m.)	12–24		0
	10–11	25–34	1
	6–9	35–49	2
	—		3
	≤5	≥50	4
A-aPO$_2$ (FiO$_2$ >50%) or PaO$_2$ (FiO$_2$ <50%) (mm Hg)	<200 or PaO$_2$ > 70		0
	—	PaO$_2$ 61–70	1
	200–349	—	2
	350–499	PaO$_2$ 55–60	3
	>500	PaO$_2$ < 55	4
Arterial pH or HCO$_3$ (mmol/L)	7.33–7.49/22–31.9		0
	—	7.5–7.59/32–40.9	1
	7.25–7.32/18–21.9	—	2
	7.15–7.24/15–17.9	7.6–7.69/41–51.9	3
	<7.15/<15	≥7.7/>52	4
Serum Na$^+$ (mmol/L)	130–149		0
	—	150–154	1
	120–129	155–159	2
	111–119	160–179	3
	<110	>180	4
Serum K$^+$ (mmol/L)	3.5–5.4		0
	3–3.4	5.5–5.9	1
	2.5–2.9	—	2
	—	6–6.9	3
	<2.5	≥7	4

Input	Measured	Measured	Points
Haematocrit (%)	30–45.9		0
	—	46–49.9	1
	20–29.9	50–59.9	2
	—	—	3
	<20	>60	4
White cell count (×10^3 cells/mm^3)	3–14.9		0
	—	15–19.9	1
	1–2.9	20–39.9	2
	—	—	3
	<1	40	4
Glasgow Coma Scale	15		0
	Subtract actual GCS from 15		0–15
	e.g. GCS 9/15 = 6 points		
Age (years)	≤44 years		0
			1
	45–54		2
	55–64		3
	65–74		4
	≥75		5
			6
Chronic health problems	None		0
	Acute renal failure		1
	Yes + elective surgery		+2
	Yes but not post-operative		+5
	Yes + emergency surgery		+6

In AIS 2005, each injury is assigned a six-digit unique numerical identifier, to the left of the decimal point. This in known as the 'pre-dot' code. There is an additional single digit to the right of the code (the 'post-dot' code), which is the AIS severity code The AIS grades each injury by severity from 1 (least severe) to 5 (critical: survival uncertain). A score of 6 is given to certain injuries termed 'maximal (currently untreatable/unsurvivable)'.

The AIS manual is divided, for ease of reference, into nine different sections based on anatomy. All injuries therefore carry a unique code that can be used for classification, for indexing in trauma registry databases and for severity.

Table B.5 Mortality Based on APACHE II Scores

APACHE II Score: Approximate Mortality Interpretation

Score	Non-operative	Post-operative
0–4	4%	1%
5–9	8%	3%
10–14	15%	7%
15–19	24%	12%
20–24	40%	30%
25–29	55%	35%
30–34	73%	73%
35–100	85%	88%

B.3.2 The Injury Severity Score (ISS)

In 1974, Baker et al. created the Injury Severity Score (ISS)[7] to relate AIS scores to patient outcomes. ISS body regions are listed in Table B.6.

The ISS is calculated by summing the square of the highest AIS scores in the three most severely injured regions. ISS scores range from 1 to 75 (since the highest AIS score for any region is 5). By convention, an AIS score of 6 (defined as a non-survivable injury) for any region becomes an ISS of 75.

The ISS only considers the single most serious injury in each region, ignoring the contribution of injury to other organs within the same region. Diverse injuries may have identical ISS scores but markedly different survival probabilities (an ISS of 25 may be obtained with isolated severe head injury or by a combination of lesser injuries across different regions). In addition, the ISS does not have the power to discriminate between the impact of similarly scored injuries to different organs, and therefore cannot identify, for example, the different impact of cerebral injury over injury to other organ systems.

Table B.6 Injury Severity Score Body Regions

Number	Region
1	Head and neck
2	Face
3	Thorax
4	Abdomen/pelvic contents
5	Extremities
6	External/skin/general

B.3.3 The New Injury Severity Score (NISS)

In response to these limitations, the ISS was modified in 1997 to become the New Injury Severity Score (NISS)[8]. NISS is calculated in the same way as ISS, but takes the three most severe injuries (i.e. the three highest AIS scores regardless of body region). The NISS is then the simple sum of the squares of these three body regions.

The NISS is able to predict survival outcomes better than the ISS. In a separate study, the NISS yielded better separation between patients with and without multiple organ failure and showed that the NISS is superior to the ISS in the prediction of multiple organ failure[9]. Although the proponents of the NISS proclaim its superiority, its use is not yet widespread.

B.3.4 Anatomic Profile (AP)

The Anatomic Profile Score (APS)[10] was introduced in 1990 to overcome some of the limitations of the ISS. In contrast to ISS, the APS allows the inclusion of more than one serious body injury per region and takes into account the primacy of central nervous system and torso injury over other injuries. The AIS scoring is used, but four values are used for injury characterization, roughly weighting the body regions. Serious trauma to the brain and spinal cord, anterior neck and chest, and all remaining injuries constitute three of the four values. The fourth value is a summary of all the remaining non-serious injuries. The APS score is the square root of the sum of the squares of all the AIS scores in a region, thus enabling the impact of multiple injuries within that region to be recognized. Component values for the four regions are summed to constitute the APS score.

A modified APS (mAPS) has recently been introduced, which is a four-number characterization of injury. The four component scores are the maximum AIS score and the square root of the sum of the squares of all AIS values for serious injury (AIS $\geq$3) in specified body regions (Table B.7). This leads to an Anatomic Profile Score, the weighted sum of the four mAPS components. The coefficients are derived from logistic regression analysis of admissions to four level-1 trauma centres (the 'controlled sites') in the Major Trauma Outcome Study.

A limitation of the use of AIS-derived scores is their cost. International Classification of Disease (ICD) taxonomy is a standard used by most hospitals and other healthcare providers to classify clinical diagnoses. Computerized mapping of ICD-9CM rubrics into AIS

Table B.7 Component Definitions of the Modified Anatomic Profile Score

Component	Body Region	Abbreviated Injury Scale Severity
mA	Head/brain	3–6
	Spinal cord	3–6
mB	Thorax	3–6
	Front of neck	3–6
mC	All other	3–6

Note: mA, mB and mC scores are derived by taking the square root of the sum of the squares for all injuries defined by each component.

body regions and severity values has been used to compute ISS, AP and NISS scores. Despite limitations, ICD–AIS conversion has been useful in population-based evaluation when AIS scoring from medical records is not possible. Outside North America, the ICD-10 is most commonly used.

B.3.5 **ICD-based Injury Severity Score (ICISS)**

Severity scoring systems also have been directly derived from ICD-coded discharge diagnoses. Most recently, the ICD-9 Severity Score (ICISS)[11] has been proposed, which is derived by multiplying survival risk ratios associated with individual ICD diagnoses. Neural networking has been employed to further improve ICISS accuracy. The ICISS has been shown to be better than ISS and to outperform the Trauma and Injury Severity Score (TRISS) in identifying outcomes and resource utilization. However, modified-AP scores, AP and NISS appear to outperform ICISS in predicting hospital mortality.

There is some confusion over which anatomical scoring system should be used; however, currently, NISS probably should be the system of choice for AIS-based scoring.

B.3.6 **Organ Injury Scaling System**

Organ Injury Scaling (OIS)[12] is a scale of anatomical injury within an organ system or body structure. The goal of OIS is to provide a common language between trauma surgeons and to facilitate research and continuing quality improvement. It is not designed to correlate with patient outcomes. The OIS tables can be found on the American Association for the Surgery of Trauma (AAST) website[12] or at the end of this chapter.

B.3.7 **Penetrating Abdominal Trauma Index (PATI)**

Moore and colleagues facilitated the identification of the patient at high risk of post-operative complications when they developed the Penetrating Abdominal Trauma Index (PATI)[13] scoring system for patients whose only source of injury was penetrating abdominal trauma. A complication risk factor was assigned to each organ system involved and then multiplied by a severity of injury estimate. Each factor was given a value ranging from 1 to 5. The complication risk designation for each organ was based on the reported incidence of post-operative morbidity associated with the particular injury.

The severity of injury was estimated by a simple modification to the AIS, ranging from 1 = minimal injury to 5 = maximal injury. The sum of the individual organ score times the risk factor comprised the final PATI score. If the PATI score is 25 or less, the risk of complications is reduced (and where it is 10 or less, there are no complications), whereas if it is greater than 25, the risks are much higher.

In a group of 114 patients with gunshot wounds to the abdomen Moore et al.[13] showed that a PATI score of more than 25 dramatically increased the risk of postoperative complications (46 per cent of patients with a PATI score of over 25 developed serious post-operative complications, compared with 7 per cent of patients with a PATI of less than 25). Further studies have validated the PATI scoring system.

B.3.8 **Revised Injury Severity Classification (RISC) II**

The first version of this score was derived from the German Trauma Registry DGU (TR-DGU) in 2003[14] and has recently updated in 2014 to RISC II[14,15].

The first version was developed and validated on 2000 patients documented between 1993 and 2000 in the TR-DGU. Eleven different data points were required from a trauma patient: new ISS, head injury, pelvic injury, age, GCS, coagulation, base deficit, haemoglobin, cardiac arrest, shock and mass transfusion. Similar as for the TRISS, the calculated score is transformed into a probability of survival $P(s)$ by the logistic function $P(s) = 1/(1 + e^{-x})$. Comparative analyses showed that the predictive performance of the RISC was better than TRISS since it contained additional predictive variables, such as initial laboratory values on admission. The RISC has been used by the TR-DGU for outcome adjustment in inter-hospital comparisons and scientific analyses since 2003.

However, the original RISC also had some limitations. Missing values were partly replaced by a specific algorithm, but the number of patients who did not receive a RISC prognosis increased to more than 15 per cent in the registry. Furthermore, observed mortality was about 2 per cent lower than the predicted RISC prognosis. Finally, additional prognostic factors had been proposed, based on recent database analyses. Thus, in 2013, an enhanced version of the RISC was developed[15].

The RISC II includes some well-known prognostic factors, like age and blood pressure, some variables already used in the original RISC (such as base deficit, haemoglobin, cardiac arrest) but also new variables like gender, pre-injury ASA, and pupil size and reactivity. It is also interesting to mention that the overall injury severity is no longer described as ISS or NISS, but as AIS severity level of the worst and the second-worst injury (plus head injury). This also allows differentiation between isolated and multiple injuries. If the injury is an isolated one, the AIS level of the second-worst injury is zero, which means that outcome prediction improves (the respective coefficient for the second-worst injury is +0.2).

RISC II attempts a new concept of treating missing values, in that there is no attempt to impute a missing value; however, the values are included in the model. Thus if a certain value is missing it will not have any influence on the outcome prediction. This is seen in Table B.8 where all categories for missing values (indicated by '???') receive 0 points in the score. No missing values will be accepted for the variables which describe the injury pattern, and age, because these elements were considered essential for any outcome estimation. Both variables (age and list of injuries as AIS codes) are also compulsory variables in the TR-DGU which means that a prognostic score could be calculated for all patients in the registry

The RISC II is based on data of 30 000 trauma cases documented in 2010 and 2011. Data from 2012 were used to validate the score. It is applied to patients with an injury of at least OIS grade 2 (thus the ISS is at least four points). The components of the RISC II are listed in Table B.8.

Validation results and comparisons with existing scores (ISS, TRISS, RISC) showed that RISC II not only could be applied to more patients but also has an improved discrimination (area under the ROS curve), precision (the predicted mortality better fits the observed one) and calibration (Hosmer-Lemeshow goodness-of-fit)[15].

B.4 CO-MORBIDITY SCORING SYSTEMS

There are several co-morbidities, which are known to affect trauma outcomes:

- Liver cirrhosis.
- Chronic obstructive pulmonary disease.
- Congenital coagulopathy.
- Diabetes.
- Congenital heart disease.
- Morbid obesity.

Specific comorbidity weighting measures are used in other disciplines (including the APACHE II); however, their use in trauma so far has not been validated:

- Charlson co-morbidity index[16]: Generally used in medical disciplines.
- TRISSCOM[17]: This adjusts the TRISS score with an age factor of 65, rather than the more common 55 years, and includes eight co-morbidities.

B.5 OUTCOME ANALYSIS

B.5.1 Functional Independence Measure (FIM) and Functional Assessment Measure (FAM)/FIM + FAM

The FIM is an 18-item global measure of disability, and can be scored alone or with the additional 12 that formulate the FAM. The FIM + FAM[18,19] is designed to measure disability in the brain-injured population. It has an ordinal scoring system for all 30 items from 1 to 7, where 1 is complete dependence, to 7, complete independence. Scoring is completed at two time points, the first 7 to 10 days after admission (admission score), and the second within 7 days of discharge (discharge score).

B.5.2 Glasgow Outcome Scale (GOS)

For head-injured patients, the level of coma on admission or within 24 hours expressed by the GCS was found to correlate with outcome. The Glasgow Outcome Scale[22] was an attempt to quantify the outcome parameters (Table B.9) for head-injured patients.

The grading of depth of coma and neurological signs was found to correlate strongly with outcome, but the

Table B.8 Components of RISC II

Variable	Value	Coefficient	Variable	Value	Coefficient
Worst Injury	AIS 3	−0.5	Sex	Female	+0.2
	AIS 4	−1.3		Male/???	0
	AIS 5	−1.7	ASA pre-trauma	1–2	+0.3
	AIS 6	−2.9		3/???	0
Second-worst injury	AIS 0–2	+0.2		4	−0.3
	AIS 3	0	Mechanism	Blunt/???	0
	AIS 4	−0.6		Penetrating	−0.6
	AIS 5	−1.4	GCS motor function	Normal	+0.6
Head injury	AIS 0-2	0		Localizes/???	0
	AIS 3–4	−0.1		No Localising	−0.4
	AIS 5–6	−0.8		None	−0.8
Age	1–5	+1.4	Systolic BP on admission	<90	−0.7
	6–10	+0.6		90–110/???	0
	11–54	0		111–50	+0.3
	55–59	−0.5		>150	0
	60–64	−0.8	CPR	No	0
	65–69	−0.9		Yes	−1.8
	70–74	−1.2	Coagulation (INR)	<1.2	+0.6
	75–79	−1.9		1.2–1.4	+0.2
	80–84	−2.4		1.4–2.4/???	0
	85+	−2.7		>2.4	−0.4
Pupil reactivity	Brisk	+0.2	Blood haemoglobin (g/dL)		
	7.0–11.9/???	0			
	Sluggish/???	0		< 7.0	−0.5
	Fixed	−1.0	Acidosis (base deficit)	<6	+0.3
Pupil size	Normal	+0.2		6–9/???	0
	Unequal	0		9–15	−0.4
	Bilat dilated	−0.5		>15	−1.5

Note: Starting with the constant value of 3.6, specific values (the coefficients) were added or subtracted, based on the observed findings, to finally give the score value. This value is then transformed into a probability of survival using the logistic function. Positive coefficients refer to an improved prognosis while negative ones worsen the prognosis.

Table B.9 Outcome Parameters

GR	Good recovery
MD	Moderate disability
SD	Severe disability
PVS	Persistent vegetative state
D	Death

low accuracy of individual signs limits their use in predicting outcomes for individuals (Table B.10).

B.5.3 **Major Trauma Outcome Study (MTOS)**

In 1982, the American College of Surgeons Committee on Trauma began the ongoing Major Trauma Outcome Study (MTOS), a retrospective, multicentre study of trauma epidemiology and outcomes.

The MTOS uses the TRISS methodology[21] to estimate the probability of survival, or $P(s)$, for a given trauma patient. The $P(s)$ is derived according to the following formula:

$$P(s) = 1/(1 + e^{-b})$$

Table B.10 Outcome Related to Signs in the First 24 Hours of Coma after Injury: Outcome Scale as Described by Glasgow Group

	Dead or Vegetative (%)	Moderate Disability or Good Recovery (%)
Pupils		
Reacting	39	50
Non-reacting	91	4
Eye movements		
Intact	33	56
Absent/bad	90	5
Motor response		
Normal	36	54
Abnormal	74	16

where e is Euler's constant (approximately 2.718282) and $b = b_0 + b_1(\text{RTS}) + b_2(\text{ISS}) + b_3(\text{age} >55)$. The b coefficients are derived by regression analysis from the MTOS database (Table B.11).

The $P(s)$ values range from zero (survival not expected) to 1.000 for a patient with a 100 per cent expectation of survival. Each patient's values can be plotted on a graph with ISS and RTS axes (Figure B.1).

The sloping line in Figure B.1 represents patients with a probability of survival of 50 per cent; these PRE charts (from PREliminary) are provided for those with blunt versus penetrating injury, and for those above versus below 55 years of age. Survivors whose coordinates are above the $P(s)50$ isobar and non-survivors below the $P(s)50$ isobar are considered atypical (statistically unexpected), and such cases are suitable for focused audit.

In addition to analyzing individual patient outcomes, TRISS allows a comparison of a study population with the huge MTOS database. The 'Z-statistic' identifies whether study group outcomes are significantly different from expected outcomes as predicted from the MTOS. The Z is the ratio $(A - E)/S$, where A = actual number of survivors, E = expected number of survivors and S = scale factor, to transform the value into a standard normal distribution. Then Z may be positive or negative, depending on whether the survival rate is greater or less than predicted by TRISS. The Z values of greater than 1.96 or less than –0.96 describe statistically significant deviation from prognosis ($P < 0.05$).

The so-called M-statistic is an injury severity match allowing a comparison of the range of injury severity in the sample population with that of the main database (i.e. the baseline group). The closer M is to 1, the better the match; the greater the disparity, the more biased Z will be. This bias can be misleading; for example, an institution with a large number of patients with low-severity injuries can falsely appear to provide a better standard of care than another institution that treats a higher number of more severely injured patients.

Table B.11 Coefficients from the Major Trauma Outcome Study Database

Blunt	Penetrating
$b_0 = -1.2470$	-0.6029
$b_1 = 0.9544$	1.1430
$b_2 = -0.0768$	-0.1516
$b_3 = -1.9052$	-2.6676

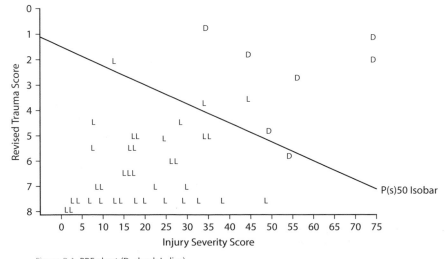

Figure B.1 PRE chart (D, dead; L, live).

The 'W-statistic', or relative outcome score, calculates the actual numbers of survivors greater (or fewer) than predicted by the MTOS, per 100 trauma patients treated. The relative outcome score can be used to compare W-values against a 'perfect outcome' of 100 per cent survival. Thus W could also be interpreted as the percentage of survivors above or below prediction. The relative outcome score may then be used to monitor improvements in trauma care delivery over time.

The TRISS has been used in numerous studies. Its value as a predictor of survival or death has been shown to be from 75 to 90 per cent as good as a perfect index, depending on the patient dataset used.

B.5.4 **A Severity Characterization of Trauma (ASCOT)**

A Severity Characterization of Trauma (ASCOT)[22,23], introduced by Champion et al. in 1990, is a scoring system that uses the APS to characterize injury in place of the ISS. Different coefficients are used for blunt and penetrating injury, and the ASCOT score is derived from the formula: $P(s) = 1/(1 + e^{-k})$. The ASCOT model coefficients are shown in Table B.12. ASCOT has been shown to outperform TRISS, particularly for penetrating injury.

Table B.12 Coefficients Derived from Major Trauma Outcome Study Data for the ASCOT Probability of Survival, $P(s)$

K-Coefficients	Type of Injury	
	Blunt	**Penetrating**
K_1	−1.157	−1.135
K_2 (RTS GCS value)	0.7705	1.0626
K_3 (RTS SBP value)	0.6583	0.3638
K_4 (RTS RR value)	0.281	0.3332
K_5 (APS head region value)	−0.3002	−0.3702
K_6 (APS thoracic region value)	−0.1961	−0.2053
K_7 (APS other serious injury value)	−0.2086	−0.3188
K_8 (age factor)	−0.6355	−0.8365

Note: APS, Anatomic Profile Score; ASCOT, A Severity Characterization of Trauma; GCS, Glasgow Coma Scale; RR, respiratory rate; RTS, Revised Trauma Score; SBP, systolic blood pressure.

B.6 **TRAUMA SCORING SYSTEMS**

Table B.13 presents a comparison of scoring systems.

B.7 **SCALING SYSTEM FOR ORGAN-SPECIFIC INJURIES**

Tables B.14 through B.45 present scaling systems for organ-specific injuries[12,26-32]:

Table B.14: Cervical vascular organ injury scale
Table B.15: Chest wall injury scale
Table B.16: Heart injury scale
Table B.17: Lung injury scale
Table B.18: Thoracic vascular injury scale
Table B.19: Diaphragm injury scale
Table B.20: Spleen injury scale
Table B.21: Liver injury scale
Table B.22: Extrahepatic biliary tree injury scale
Table B.23: Pancreas injury scale
Table B.24: Oesophagus injury scale
Table B.25: Stomach injury scale
Table B.26: Duodenum injury scale
Table B.27: Small bowel injury scale
Table B.28: Colon injury scale
Table B.29: Rectum injury scale
Table B.30: Abdominal vascular injury scale
Table B.31: Adrenal organ injury scale
Table B.32: Kidney injury scale
Table B.33: Ureter injury scale
Table B.34: Bladder injury scale
Table B.35: Urethra injury scale
Table B.36: Uterus (non-pregnant) injury scale
Table B.37: Uterus (pregnant) injury scale
Table B.38: Fallopian tube injury scale
Table B.39: Ovary injury scale
Table B.40: Vagina injury scale
Table B.41: Vulva injury scale
Table B.42: Testis injury scale
Table B.43: Scrotum injury scale
Table B.44: Penis injury scale
Table B.45: Peripheral vascular organ injury scale

In these tables, ICD refers to the *International Classification of Diseases* (ICD9-CM and ICD-10, 2015 edition) and AIS refers to the Abbreviated Injury Scale 2005 (2008 update) of the American Association for the Advancement of Automotive Medicine[6].

Where necessary, in the ICD-10 system, a *fifth* digit is used as follows:

Closed injury: 0
Open injury: 1

Table B.13 Comparison of Scoring Systems

Scoring System	Year	Predicts What?	How Calculated?	Score Range/ Interpretation	Benefits	Limitations
Physiological Scoring Systems						
GCS	1977	Brain function patient survival	Based on higher cerebral response to stimulation (eyes, motor and verbal)	Range from 3/15 (no or minimal neurological function) to 15/15 (normal or near-normal neurological function	Simple and easy to calculate	The best available score needs to be used, otherwise scale is inaccurate
PTS	1988	Facilitates triage; measure of mortality risk	Sum of six physiological scores	Range from 2 (best) to –1 (worst)	Used as a trigger to refer a child to a trauma centre	Not widely used
RTS	1989	Patient survival		Range from 0 (severe physiological derangement) to 7.84 (no physiological derangement)	Provides physiological assessment of the patient, high association with mortality; superior to TRISS and ISS in predicting mortality in the ICU	Incubation and sedation prior to arrival alter accuracy
APACHE-II	1985	Patient survival and disease severity	Based on the worst 12 routine physiological measurements, in the first 24 hours of ICU admission, as well as age and chronic health conditions	Range from 0 (very low risk of mortality) to 71 (very high risk of mortality); scores of greater than 15 are considered moderate to severe risk	Superior to TRISS and ISS in predicting mortality in the ICU; generally now Web-based entry and calculation	ICU specific; use limited by missing data; time-consuming and complex to calculate
Anatomical Scoring Systems						
AIS	1971	Patient survival			Developed to classify severity of injury, but validated to measure probability of death	Does not predict functional impairment
ISS	1974	Patient survival	Body divided into six anatomical regions, each of which is given a score; highest three scores are squared and summed	44 possible scores, ranging from 1 (less severe) to 75 (unsurvivable)	Most widely used trauma severity score; relates AIS to patient outcomes	No physiological predictors; does not account for more than one injury in the same region; complex
NISS	1997	Patient survival	Sum of the squares of the three most severe AIS severities, regardless of body region	As for ISS	Addresses multiple occurrence of serious injury within body region; slight predictive advantage over ISS and ICISS	Not widely used; complex
APS	1990	Patient survival	Three 'modified components' are scored based on AIS, and weighted to form a single APS	Range varies; higher numbers have worse prognosis	Based on location and severity of trauma	Not widely used; complex
ICISS	1996	Patient survival	Computed directly from ICD-9 codes into a survival risk ratio (SRR)	Range from 0 (unsurvivable) to 1 (high chance of survival)	Not based on AIS/ISS; no specialised training required; outperforms ISS	Not widely used; based on ICD-9 codes only; may reflect hospital rather than injury survival
ICDMAP-90	1997	Injury severity	Translates ICD-9 discharge diagnosis codes into an ISS, ISS and APS	Variability in ICD/AIS scores	Similar to ICISS; conservative estimates of injury severity	Not widely used; based on ICD-9 codes only
TRAIS	2003	Patient survival	Same as ICISS, but uses AIS descriptor codes	Range from 0 (unsurvivable) to 1 (high chance of survival)	Similar to ICISS; outpredicts ISS, NISS and APS	Not widely used

Table B.13 Comparison of Scoring Systems – *continued*

Scoring System	Year	Predicts What?	How Calculated?	Score Range/ Interpretation	Benefits	Limitations
OIS	1987	Anatomic injury	Anatomic injury	Ranges from grade 1 (minor injury) to grade 5 (major injury) and grade 6 (fatal injury)	Standardized severity of injury; widely used	No predictability of mortality when used in isolation
RISC II	2014	Patient survival	Based on German Trauma Registry	Uses multiple coefficients based on injury, age and physiology	Validation results and comparisons with existing scores showed that RISC II had improved discrimination, predicted mortality and calibration	Not widely used outside the Federal Republic of Germany
Co-morbidity Scoring Systems						
Charlson	1987	Patient survival	Score consists of 19 possible co-morbid conditions, each allocated a weight of 1–6 based on the relative risk of 1 year mortality; values are summed	Range from 0 (low chance of death) to 37 (high chance of death)	Validated in internal medicine patients only	Not trauma specific, and not generally used for the trauma patient; adapted for ICD-9 codes only
TRISSCOM	2004	Patient survival	Similar to TRISS with adjustments for age (dichotomised to 65 rather than 55) and with the addition of eight co-morbidity variables	Scores range from 0 (unsurvivable) to 1 (high likelihood of survival)	Reflects the ageing population	Not widely used; no severity weighting on co-morbidities
Combination Scoring Systems						
TRISS	1987	Patient survival	Combines ISS, RTS and age; regression coefficients derived from MTOS database	Scores run from 0 (unsurvivable) to 1 (high likelihood of survival)	Separate coefficients/ probabilities for patients with blunt and penetrating injuries	Requires multiple variables
ASCOT	1990	Patient survival	Uses APS to define injury severity	Range varies	As for TRISS with better predictive values for penetrating trauma	Requires multiple variables
Outcome-based Analysis						
FIM/FAM	2000	Outcome following brain injury	Two scores – an admission score and a discharge score	30 data points, each of which can be scored from 1 (fully dependent) to 7 (fully independent)	Allows objective assessment to assess recovery, and the setting of goals	Proprietary score therefore expensive; widely used in rehabilitation centres
GOS	1975	For outcome following head injury	The level of coma on admission correlates with outcome; the GOS attempts to quantify this	Grading is made between a good recovery to death	Grading of coma correlates strongly with outcome	Low accuracy of individual signs
MTOS	1982	Probability of survival	ISS methodology for a given trauma patient using coefficients representing RTS, ISS and age	The predictability of survival can be calculated	Allows a comparison of the study population by a huge database, with individuals or hospitals	Complex to calculate

Note: AIS: Abbreviated Injury score; APACHE-II: Acute Physiologic and Chronic Health Evaluation II; APS: Anatomic Profile Score; ASCOT: A Severity Characterisation of Trauma; Charlson: Charlson Comorbidity Index (CCI); FIM: Functional Independence Measure; FAM: Functional Assessment Measure; GCS: Glasgow Coma Scale; GOS: Glasgow Outcome Scale; ICDMAP-90: International Classification of Disease 'map' – 1990; ICISS: International Classification of Disease Injury Severity Score; ISS: Injury Severity Score; MTOS: Major Trauma Outcome Study; NISS: New Injury Severity Score; OIS: American Association for the Surgery of Trauma Organ Injury Scale; PTS: Paediatric Trauma Score; RISC II: Revised Injury Severity Classification II; RTS: Revised Trauma Score; TRAIS: Trauma Registry Abbreviated Injury Score; TRISS: Trauma and Injury Severity Score; TRISSCOM: Trauma and Injury Severity Score Comorbidity.

Source: Table modified from Becher RD, Meredith JW, Kilgo P, in Mattox KL, Moore EE, Feliciano DV, Eds., *Trauma*, 7th ed., NcGraw-Hill, New York, NY, 80–82, 2012. With permission.

Table B.14 Cervical Vascular Organ Injury Scale

Grade[a]	Description of Injury	ICD-9	ICD-10	AIS-2005
I	Thyroid vein	900.8	S15.8	
	Common facial vein	900.8	S15.8	
	External jugular vein	900.81	S15.2	1–3
	Non-named arterial/venous branches	900.9	S15.9	
II	External carotid arterial branches (ascending pharyngeal, superior thyroid, lingual, facial, maxillary, occipital, posterior auricular)	900.8	S15.0	1–3
	Thyrocervical trunk or primary branches	900.8	S15.8	1–3
	Internal jugular vein	900.1	S15.3	1–3
III	External carotid artery	900.02	S15.0	2–3
	Subclavian vein	901.3	S25.3	3–4
	Vertebral artery	900.8	S15.1	2–4
IV	Common carotid artery	900.01	S15.0	3–5
	Subclavian artery	901.1	S25.1	3–4
V	Internal carotid artery (extracranial)	900.03	S15.0	3–5

[a]Increase one grade for multiple grade III or IV injuries involving more than 50 per cent of the vessel circumference. Decrease one grade for less than 25 per cent vessel circumference disruption for grade IV or V.

Source: From Moore EE, Malangoni MA, Cogbill TH, Peterson NE, Champion HR, Shackford SR, *J Trauma,* 41, 523–524, 1996. With permission.

Table B.15 Chest Wall Injury Scale

Grade[a]	Injury Type	Description of Injury	ICD-9	ICD-10	AIS-2005
I	Contusion	Any size	911.0/922.1	S20.2	1
	Laceration	Skin and subcutaneous	875.0	S20.4	1
	Fracture	<3 ribs, closed;	807.01/807.02	S22.3	1–2
		non-displaced, clavicle closed	810.00/810.03	S42.0	2
II	Laceration	Skin, subcutaneous and muscle	875.1	S20.4	2
	Fracture	≥3 adjacent ribs, closed	807.03/807.08	S22.4	1
		Open or displaced clavicle	810.10/810.13	S42.0	2–3
		Non-displaced sternum, closed	807.2	S22.2	2
		Scapular body, open or closed	811.00/811.18	S42.1	2
III	Laceration	Full thickness including pleural penetration – front	862.29	S21.1	2
		Full thickness including pleural penetration – back	862.29	S21.2	2
	Fracture	Open or displaced sternum	807.2	S22.2	2
		Flail sternum	807.3	S22.2	2
		Unilateral flail segment (<3 ribs)	807.4	S22.5	3–4
IV	Laceration	Avulsion of chest wall tissues with underlying rib fractures	807.10/807.18	S22.8	4
	Fracture	Unilateral flail chest (≥3 ribs)	807.4	S22.5	3–4
V	Fracture	Bilateral flail chest (≥3 ribs on both sides)	807.4	S22.5	5

[a]Upgrade by one grade for bilateral injuries.

Note: This scale is confined to the chest wall alone and does not reflect associated internal or abdominal injuries. Therefore, further delineation of upper versus lower or anterior versus posterior chest wall was not considered, and a grade VI was not warranted. Specifically, thoracic crush was not used as a descriptive term; instead, the geography and extent of fractures and soft tissue injury were used to define the grade.

Source: From Moore EE, Cogbill TH, Jurkovich GJ, *J Trauma,* 33, 337–338, 1992. With permission.

Table B.16 Heart Injury Scale

Grade[a]	Description of Injury	ICD-9	ICD-10	AIS-2005
I	Blunt cardiac injury with minor ECG abnormality (non-specific ST or T wave changes, premature arterial or ventricular contraction or persistent sinus tachycardia)	861.01	S26.0	3
	Blunt or penetrating pericardial wound without cardiac injury, cardiac tamponade or cardiac herniation			
II	Blunt cardiac injury with heart block (right or left bundle branch, left anterior fascicular or atrioventricular) or ischaemic changes (ST depression or T wave inversion) without cardiac failure	861.01	S26.0	3
	Penetrating tangential myocardial wound up to, but not extending through, endocardium, without tamponade	861.12	S26.0	3
III	Blunt cardiac injury with sustained (≥6 beats/min) or multifocal ventricular contractions	861.01	S26.0	3–4
	Blunt or penetrating cardiac injury with septal rupture, pulmonary or tricuspid valvular incompetence, papillary muscle dysfunction or distal coronary arterial occlusion without cardiac failure	861.01	S26.0	3–4
	Blunt pericardial laceration with cardiac herniation	861.01	S26.0	3–4
	Blunt cardiac injury with cardiac failure	861.01	S26.0	3–4
	Penetrating tangential myocardial wound up to, but extending through, endocardium, with tamponade	861.12	S26.0	3
IV	Blunt or penetrating cardiac injury with septal rupture, pulmonary or tricuspid valvular incompetence, papillary muscle dysfunction or distal coronary arterial occlusion producing cardiac failure	861.12	S26.0	3
	Blunt or penetrating cardiac injury with aortic mitral valve incompetence	861.03	S26.0	5
	Blunt or penetrating cardiac injury of the right ventricle, right atrium or left atrium	861.03	S26.0	5
V	Blunt or penetrating cardiac injury with proximal coronary arterial occlusion	861.03	S26.0	5
	Blunt or penetrating left ventricular perforation	861.13	S26.0	5
	Stellate wound with <50 per cent tissue loss of the right ventricle, right atrium or left atrium	861.03	S26.0	5
VI	Blunt avulsion of the heart; penetrating wound producing >50 per cent tissue loss of a chamber	861.13	S26.0	6

[a]Advance one grade for multiple wounds to a single chamber or multiple chamber involvement.

Note: With ICD-10, use supplementary character: 0 = without an open wound into the thoracic cavity; 1 = with an open wound into the thoracic cavity.

Source: From Moore EE, Malangoni MA, Cogbill TH, et al., *J Trauma*, 36, 299–300, 1994. With permission.

Table B.17 Lung Injury Scale

Grade[a]	Injury Type	Description of Injury	ICD-9	ICD-10	AIS-2005
I	Contusion	Unilateral, <1 lobe	861.12/861.31	S27.3	3
II	Contusion	Unilateral, single lobe	861.20/861.30	S27.3	3
	Laceration	Simple pneumothorax	860.0/1/4/5	S27.0	3
III	Contusion	Unilateral, >1 lobe	861.20/861.30	S27.3	3
	Laceration	Persistent (>72-h) air leak from distal airway	860.0/1/4/5	S27.3	3–4
	Haematoma	Non-expanding intraparenchymal	862.0/861.30	S27.3	
IV	Laceration	Major (segmental or lobar) air leak	862.21/861.31	S27.4	4–5
	Haematoma	Expanding intraparenchymal		S25.4	
	Vascular	Primary branch intrapulmonary vessel disruption	901.40	S25.4	3–5
V	Vascular	Hilar vessel disruption	901.41/901.42	S25.4	4
VI	Vascular	Total uncontained transection of pulmonary hilum	901.41/901.42	S25.4	4

[a]Advance one grade for bilateral injuries up to grade III.

Note: Haemothorax is scored under the thoracic vascular injury scale. With ICD-10, use supplementary character: 0 = without an open wound into the thoracic cavity; 1 = with an open wound into the thoracic cavity.

Source: From Moore EE, Malangoni MA, Cogbill TH, et al., *J Trauma*, 36, 299–300, 1994. With permission.

Table B.18 Thoracic Vascular Injury Scale

Grade[a]	Description of Injury	ICD-9	ICD-10	AIS-2005
I	Intercostal artery/vein	901.81	S25.5	2–3
	Internal mammary artery/vein	901.82	S25.8	2–3
	Bronchial artery/vein	901.89	S25.4	2–3
	Oesophageal artery/vein	901.9	S25.8	2–3
	Hemiazygos vein	901.89	S25.8	2–3
	Unnamed artery/vein	901.9	S25.9	2–3
II	Azygos vein	901.89	S25.8	2–3
	Internal jugular vein	900.1	S15.3	2–3
	Subclavian vein	901.3	S25.3	3–4
	Innominate vein	901.3	S25.3	3–4
III	Carotid artery	900.01	S15.0	3–5
	Innominate artery	901.1	S25.1	3–4
	Subclavian artery	901.1	S25.1	3–4
IV	Thoracic aorta, descending	901.0	S25.0	4–5
	Inferior vena cava (intrathoracic)	902.10	S35.1	3–4
	Pulmonary artery, primary intraparenchymal branch	901.41	S25.4	3
	Pulmonary vein, primary intraparenchymal branch	901.42	S25.4	3
V	Thoracic aorta, ascending and arch	901.0	S25.0	5
	Superior vena cava	901.2	S25.2	3–4
	Pulmonary artery, main trunk	901.41	S25.4	4
	Pulmonary vein, main trunk	901.42	S25.4	4
VI	Uncontained total transection of thoracic aorta or pulmonary hilum	901.0	S25.0	5
	Uncontained total transection of pulmonary hilum	901.41/901.42	S25.4	5

[a]Increase one grade for multiple grade III or IV injuries if more than 50 per cent of the circumference. Decrease one grade for grade IV injuries if less than 25 per cent of the circumference.

Source: From Moore EE, Malangoni MA, Cogbill TH, et al., *J Trauma*, 36, 299–300, 1994. With permission.

Table B.19 Diaphragm Injury Scale

Grade[a]	Description of Injury	ICD-9	ICD-10	AIS-2005
I	Contusion	862.0	S27.8	2
II	Laceration <2 cm	862.1	S27.8	3
III	Laceration 2–10 cm	862.1	S27.8	3
IV	Laceration >10 cm with tissue loss ≤25 cm²	862.1	S27.8	3
V	Laceration with tissue loss >25 cm²	862.1	S27.8	3

[a]Advance one grade for bilateral injuries up to grade III.

Source: From Moore EE, Malangoni MA, Cogbill TH, et al., *J Trauma*, 36, 299–300, 1994. With permission.

Table B.20 Spleen Injury Scale (1994 Revision)

Grade[a]	Injury Type	Description of Injury	ICD-9	ICD-10	AIS-2005
I	Haematoma	Subcapsular, <10% surface area	865-01/865.11	S36.0	2
	Laceration	Capsular tear, <1 cm parenchymal depth	865.02/865.12	S36.0	2
II	Haematoma	Subcapsular, 10–50% surface area; intraparenchymal, <5 cm in diameter	865.01/865.11	S36.0	2
	Laceration	Capsular tear, 1–3 cm parenchymal depth that does not involve a trabecular vessel	865.02/865.12	S36.0	2
III	Haematoma	Subcapsular, >50% surface area or expanding; ruptured subcapsular or parenchymal haematoma; intraparenchymal haematoma ≥ 5 cm or expanding	865.03	S36.0	3
	Laceration	>3 cm parenchymal depth or involving trabecular vessels	865.03	S36.0	3
IV	Laceration	Laceration involving segmental or hilar vessels producing major devascularization (>25% of spleen)	865.13	S36.0	4
V	Laceration	Completely shattered spleen	865.04	S36.0	5
	Vascular	Hilar vascular injury with devascularized spleen	865.14	S36.0	5

[a]Advance one grade for multiple injuries up to grade III.

Note: With ICD-10, use supplementary character: 0 = without an open wound into the abdominal cavity; 1 = with an open wound into the abdominal cavity.

Source: Moore EE, Cogbill TH, Jurkovich GJ, Shackford SR, Malangoni MA, Champion HR, *J Trauma*, 38, 323–324, 1995. With permission.

Table B.21 Liver Injury Scale (1994 Revision)

Grade[a]	Type of Injury	Description of Injury	ICD-9	ICD-10	AIS-2005
I	Haematoma	Subcapsular, <10% surface area	864.01/864.11	S36.1	2
	Laceration	Capsular tear, <1 cm parenchymal depth	864.02/864.12	S36.1	2
II	Haematoma	Subcapsular, 10–50% surface area: intraparenchymal <10 cm in diameter	864.01/864.11	S36.1	2
	Laceration	Capsular tear 1–3 cm, parenchymal depth, <10 cm in length	864.03/864.13	S36.1	2
III	Haematoma	Subcapsular, >50% surface area or]ruptured subcapsular or parenchymal haematoma; intraparenchymal haematoma >10 cm or expanding	864.04/864.14	S36.1	3
	Laceration	3 cm parenchymal depth	864.04/864.14	S36.1	3
IV	Laceration	Parenchymal disruption involving 25–75% hepatic lobe or 1–3 Couinaud's segments within a single lobe	864.04/864.14	S36.1	4
V	Laceration	Parenchymal disruption involving >75% of hepatic lobe or >3 Couinaud's segments within a single lobe	864.04/864.14	S36.1	5
VI	Vascular	Juxtahepatic venous injuries; i.e. retrohepatic vena cava/central major hepatic veins	864.04/864.14	S36.1	5
	Vascular	Hepatic avulsion	864.04/864.14	S36.1	5

[a]Advance one grade for multiple injuries up to grade III.

Note: With ICD-10, use supplementary character: 0 = without an open wound into the abdominal cavity; 1 = with an open wound into the abdominal cavity.

Source: From Moore EE, Cogbill TH, Jurkovich GJ, Shackford SR, Malangoni MA, Champion HR, *J Trauma*, 38, 323–324, 1995. With permission.

Table B.22 Extrahepatic Biliary Tree Injury Scale

Grade[a]	Description of Injury	ICD-9	ICD-10	AIS-2005
I	Gallbladder contusion/haematoma	868.02	S36.1	2
	Portal triad contusion	868.02	S36.1	2
II	Partial gallbladder avulsion from liver bed; cystic duct intact	868.02	S36.1	2
	Laceration or perforation of the gallbladder	868.12	S36.1	2
III	Complete gallbladder avulsion from liver bed	868.02	S36.1	3
	Cystic duct laceration	868.12	S36.1	3
IV	Partial or complete right hepatic duct laceration	868.12	S36.1	3
	Partial or complete left hepatic duct laceration	868.12	S36.1	3
	Partial common hepatic duct laceration (<50%)	868.12	S36.1	3
	Partial common bile duct laceration (<50%)	868.12	S36.1	3
V	>50% transection of common hepatic duct	868.12	S36.1	3–4
	>50% transection of common bile duct	868.12	S36.1	3–4
	Combined right and left hepatic duct injuries	868.12	S36.1	3–4
	Intraduodenal or intrapancreatic bile duct injuries	868.12	S36.1	3–4

[a]Advance one grade for multiple injuries up to grade III.

Note: With ICD-10, use supplementary character: 0 = without an open wound into the abdominal cavity; 1 = with an open wound into the abdominal cavity.

Source: From Moore EE, Jurkovich GJ, Knudson MM, et al., *J Trauma*, 39:1069–1070, 1995. With permission.

Table B.23 Pancreas Injury Scale

Grade[a]	Type of Injury	Description of Injury	ICD-9	ICD-10	AIS-2005
I	Haematoma	Minor contusion without duct injury	863.81/863.84	S36.2	2
	Laceration	Superficial laceration without duct injury	863.81/863.84	S36.2	2
II	Haematoma	Major contusion without duct injury or tissue loss	863.81/863.84	S36.2	2
	Laceration	Major laceration without duct injury or tissue loss	863.92/863.94	S36.2	3
III	Laceration	Distal transection or parenchymal injury with duct injury	863.91	S36.2	3
IV	Laceration	Proximal transection or parenchymal injury involving ampulla	863.91	S36.2	4
V	Laceration	Massive disruption of pancreatic head		S36.2	5

[a]Advance one grade for multiple injuries up to grade III.

Notes: With ICD-10, use supplementary character: 0 = without an open wound into the abdominal cavity; 1 = with an open wound into the abdominal cavity. 863.51,863.91: head; 863.99,862.92: body; 863.83,863.93: tail. The proximal pancreas is to the patient's right of the superior mesenteric vein.

Source: From Moore EE, Cogbill TH, Malangoni MA, Jurkovich GJ, Shackford SR, Champion HR, *J Trauma*, 30, 1427–1429, 1990. With permission.

Table B.24 Oesophagus Injury Scale

Grade[a]	Type of Injury	Description of Injury	ICD-9	ICD-10	AIS-2005
I	Contusion	Contusion/haematoma (cervical oesophagus)	862.22/826.32	S10.0	2
		Contusion/haematoma (thoracic oesophagus)	862.22/826.32	S27.8	3
		Contusion/haematoma (abdominal oesophagus)	862.22/862.32	S36.8	3
II	Laceration	Partial thickness laceration	862.22/826.32	S10.0/S27.8/S36.8	4
III	Laceration	Laceration <50% circumference	862.22/826.32	S10.0/S27.8/S36.8	4
IV	Laceration	Laceration >50% circumference	862.22/826.32	S10.0/S27.8/S36.8	5
V	Tissue loss	Segmental loss or devascularization <2 cm	862.22/826.32	S10.0/S27.8/S36.8	5
	Tissue loss	Segmental loss or devascularization >2 cm	862.22/826.32	S10.0/S27.8/S36.8	

[a]Advance one grade for multiple lesions up to grade III.

Note: With ICD-10, use fifth character supplementary character: 0 = without an open wound into the abdominal or thoracic cavity; 1 = with an open wound into the abdominal or thoracic cavity. S10.0: cervical oesophagus; S27.8: thoracic oesophagus; S36.8: abdominal oesophagus.

Source: From Moore EE, Cogbill TH, Malangoni MA, Jurkovich GJ, Shackford SR, Champion HR, *J Trauma*, 30, 1427–1429, 1990. With permission.

Table B.25 Stomach Injury Scale

Grade[a]	Type of Injury	Description of Injury	ICD-9	ICD-10	AIS-2005
I	Contusion	Contusion/haematoma	863.0/863.1	S36.3	2
	Laceration	Partial thickness laceration	863.0/863.1	S36.3	2
II	Laceration	<2 cm in gastro-oesophageal junction or pylorus	863.0/863.1	S36.3	3
		<5 cm in proximal 1/3 stomach	863.0/863.1	S36.3	3
		<10 cm in distal 2/3 stomach	863.0/863.1	S36.3	3
III	Laceration	>2 cm in gastro-oesophageal junction or pylorus	863.0/863.1	S36.3	3
		>5 cm in proximal 1/3 stomach	863.0/863.1	S36.3	3
		>10 cm in distal 2/3 stomach	863.0/863.1	S36.3	3
IV	Tissue loss	Tissue loss or devascularization <2/3 stomach	863.0/863.1	S36.3	4
V	Tissue loss	Tissue loss or devascularization >2/3 stomach	863.0/863.1	S36.3	4

[a]Advance one grade for multiple lesions up to grade III.

Note: With ICD-10, use supplementary character: 0 = without an open wound into the abdominal cavity; 1 = with an open wound into the abdominal cavity.

Source: From Moore EE, Cogbill TH, Malangoni MA, Jurkovich GJ, Shackford SR, Champion HR, *J Trauma*, 30, 1427–1429, 1990. With permission.

Table B.26 Duodenum Injury Scale

Grade[a]	Type of Injury	Description of Injury	ICD-9	ICD-10	AIS-2005
I	Haematoma	Involving single portion of duodenum	863.21	S36.4	2
	Laceration	Partial thickness, no perforation	863.21	S36.4	3
II	Haematoma	Involving more than one portion	863.21	S36.4	2
	Laceration	Disruption <50% of circumference	863.31	S36.4	4
III	Laceration	Disruption 50–75% of circumference of D2	863.31	S36.4	4
		Disruption 50–100% of circumference of D1, D3 or D4	863.31	S36.4	4
IV	Laceration	Disruption >75% of circumference of D2	863.31	S36.4	5
		Involving ampulla or distal common bile duct	863.31	S36.4	5
V	Laceration	Massive disruption of duodenopancreatic complex	863.31	S36.4	5
	Vascular	Devascularization of duodenum	863.31	S36.4	5

[a]Advance one grade for multiple injuries up to grade III.

Note: With ICD-10, use supplementary character: 0 = without an open wound into the abdominal cavity; 1 = with an open wound into the abdominal cavity. D1, first portion of duodenum; D2, second portion of duodenum; D3, third portion of duodenum; D4, fourth portion of duodenum.

Source: From Moore EE, Cogbill TH, Malangoni MA, Jurkovich GJ, Shackford SR, Champion HR, *J Trauma*, 30, 1427–1429, 1990. With permission.

Table B.27 Small Bowel Injury Scale

Grade[a]	Type of Injury	Description of Injury	ICD-9	ICD-10	AIS-2005
I	Haematoma	Contusion or haematoma without devascularization	863.20	S36.4	2
	Laceration	Partial thickness, no perforation	863.20	S36.4	2
II	Laceration	Laceration <50% of circumference	863.30	S36.4	3
III	Laceration	Laceration ≥50% of circumference without transection	863.30	S36.4	3
IV	Laceration	Transection of the small bowel	863.30	S36.4	4
V	Laceration	Transection of the small bowel with segmental tissue loss	863.30	S36.4	4
	Vascular	Devascularized segment	863.30	S36.4	4

[a]Advance one grade for multiple injuries up to grade III.

Note: With ICD-10, use supplementary character: 0 = without an open wound into the abdominal cavity; 1 = with an open wound into the abdominal cavity.

Source: From Moore EE, Cogbill TH, Malangoni MA, Jurkovich GJ, Shackford SR, Champion HR, *J Trauma*, 30, 1427–1429, 1990. With permission.

Table B.28 Colon Injury Scale

Grade[a]	Type of Injury	Description of Injury	ICD-9	ICD-10	AIS-2005
I	Haematoma	Contusion or haematoma without devascularization	863.40–863.44	S36.5	2
	Laceration	Partial thickness, no perforation	863.40–863.44	S36.5	2
II	Laceration	Laceration <50% of circumference	863.50–863.54	S36.5	3
III	Laceration	Laceration ≥50% of circumference without transection	863.50–863.54	S36.5	3
IV	Laceration	Transection of the colon	863.50–863.54	S36.5	4
V	Laceration	Transection of the colon with segmental tissue loss	863.50–863.54	S36.5	4

[a]Advance one grade for multiple injuries up to grade III.

Note: With ICD-9, 863.40/863.50 = non-specific site in colon; 863.41/863.51 = ascending colon; 863.42/863.52 = transverse colon; 863.43/863.53 = descending colon; 863.44/863.54 = sigmoid colon. With ICD-10, use supplementary character: 0 = without an open wound into the abdominal cavity; 1 = with an open wound into the abdominal cavity.

Source: From Moore EE, Cogbill TH, Malangoni MA, Jurkovich GJ, Shackford SR, Champion HR, *J Trauma*, 30, 1427–1429, 1990. With permission.

Table B.29 Rectum Injury Scale

Grade[a]	Type of Injury	Description of Injury	ICD-9	ICD-10	AIS-2005
I	Haematoma	Contusion or haematoma without devascularization	863.45	S36.6	2
	Laceration	Partial-thickness laceration	863.45	S36.6	2
II	Laceration	Laceration <50% of circumference	863.55	S36.6	3
III	Laceration	Laceration ≥50% of circumference	863.55	S36.6	4
IV	Laceration	Full-thickness laceration with extension into the perineum	863.55	S36.6	5
V	Vascular	Devascularized segment	863.55	S36.6	5

[a]Advance one grade for multiple injuries up to grade III.

Note: With ICD-10, use supplementary character: 0 = without an open wound into the abdominal cavity; 1 = with an open wound into the abdominal cavity.

Source: From Moore EE, Cogbill TH, Malangoni MA, Jurkovich GJ, Shackford SR, Champion HR, *J Trauma*, 30, 1427–1429, 1990. With permission.

Table B.30 Abdominal Vascular Injury Scale

Grade[a]	Description of Injury	ICD-9	ICD-10	AIS-2005
I	Non-named superior mesenteric artery or superior mesenteric vein branches	902.20/.39	S35.2	NS
	Non-named inferior mesenteric artery or inferior mesenteric vein branches	902.27/.32	S35.2	NS
	Phrenic artery or vein	902.89	S35.8	NS
	Lumbar artery or vein	902.89	S35.8	NS
	Gonadal artery or vein	902.89	S35.8	NS
	Ovarian artery or vein	902.81/902.82	S35.8	NS
	Other non-named small arterial or venous structures requiring ligation	902.80	S35.9	NS
II	Right, left or common hepatic artery	902.22	S35.2	3
	Splenic artery or vein	902.23/902.34	S35.2	3
	Right or left gastric arteries	902.21	S35.2	3
	Gastroduodenal artery	902.24	S35.2	3
	Inferior mesenteric artery/trunk or inferior mesenteric vein/trunk	902.27/902.32	S35.2	3
	Primary named branches of mesenteric artery (e.g. ileocolic artery) or mesenteric vein	902.26/902.31	S35.2	3
	Other named abdominal vessels requiring ligation or repair	902.89	S35.8	3
III	Superior mesenteric vein, trunk and primary subdivisions	902.31	S35.3	3
	Renal artery or vein	902.41/902.42	S35.4	3
	Iliac artery or vein	902.53/902.54	S35.5	3
	Hypogastric artery or vein	902.51/902.52	S35.5	3
	Vena cava, infrarenal	902.10	S35.1	3
IV	Superior mesenteric artery, trunk	902.25	S35.2	3
	Coeliac axis proper	902.24	S35.2	3
	Vena cava, suprarenal and infrahepatic	902.10	S35.1	3
	Aorta, infrarenal	902.00	S35.0	4
V	Portal vein	902.33	S35.3	3
	Extraparenchymal hepatic vein only	902.11	S35.1	3
	Extraparenchymal hepatic veins + liver	902.11	S35.1	5
	Vena cava, retrohepatic or suprahepatic	902.19	S35.1	5
	Aorta suprarenal, subdiaphragmatic	902.00	S35.0	4

[a]This classification system is applicable to extraparenchymal vascular injuries. If the vessel injury is within 2 cm of the organ parenchyma, refer to the specific organ injury scale. Increase one grade for multiple grade III or IV injuries involving >50 per cent of the vessel circumference. Downgrade one grade if <25 per cent of the vessel circumference laceration for grades IV or V.

Note: With ICD-10, use supplementary character: 0 = without an open wound into the abdominal cavity; 1 = with an open wound into the abdominal cavity. NS, not scored.

Source: From Moore EE, Cogbill TH, Jurkovich GJ, *J Trauma*, 33, 337–338, 1992. With permission.

Table B.31 Adrenal Organ Injury Scale

Grade[a]	Description of Injury	ICD-9	ICD-10	AIS-2005
I	Contusion	868.01/.11	S37.9	1
II	Laceration involving only cortex (<2 cm)	868.01/.11	S37.8	1
III	Laceration extending into medulla (≥2 cm)	868.01/.11	S37.8	2
IV	>50% parenchymal destruction	868.01/.11	S37.8	2
V	Total parenchymal destruction (including massive intraparenchymal haemorrhage) Avulsion from blood supply	868.01/.11	S37.8	3

[a]Advance one grade for bilateral lesions up to grade V.

Note: With ICD-10, use supplementary character: 0 = without an open wound into the abdominal cavity; 1 = with an open wound into the abdominal cavity.

Source: From Moore EE, Malangoni MA, Cogbill TH, Peterson NE, Champion HR, Shackford SR. Organ Injury Scaling VII: Cervical Vascular, Peripheral Vascular, Adrenal, Penis, Testis and Scrotum. *J Trauma*: 1996; 41(3):523–4.

Table B.32 Kidney Injury Scale

Grade[a]	Type of Injury	Description of Injury	ICD-9	ICD-10	AIS-2005
I	Contusion	Microscopic or gross haematuria, urological studies normal	866.00/866.01	S37.0	2
	Haematoma	Subcapsular, non-expanding without parenchymal laceration	866.01	S37.0	2
II	Haematoma	Non-expanding perirenal haematoma confined to renal retroperitoneum	866.01	S37.0	2
	Laceration	<1.0 cm parenchymal depth of renal cortex without urinary extravasation	866.11	S37.0	2
III	Laceration	>1.0 cm parenchymal depth of renal cortex without collecting system rupture or urinary extravasation	866.11	S37.0	3
IV	Laceration	Parenchymal laceration extending through renal cortex, medulla and collecting system	866.02/866.12	S37.0	4
	Vascular	Main renal artery or vein injury with contained haemorrhage	866.03/866.11	S37.0	4
V	Laceration	Completely shattered kidney	866.04/866.14	S37.0	5
	Vascular	Avulsion of renal hilum that devascularizes kidney	866.13	S37.0	5

[a]Advance one grade for bilateral injuries up to grade III.

Note: With ICD-10, use supplementary character: 0 = without an open wound into the abdominal cavity; 1 = with an open wound into the abdominal cavity.

Source: From Moore EE, Shackford SR, Pachter HL, et al., *J Trauma*, 9, 1664–1666, 1989. With permission.

Table B.33 Ureter Injury Scale

Grade[a]		Description of Injury	ICD-9	ICD-10	AIS-2005
I	Haematoma	Contusion or haematoma without devascularization	867.2/867.3	S37.1	2
II	Laceration	<50% transection	867.2/867.3	S37.1	2
III	Laceration	≥50% transection	867.2/867.3	S37.1	3
IV	Laceration	Complete transection with <2 cm devascularization	867.2/867.3	S37.1	3
V	Laceration	Avulsion with >2 cm devascularization	867.2/867.3	S37.1	3

[a]Advance one grade for bilateral up to grade III.

Note: With ICD-10, use supplementary character: 0 = without an open wound into the abdominal cavity; 1 = with an open wound into the abdominal cavity.

Source: From Moore EE, Cogbill TH, Jurkovich GJ, *J Trauma*, 33, 337–338, 1992. With permission.

Table B.34 Bladder Injury Scale

Grade[a]	Injury Type	Description of Injury	ICD-9	ICD-10	AIS-2005
I	Haematoma	Contusion, intramural haematoma	867.0/867.1	S37.2	2
	Laceration	Partial thickness	867.0/867.1	S37.2	3
II	Laceration	Extraperitoneal bladder wall laceration <2 cm	867.0/867.1	S37.2	4
VIII	Laceration	Extraperitoneal (≥2 cm) or intraperitoneal (<2 cm) bladder wall laceration	867.0/867.1	S37.2	4
IV	Laceration	Intraperitoneal bladder wall laceration ≥2 cm	867.0/867.1	S37.2	4
V	Laceration	Intraperitoneal or extraperitoneal bladder wall laceration extending into the bladder neck or ureteral orifice (trigone)	867.0/867.1	S37.2	4

[a]Advance one grade for multiple lesions up to grade III.

Note: With ICD-10, use supplementary character: 0 = without an open wound into the pelvic cavity; 1 = with an open wound into the pelvic cavity.

Source: From Moore EE, Cogbill TH, Jurkovich GJ, J Trauma, 33, 337–338, 1992. With permission.

Table B.35 Urethra Injury Scale

Grade[a]	Injury Type	Description of Injury	ICD-9	ICD-10	AIS-2005
I	Contusion	Blood at urethral meatus; urethrography normal	867.0/867.1	S37.3	2
II	Stretch injury	Elongation of urethra without extravasation on urethrography	867.0/867.1	S37.3	2
III	Partial disruption	Extravasation of urethrography contrast at injury site with visualization in the bladder	867.0/867.1	S37.3	2
IV	Complete disruption	Extravasation of urethrography contrast at injury site without visualization in the bladder; <2 cm of urethra separation	867.0/867.1	S37.3	3
V	Complete disruption	Complete transaction with ≥2 cm urethral separation, or extension into the prostate or vagina	867.0/867.1	S37.3	4

[a]Advance one grade for bilateral injuries up to grade III.

Note: With ICD-10, use supplementary character: 0 = without an open wound into the pelvic cavity; 1 = with an open wound into the pelvic cavity.

Source: From Moore EE, Cogbill TH, Jurkovich GJ, J Trauma, 33, 337–338, 1992. With permission.

Table B.36 Uterus (Non-pregnant) Injury Scale

Grade[a]	Description of Injury	ICD-9	ICD-10	AIS-2005
I	Contusion/haematoma	867.4/867.5	S37.6	2
II	Superficial laceration (<1 cm)	867.4/867.5	S37.6	2
III	Deep laceration (≥1 cm)	867.4/867.5	S37.6	3
IV	Laceration involving the uterine artery	902.55	S37.6	3
V	Avulsion/devascularization	867.4/867.5	S37.6	3

[a]Advance one grade for multiple injuries up to grade III.

Note: With ICD-10, use supplementary character: 0 = without an open wound into the pelvic cavity; 1 = with an open wound into the pelvic cavity.

Source: From Moore EE, Jurkovich GJ, Knudson MM, et al., J Trauma, 39, 1069–1070, 1995. With permission.

Table B.37 Uterus (Pregnant) Injury Scale

Grade[a]	Description of Injury	ICD-9	ICD-10	AIS-2005
I	Contusion or haematoma (without placental abruption)	867.4/867.5	S37.6	2
II	Superficial laceration (<1 cm) or partial placental abruption <25%	867.4/867.5	S37.6	3
III	Deep laceration (≥1 cm) occurring in second trimester or placental abruption >25% but <50%	867.4/867.5	S37.6	3
	Deep laceration (≥1 cm) in third trimester	867.4/867.5	S37.6	4
IV	Laceration involving uterine artery	902.55	S37.6	4
	Deep laceration (≥1 cm) with >50% placental abruption	867.4/867.5	S37.6	4
V	Uterine rupture			
	• Second trimester	867.4/867.5	S37.6	4
	• Third trimester	867.4/867.5	S37.6	5
	Complete placental abruption	867.4/867.5	S37.6	4–5

[a]Advance one grade for multiple injuries up to grade III.

Note: With ICD-10, use supplementary character: 0 = without an open wound into the pelvic cavity; 1 = with an open wound into the pelvic cavity.

Source: From Moore EE, Jurkovich GJ, Knudson MM, et al., *J Trauma*, 39, 1069–1070, 1995. With permission.

Table B.38 Fallopian Tube Injury Scale

Grade[a]	Description of Injury	ICD-9	ICD-10	AIS-2005
I	Haematoma or contusion	867.6/867.7	S37.5	2
II	Laceration <50% circumference	867.6/867.7	S37.5	2
III	Laceration ≥50% circumference	867.6/867.7	S37.5	2
IV	Transection	867.6/867.7	S37.5	2
V	Vascular injury; devascularized segment	902.89	S35.8	2

[a]Advance one grade for bilateral injuries up to grade III.

Note: With ICD-10, use supplementary character: 0 = without an open wound into the abdominal or pelvic cavity; 1 = with an open wound into the abdominal or pelvic cavity.

Source: From Moore EE, Jurkovich GJ, Knudson MM, et al., *J Trauma*, 39, 1069–1070, 1995. With permission.

Table B.39 Ovary Injury Scale

Grade[a]	Description of Injury	ICD-9	ICD-10	AIS-2005
I	Contusion or haematoma	867.6/867.7	S37.4	1
II	Superficial laceration (depth <0.5 cm)	867.6/867.7	S37.4	2
III	Deep laceration (depth ≥0.5 cm)	867.8/867.7	S37.4	3
IV	Partial disruption or blood supply	902.81	S35.8	3
V	Avulsion or complete parenchymal destruction	902.81	S37.4	3

[a]Advance one grade for bilateral injuries up to grade III.

Note: With ICD-10, use supplementary character: 0 = without an open wound into the abdominal or pelvic cavity; 1 = with an open wound into the abdominal or pelvic cavity.

Source: From Moore EE, Jurkovich GJ, Knudson MM, et al., *J Trauma*, 39, 1069–1070, 1995. With permission.

Table B.40 Vagina Injury Scale

Grade[a]	Description of Injury	ICD-9	ICD-10	AIS-2005
I	Contusion or haematoma	922.4	S30.2	1
II	Laceration, superficial (mucosa only)	878.6	S31.4	1
III	Laceration, deep into fat or muscle	878.6	S31.4	2
IV	Laceration, complex, into cervix or peritoneum	868.7	S31.4	3
V	Injury into adjacent organs (anus, rectum, urethra, bladder)	878.7	S39.7	3

[a]Advance one grade for multiple injuries up to grade III.

Note: With ICD-10, use supplementary character: 0 = without an open wound into the abdominal or pelvic cavity; 1 = with an open wound into the abdominal or pelvic cavity.

Source: From Moore EE, Jurkovich GJ, Knudson MM, et al., *J Trauma*, 39, 1069–1070, 1995. With permission.

Table B.41 Vulva Injury Scale

Grade[a]	Description of Injury	ICD-9	ICD-10	AIS-2005
I	Contusion or haematoma	922.4	S30.2	1
II	Laceration, superficial (skin only)	878.4	S31.4	1
III	Laceration, deep (into fat or muscle)	878.4	S31.4	2
IV	Avulsion; skin, fat or muscle	878.5	S38.2	3
V	Injury into adjacent organs (anus, rectum, urethra, bladder)	878.5	S39.7	3

[a]Advance one grade for multiple injuries up to grade III.

Source: From Moore EE, Jurkovich GJ, Knudson MM, et al., *J Trauma*, 39, 1069–1070, 1995. With permission.

Table B.42 Testis Injury Scale

Grade[a]	Description of Injury	ICD-9	ICD-10	AIS-2005
I	Contusion/haematoma	911.0–922.4	S30.2	1
II	Subclinical laceration of tunica albuginea	922.4	S31.3	1
III	Laceration of tunica albuginea with <50% parenchymal loss	878.2	S31.3	2
IV	Major laceration of tunica albuginea with ≥50% parenchymal loss	878.3	S31.3	2
V	Total testicular destruction or avulsion	878.3	S38.2	2

[a]Advance one grade for bilateral lesions up to grade V.

Source: From Moore EE, Malangoni MA, Cogbill TH, Peterson NE, Champion HR, Shackford SR, *J Trauma*, 41, 523–524, 1996. With permission.

Table B.43 Scrotum Injury Scale

Grade	Description of Injury	ICD-9	ICD-10	AIS-2005
I	Contusion	922.4	S30.2	1
II	Laceration <25% of scrotal diameter	878.2	S31.2	1
III	Laceration ≥25% of scrotal diameter	878.3	S31.3	2
IV	Avulsion <50%	878.3	S38.2	2
V	Avulsion ≥50%	878.3	S38.2	2

Source: From Moore EE, Malangoni MA, Cogbill TH, Peterson NE, Champion HR, Shackford SR, *J Trauma*, 41, 523–524, 1996. With permission.

Table B.44 Penis Injury Scale

Grade[a]	Description of Injury	ICD-9	ICD-10	AIS-2005
I	Cutaneous laceration/contusion	911.0/922.4	S30.2/31/2	1
II	Buck fascia (cavernosum) laceration without tissue loss	878.0	S37.8	1
III	Cutaneous avulsion	878.1	S38.2	3
	Laceration through glans/meatus			
	Cavernosal or urethral defect <2 cm			
IV	Partial penectomy	878.1	S38.2	3
	Cavernosal or urethral defect ≥2 cm			
V	Total penectomy	876.1	S38.2	3

[a]Advance one grade for multiple injuries up to grade III.

Source: From Moore EE, Malangoni MA, Cogbill TH, Peterson NE, Champion HR, Shackford SR, *J Trauma*, 41, 523–524, 1996. With permission.

Table B.45 Peripheral Vascular Organ Injury Scale

Grade[a]	Description of Injury	ICD-9	ICD-10	AIS-2005
I	Digital artery/vein	903.5	S65.5	1–3
	Palmar artery/vein	903.4	S65.3	1–3
	Deep palmar artery/vein	904.6	S65.3	1–3
	Dorsalis pedis artery	904.7	S95.0	1–3
	Plantar artery/vein	904.5	S95.1	1–3
	Non-named arterial/venous branches	903.8/904.7	S55.9/S85.9	1–3
II	Basilic/cephalic vein	903.8	S45.8/S55.8	1–3
	Saphenous vein	904.3	S75.2	1–3
	Radial artery	903.2	S55.1	1–3
	Ulnar artery	903.3	S55.0	1–3
III	Axillary vein	903.02	S45.1	2–3
	Superficial/deep femoral vein	903.02	S75.1	2–3
	Popliteal vein	904.42	S85.5	2–3
	Brachial artery	903.1	S45.1	2–3
	Anterior tibial artery	904.51/904.52	S85.1	1–3
	Posterior tibial artery	904.53/904.54	S85.1	1–3
	Peroneal artery	904.7	S85.2	1–3
	Tibioperoneal trunk	904.7	S85.2	2–3
IV	Superficial/deep femoral artery	904.1/904.7	S75.0	3–4
	Popliteal artery	904.41	S85.0	2–3
V	Axillary artery	903.01	S45.0	2–3
	Common femoral artery	904.0	S75.0	3–4

[a]Increase one grade for multiple grade III or IV injuries involving >50 per cent of the vessel circumference. Decrease one grade for <25 per cent disruption of the vessel circumference for grades IV or V.

Source: From Moore EE, Malangoni MA, Cogbill TH, Peterson NE, Champion HR, Shackford SR, *J Trauma*, 41, 523–524, 1996. With permission.

B.8 SUMMARY

Trauma scoring systems and allied methods of analyzing outcomes after trauma are steadily evolving and have become increasingly sophisticated over recent years.

Trauma scoring systems are designed to facilitate pre-hospital triage, identify trauma patients whose outcomes are statistically unexpected for quality assurance analysis, allow an accurate comparison of different trauma populations and organize and improve trauma systems. They are vital for the scientific study of the epidemiology and the treatment of trauma and may even be used to define resource allocation and reimbursement in the future.

Trauma scoring systems that measure outcome solely in terms of death or survival are at best blunt instruments. Despite the existence of several scales (Quality of Well-being Scale, Sickness Impact Profile, etc.), further efforts are needed to develop outcome measures that are able to evaluate the multiplicity of outcomes across the full range of diverse trauma populations.

Despite the profusion of acronyms, scoring systems are a vital component of trauma care-delivery systems. The effectiveness of well-organized, centralized, multidisciplinary trauma centres in reducing the mortality and morbidity of injured patients is well documented. Further improvement and expansion of trauma care can only occur if developments are subjected to scientifically rigorous evaluation. Thus, trauma scoring systems play a central role in the provision of trauma care today and for the future.

REFERENCES

1. Teasdale G, Jennet B: Assessment of coma and impaired consciousness: a practical scale. *Lancet*. 1974;ii:81–84.
2. Tepas JJ 3rd, Ramenofsky ML, Mollitt DL, Gans BM, DiScala C. The Paediatric Trauma Score as a predictor of injury severity: an objective assessment. *J Trauma*. 1988;28:425–429.
3. Champion HR, Sacco WJ, Copes WS, Gann DS, Gennarelli TA, Flanagan ME. A revision of the Trauma Score. *J Trauma*. 1989;29:623–629.
4. Knaus EA, Draper EA, Wagner DP, et al. APACHE II: A severity of disease classification system. *Crit Care Med* 1985;13(10):818–829.
5. Calculation of the APACHE II Score. htpp://www.mdcalc.com/apache-ii-score-for-icu-mortality. Accessed December 2014.
6. American Association for the Advancement of Automotive Medicine. *The Abbreviated Injury Scale: 2005 – Update 2008 Revision*. Barrington, IL: AAAM, 2008. http://www.AAAM.org.
7. Baker SP, O'Neill B, Haddon W, Long WB. The Injury Severity Score: a method for describing patients with multiple injuries and evaluating emergency care. *J Trauma*. 1974;14:187–196.
8. Osler T, Baker SP, Long W. A modification of the Injury Severity Score that both improves accuracy and simplifies scoring. *J Trauma*. 1997;43:922–926.
9. Balogh Z, Offner PJ, Moore EE, Biffl WL. NISS predicts postinjury multiple organ failure better than the ISS. *J Trauma*. 2000;48:624–628.
10. Copes WS, Champion HR, Sacco WJ, et al. Progress in characterising anatomical injury. *J Trauma*. 1990;30(10):1200–1207.
11. Osler T, Rutledge R, Deis J, Bedrick E. ICISS: an international classification of disease-9 based injury severity score. *J Trauma*. 1997;41:380–388.
12. Organ Injury Scale of the American Association for the Surgery of Trauma (OIS-AAST). http://www.aast.org. Accessed December 2010.
13. Moore EE, Dunn EL, Moore JB, et al. Penetrating Abdominal Trauma Index. *J Trauma*. 1981;21:439–445.
14. Lefering R. Development and validation of the Revised Injury Severity Classification (RISC) score for severely injured patients. *Eur J Trauma Emerg Surg*. 2009;35:437–447.
15. Lefering R, Huber-Wagner S, Nienaber U, et al. Update of the trauma risk adjustment model of the Trauma Register DGU: the Revised Injury Severity Classification, version II. *Crit Care*. 2014;18(5):476(epub).
16. Gabbe BJ, Magtengaard K, Osler T, et al. Is the Charlson Comorbidity Index (CCI) useful for predicting trauma outcomes? *Acad Emerg Med*. 2005;12(4);318–321.
17. Bergeron E, Rossignol M, Osler T, et al. Improving the TRISS methodology by restructuring age categories and adding comorbidities. *J Trauma*. 2004;5(4):760–767.
18. Turner-Stokes L, Nyein K, Turner-Stokes T, et al. The UK FIM+FAM Functional Assessment Measure. *Clin Rehabil*. 1999;13(4):277–287.
19. Wright J. The Functional Assessment Measure. The Center for Outcome Measurement in Brain Injury. http://www.tbims.org/combi/FAM. Accessed December 2014.
20. Jennet B, Bond MR. Assessment of outcome: a practical scale. *Lancet*. 1975;i:480–487.
21. Boyd CR, Tolson MA, Copes WS. Evaluating trauma care: the TRISS model. *J Trauma*. 1987;27:370–378.
22. Champion HR, Copes WS, Sacco WJ, et al. A new characterisation of injury severity. *J Trauma*. 1990;30:539–546.

23. Champion HR, Copes WS, Sacco WJ, et al. Improved predictions from A Severity Characterization of Trauma (ASCOT) over Trauma and Injury Severity Score (TRISS): results of an independent evaluation. *J Trauma*. 1996;40:42–48.

24. World Health Organization. ICD-9CM. *International Classification of Diseases, Ninth Revision, Clinical Modification*. Center for Disease Control and Prevention, Hyattsville, MD. http://www.cdc.gov/nchs/icd.htm. Accessed December 2014.

25. World Health Organization. *ICD-10 Codes*. 2015 version online. http://www.who.int/classifications/icd/en/. Accessed December 2014.

26. Moore EE, Malangoni MA, Cogbill TH, Peterson NE, Champion HR, Shackford SR. Organ injury scaling VII: cervical vascular, peripheral vascular, adrenal, penis, testis and scrotum. *J Trauma*. 1996;41:523–524.

27. Moore EE, Cogbill TH, Jurkovich GJ. Organ injury scaling III: chest wall, abdominal vascular, ureter, bladder and urethra. *J Trauma*. 1992;33:337–338.

28. Moore EE, Malangoni MA, Cogbill TH, et al. Organ injury scaling IV: thoracic, vascular, lung, cardiac and diaphragm. *J Trauma*. 1994;36:299–300.

29. Moore EE, Cogbill TH, Jurkovich GJ, Shackford SR, Malangoni MA, Champion HR. Organ injury scaling: spleen and liver (1994 Revision). *J Trauma*. 1995;38:323–324.

30. Moore EE, Jurkovich GJ, Knudson MM, et al. Organ injury scaling VI: extrahepatic biliary, oesophagus, stomach, vulva, vagina, uterus (non-pregnant), uterus (pregnant), fallopian tube, and ovary. *J Trauma*. 1995;39:1069–1070.

31. Moore EE, Cogbill TH, Malangoni MA, Jurkovich GJ, Shackford SR, Champion HR. Organ injury scaling: pancreas, duodenum, small bowel, colon and rectum. *J Trauma*. 1990;30:1427–1429.

32. Moore EE, Shackford SR, Pachter HL, et al. Organ injury scaling: spleen, liver and kidney. *J Trauma*. 1989;9:1664–1666.

Appendix C
The Definitive Surgical Trauma Care Course: Course Requirements and Syllabus

International Association for Trauma
Surgery and Intensive Care
IATSIC Secretariat
International Society of Surgery
Seltisbergerstrasse 16
CH-4419 Lupsingen
Switzerland
Phone: +41 61 81 59 666
Fax: +41 61 81 14 775
E-mail: Iatsic@iss-sic.ch
URL: www.iatsic.org

C.1 BACKGROUND

Injury (trauma) remains a major healthcare problem throughout the world. In addition to improving awareness of trauma prevention and management, improved application of surgical skills is expected to save further lives and contribute to minimizing disability. It is widely recognized that training of surgeons in the management of trauma is substantially deficient because of:

- Limited exposure within individual training programmes to the types of patient required to develop the appropriate level of skills.
- Traditional trauma surgical training, which has been organ-specific.

Consequently, surgeons can finish their training with suboptimal skills in this field, where there is often little time to contemplate an appropriate course of action.

Through the early 1990s, it became apparent to a number of surgeons familiar with trauma management around the world that there was a specific need for surgical training in the technical aspects of the operative care of trauma patient, with particular emphasis on those who were close to completing, or had recently completed, their training. This course had its origins during a meeting in October 1993 between Drs Howard Champion (USA), David Mulder (Canada), Donald Trunkey (USA), Stephen Deane (Australia) and Abe Fingerhut (France).

This post-graduate surgical course, developed in collaboration with professional educators, assumes competence with assessment and resuscitative measures that have become standardized through the Advanced Trauma Life Support® (ATLS) course of the American College of Surgeons. It draws on the specialist surgical training of all course participants and reviews, strengthens and organizes the performance of established and new procedures specially required in trauma surgery. It is expected that the course will have special relevance for surgeons in countries where major trauma rates are high, and for rapidly mobilized medical units in areas of conflict. It is also likely to be valuable in developing countries where education and physical resources are limited.

C.2 COURSE DEVELOPMENT AND TESTING

There have been many attempts to test the concept:

- Dr Fingerhut's laparoscopic trauma surgical training course, which he had run for two previous years at the European Surgical Education Centre in Paris, was modified to incorporate these concepts. This two-day course consisted of didactic sessions in the morning and animal laboratory sessions in the afternoon. Evaluation responses were excellent.

- The Uniformed Services University of the Health Sciences, Bethesda, Maryland, USA, started a similar course in August 1994. Dr Don Jenkins has now put over 100 military surgeons through the course in the United States, and he is currently working on bringing the course to Chile.
- There was a Swedish Trauma Surgery Course which Drs Trunkey, Fingerhut and Champion attended in Sweden in November 1994. This was run by Dr Sten Lennquist. The course was four days of didactic teaching and one day of practical work.
- In Sydney in May 1996, a very successful pilot course was organized at Prince Henry Hospital. The international faculty at that course included Don Trunkey, Abe Fingerhut and Howard Champion. The course was a tremendous success, and successful courses have since been held worldwide.
- Following courses in Australia, Austria and South Africa, a standardized manual and slide set were developed in 1999.
- The course is revised every four years, with updated material, in order to stay current and to recognize the rapid improvements in trauma care globally.

C.3 COURSE DETAILS

C.3.1 Ownership

The Definitive Surgical Trauma Care™ (DSTC) course is a registered trademark of the International Association for Trauma Surgery and Intensive Care (IATSIC). IATSIC is an Integrated Society of the International Society of Surgery/Société Internationale de Chirugie (ISS–SIC) based in Lupsingen, Switzerland. Only courses recognized by IATSIC may be called DSTC courses.

C.3.2 Mission Statement

The DSTC course is designed to train participants in the techniques required for the surgical care of the trauma patient. This is done by a combination of lectures, demonstrations, case discussions and practical sessions, utilizing animal tissue and human (cadaver or prosected) tissue if available.

C.3.3 Application to Hold a Course

Application can be made to IATSIC for recognition of a course. Provided the minimum requirements for the course have been met, as laid down below, IATSIC will recognize the course, which will then be entitled to be called a DSTC course and carry the IATSIC logo. The initial course to be presented will be the course prescribed by IATSIC, and no changes may be made to the course material or syllabus.

C.3.4 Eligibility to Present

C.3.4.1 LOCAL ORGANIZATIONS

The DSTC course can be presented by any tertiary academic institution or recognized surgical organization.

C.3.4.2 NATIONAL ORGANIZATIONS

National organizations can present the course in their own country on behalf of IATSIC. A memorandum of understanding will be signed with IATSIC. Following the presentation of the first two courses, the national organization shall have the right to modify the course to enhance its relevance to local conditions, although still respecting the core curriculum.

C.3.5 Course Materials and Overview

The course takes place over three days with the following course materials:

- The content of the course will, as a minimum, contain the core curriculum, as laid down in the IATSIC DSTC manual (see Appendix D). Additional material and modules may be included at the discretion of the local organizers, provided such material is not in conflict with the core curriculum.
- Additional 'add-on' modules may be presented at the discretion of the local organizers.
- The course will use a specific set of slides and the DSTC course manual.
- IATSIC is able to furnish the IATSIC DSTC course manual and course materials (including slides on PowerPoint), if requested, at a substantial discount. However, provided the minimum core syllabus is adhered to, a local course manual and material can be used.

C.3.6 **Course Director**

In addition to the requirements below, the course director must be a full, current member of IATSIC. For an inaugural course, the course director must be a member of the IATSIC Executive Committee.

C.3.7 **Course Faculty**

- Course faculty will be divided into:
  · Local faculty
  · International faculty
  · Guest lecturers
- Course faculty members must have attended a DSTC course.
- Course faculty members must have completed an ATLS Instructor course, Royal College of Surgeons 'Train the Trainers' course or an equivalent instructor training course.
- Course international faculty must be members of IATSIC.
- Additional guest lecturers with particular expertise in a subject are permitted.
- Details of all faculty members with confirmation of the above, and full Ethics Committee approval, must be lodged with IATSIC at least three months prior to the prior to commencement of the course.
- The recommended student:instructor ratio should ideally be 4:1, not including the course director.

C.3.8 **Course Participants**

- All course participants must be licensed medical practitioners.
- Attendance at the entire course is mandatory.
- The level of applicants can be decided locally, provided that the participants are licensed medical practitioners, and are *actively involved in the surgical decision making and surgery* of the trauma patient.
- An entrance examination can be used if needed. An exit examination is not mandatory.

C.3.9 **Practical Skill Stations**

Practical skills may be demonstrated on different material, depending on the local constraints. The practical component of the course *must* include an animal laboratory. However, the use of cadavers is optional and dependent on local conditions. Full local ethical committee certificates of approval for all animal and other tissue work, and any other legal necessary approvals, *must* be obtained and must be submitted to IATSIC *before* a course can be approved or held.

C.3.10 **Course Syllabus**

In order for IATSIC to recognize the course as a valid DSTC course, the course must meet or exceed the minimum requirements of the core curriculum. The core curriculum and 'modules' are contained in this manual. The course consists of:

- Core knowledge.
- Surgical skills (see Appendix D).
- Additional modules, which may be added as required, at the discretion of the local organizing committee and as required for local needs.
- Where human material is available for dissection, the course is often enhanced by presentation in association with the American College of Surgeons (ACS) or the ACS Course in Advanced Surgical Skills for Exposure in Trauma (ASSET).

C.3.11 **Course Certification**

- Participants are required to attend the entire course.
- Certification of attendance and completion of the course can be issued.
- The certificates of the courses will be numbered.
- Details of the course, final faculty and participants, as well as a course evaluation, must be submitted to IATSIC after the course.

C.4 **IATSIC RECOGNITION**

Application for recognition of individual courses should be made to IATSIC. IATSIC-recognized courses may carry the endorsement logos of IATSIC and the ISS-SIC and will be entitled to be called DSTC courses.

The DSTC course is the intellectual property and a registered trademark of IATSIC, and IATSIC is an Integrated Society of the ISS–SIC based in Lupsingen, Switzerland. Although it may carry the endorsement (support) of other bodies, this does not imply that other organizations may operate or control the DSTC course in any way.

The DSTC course is designed to train medical practitioners in the techniques required for the definitive surgical care of the trauma patient. This is done by a combination of lectures, demonstrations, case discussions and practical sessions.

The registration and control of the DSTC courses will be controlled by the DSTC Sub-Committee on behalf of IATSIC. While it is desirable that national courses be controlled by a national organization, there will be no restriction on local courses provided that international DSTC criteria are met. Application to hold a course must be made through IATSIC.

Only courses recognized by IATSIC may be called DSTC courses.

C.5 **COURSE INFORMATION**

Course information is obtainable from IATSIC.

Appendix D
Definitive Surgical Trauma Care Course – Core Surgical Skills

D.1 THE NECK

D.1.1. Standard neck (pre-sternomastoid) incision
D.1.2. Control and repair of the carotid vessels
    D.1.2.1. Zone II
    D.1.2.2. Extension into zone III
    D.1.2.3. Division of the digastric muscle and subluxation or division of the mandible
    D.1.2.4. Extension into zone I
D.1.3. Extension by supraclavicular incision
    D.1.3.1. Ligation of the proximal internal carotid artery
    D.1.3.2. Repair with a divided external carotid artery
D.1.4. Access to, control of and ligation of the internal jugular vein
D.1.5. Access to and repair of the trachea
D.1.6. Access to and repair of the cervical oesophagus

D.2 THE CHEST

D.2.1. Incisions
    D.2.1.1. Anterolateral thoracotomy
    D.2.1.2. Sternotomy
    D.2.1.3. 'Clamshell' bilateral thoracotomy incision
D.2.2. Thoracotomy
    D.2.2.1. Exploration of the thorax
    D.2.2.2. Ligation of the intercostal and internal mammary vessels
    D.2.2.3. Emergency department (resuscitative) thoracotomy
        D.2.2.3.1. Supradiaphragmatic control of the aorta
        D.2 2.3.2. Control of the pulmonary hilum
        D.2.2.3.3. Internal cardiac massage
D.2.3. Pericardiotomy
    D.2.3.1. Preservation of the phrenic nerve
    D.2.3.2. Access to the pulmonary veins
D.2.4. Access to and repair of the thoracic aorta
D.2.5. Lung wounds
    D.2.5.1. Oversewing
    D.2.5.2. Stapling
    D.2.5.3. Partial lung resection
    D.2.5.4. Tractectomy
    D.2.5.5. Lobectomy
D.2.6. Access to and repair of the thoracic oesophagus
D.2.7. Access to and repair of the diaphragm
D.2.8. Compression of the left subclavian vessels from below
D.2.9. Left anterior thoracotomy
    D.2.9.1. Visualization of the supra-aortic vessels
D.2.10. Heart repair
    D.2.10.1. Finger control
    D.2.10.2. Involvement of the coronary vessels
D.2.11. Insertion of a shunt

D.3 THE ABDOMINAL CAVITY

D.3.1. Midline laparotomy
    D.3.1.1. How to explore (priorities)
    D.3.1.2. Packing
    D.3.1.3. Localization of retroperitoneal haematomas – when to explore?
    D.3.1.4. Damage control
        D.3.1.4.1. Techniques
        D.3.1.4.2. Abdominal closure
    D.3.1.5. Extension of laparotomy incision
        D.3.1.5.1. Lateral extension

D.3.1.5.2. Sternotomy
D.3.1.6. Cross-clamping of the aorta at the diaphragm (division at the left crus)
D.3.2. Left visceral medial rotation
D.3.2.1. Reflection of the left (descending) colon medially
D.3.2.2. Reflection of the pancreas and spleen towards the midline
D.3.3. Right visceral medial rotation
D.3.3.1. Kocher manoeuvre
D.3.3.2. Reflection of the right (ascending) colon medially
D.3.4. Abdominal oesophagus
D.3.4.1. Mobilization
D.3.4.2. Repair
D.3.4.2.1. Simple
D.3.4.2.2. Mobilization of the fundus to reinforce sutures
D.3.5. Stomach
D.3.5.1. Mobilization
D.3.5.2. Access to vascular control
D.3.5.3. Repair of anterior and posterior wounds
D.3.5.4. Pyloric exclusion
D.3.5.5. Distal gastrectomy
D.3.6. Bowel
D.3.6.1. Resection
D.3.6.2. Small and large bowel anastomosis
D.3.6.3. Staple colostomy
D.3.6.4. Ileostomy technique

D.4 THE LIVER

D.4.1. Mobilization (falciform, suspensory, triangular and coronary ligaments)
D.4.2. Liver packing
D.4.3. Hepatic isolation
D.4.3.1. Control of the infrahepatic inferior vena cava
D.4.3.2. Control of the suprahepatic superior vena cava
D.4.3.3. Pringle manoeuvre
D.4.4. Repair of parenchymal laceration
D.4.5. Technique of finger fracture
D.4.6. Tractotomy
D.4.7. Packing for injury to hepatic veins
D.4.8. Hepatic resection
D.4.9. Non-anatomical partial resection
D.4.10. Use of tissue adhesives

D.4.11. Tamponade for penetrating injury (Foley/Penrose drains, Sengstaken tube)

D.5 THE SPLEEN

D.5.1. Mobilization
D.5.2. Suture
D.5.3. Use of tissue adhesives
D.5.4. Partial splenectomy
D.5.4.1. Sutures
D.5.4.2. Staples
D.5.5. Total splenectomy

D.6 THE PANCREAS

D.6.1. Mobilization of the tail of the pancreas
D.6.2. Mobilization of the head of the pancreas
D.6.3. Localization of the main duct and its repair
D.6.4. Distal pancreatic resection
D.6.4.1. Stapler
D.6.4.2. Oversewing
D.6.5. Use of tissue adhesives
D.6.6. Access to the mesenteric vessels (division of the pancreas)

D.7 THE DUODENUM

D.7.1. Mobilization of the duodenum
D.7.1.1. Kocher manoeuvre (rotation of the duodenum)
D.7.1.2. Division of the ligament of Treitz
D.7.1.3. Repair of the duodenum

D.8 THE GENITOURINARY SYSTEM

D.8.1. Kidney
D.8.1.1. Mobilization
D.8.1.2. Vascular control
D.8.1.3. Repair
D.8.1.4. Partial nephrectomy
D.8.1.5. Nephrectomy
D.8.2. Ureter
D.8.2.1. Mobilization
D.8.2.2. Stenting
D.8.2.3. Repair

D.8.3. Bladder

D.8.3.1. Repair of intraperitoneal rupture

D.8.3.2. Repair of extraperitoneal rupture

D.9 ABDOMINAL VASCULAR INJURIES

D.9.1. Exposure and control

D.9.1.1. Aorta and its branches

D.9.1.1.1. Exposure

D.9.1.1.2. Repair

D.9.1.1.3. Shunt

D.9.1.2. Inferior vena cava

D.9.1.2.1. Suprahepatic inferior vena cava

D.9.1.2.2. Infrahepatic inferior vena cava

D.9.1.2.3. Control of haemorrhage with swabs

D.9.1.2.4. Repair both anteriorly and posteriorly, through an anterior wound

D.9.1.2.5. Shunting

D.9.2. Pelvis

D.9.2.1. Control of the pelvic vessels

D.9.2.1.1. Extraperitoneal packing

D.9.2.1.2. Suture of artery and vein

D.9.2.1.3. Ligation of artery and vein

D.9.2.1.4. Packing/anchor ligation of the sacral vessels

D.10 PERIPHERAL VASCULAR INJURIES

D.10.1. Extremities: vascular access

D.10.1.1. Axillary

D.10.1.2. Brachial

D.10.1.3. Femoral

D.10.1.4. Popliteal

D.10.2. Fasciotomy

D.10.2.1. Upper limb

D.10.2.2. Lower limb

Appendix E
Briefing for Operating Room Scrub Nurses

E.1 INTRODUCTION

Damage control techniques for the management of the major trauma patient are now accepted concepts and include temporizing measures to prevent a cold, acidotic and coagulopathic patient from further deterioration and eventual death. Some personnel working in the operating room/theatre (OR/OT) environment may not have had previous exposure to these techniques, especially in countries where trauma volumes are limited and major trauma is a stressful rarity. This appendix is intended to help prepare the team for the imminent arrival and intraoperative management of the major trauma patient. Good communication is the key to success. Anticipate and think laterally.

The aspects of care referred to in this section are as follows:

- Preparation.
- Cleaning and draping.
- Instruments and issues of technique.
- Special tools and equipment – including improvised gadgets.
- Medico-legal aspects.
- Communication.

E.2 PREPARING THE OPERATING ROOM

As has been mentioned, patients with major trauma are complex in that they have deranged physiology and may have complex injuries with competing priorities for treatment. Optimizing the OR before the patient arrives and planning ahead for every eventuality is what will make the difference between a stressful, chaotic experience for all concerned, and a planned environment where every member of the team has a role and acknowledges the strength of all the members of the team.

E.2.1 Environment

Because of the underlying coagulopathy and hypothermia, the patient needs to be prevented from further heat loss at all costs to maximize haemostasis:

- The internal temperature of the operating room/theatre (OR/OT) should be set to at least 27°C and maintained at this level[1].
- Fluid and blood should be warmed before and during administration, using devices such as a Level 1 (Smiths Medical, St. Paul, MN) or Ranger (3M Medical, St. Paul, MN) device, which allows for rapid infusion without sacrificing adequate heat transmission to the fluid. Ideally, the temperature should be set at 41°C.
- Patient warming devices should be present and readied for use. These can include a circulating warm fluid underlay or warm air circulation device (e.g. Bair Hugger (3M Medical), which must be directly in contact with the skin and not over a bed sheet.

E.2.2 Blood Loss

Because of the propensity for massive blood loss, one should consider activating and priming a cell-saving device of some description. Blood from the chest drain need not be washed and can be autotransfused directly provided that normal saline (0.9 per cent) has been used in the collection device and not water.

E.2.3 **Instruments**

- Now is the time to request extra instrument packs and obtain packs of sponges/swabs as these will be rapidly required in large numbers.
- A trolley with multiple drawers with pre-packed equipment may be a useful option[2].
- Equipment for thoracotomy and vascular access/ repair should be mandatory and a large selection of sutures, staplers and drains should be available including items for unusual uses, such as a Sengstaken-Blakemore tube.

E.2.4 **Cleaning**

With damage control surgery, there is less time than usual to provide a truly sterile field, and alternate methods should be used to achieve the same result. It is often said that 'sterility is a luxury in trauma':

- Typically, either an iodophore- or a chlorhexidine-based skin preparation is utilized, and this applies equally to the trauma patient. One should not use both types as they may inactivate each other. Chlorhexidine-based solutions are the current solution of choice[3,4].
- The method of application may, however, vary. One option, utilized in a number of prominent North American centres, is the use of a spray bottle to apply the preparation solution. This has been shown to be as effective as traditional circular sponging techniques[4,5].
- Cleaning should be extended widely beyond the expected bounds of the operative field, and the recommendation is to clean from neck to knees, as this allows for extension from abdomen to chest or for vein harvest from the saphenous veins.

E.2.5 **Draping**

Draping is also along unconventional lines, and this ensures that the surgeons can have ready access to more than just the area of single focus, which is usual for when elective surgery is performed.

- Drape widely using drapes that attach to the skin or fix them with skin staples, laterally from the neck, lateral to the chest at the mid-axillary lines and along the same plane to the knees. The

genitalia are covered with a small drape or an opened swab (Figure E.1).
- Prevent further heat loss by covering the areas not initially needed for surgical access with sterile drapes. For example, if the abdomen is the default operation, cover the chest and legs with drapes that are easily removed if access to those regions is required.

Figure E.1 Draping required for a trauma laparotomy.

E.2.6 **Adjuncts**

As far as pre-planning for the actual procedure is concerned, one can only recommend that the OR team 'anticipate' all eventualities. Remember, too, that as there is little time to spare, the risk of injury to operative team members is high, and all precautions should be taken to ensure maximal protection.

- Although there is no good evidence that masks, overshoes and caps protect the patient from infection during surgery, standard precautions should be maintained to protect the team members. The OR nurse should ensure that all staff in the 'sterile area' are appropriately attired.

- Place the scalpel in a receiver (kidney-bowl) for the surgeon to take and replace. The body cavities should be opened primarily with a scalpel and heavy (Mayo) scissors.
- Have 20–30 large *dry* swabs or sponges ready for the surgeon to perform rapid packing. These are best passed 'folded' initially, unless the surgeon specifies otherwise, as for definitive packing, swabs should be used *folded* in layers.
- The suction devices should be ready and should preferably be routed to the cell-saver device. It is useful for there to be *two* suction devices at the table.
- An electrocautery machine should be available, but there is no time for small vessel haemostasis at this point, and this will most likely be used later.

E.3 SURGICAL PROCEDURE

E.3.1 Instruments

The instrument sets one should have at the ready are as follows:

- A thoracotomy tray ready in the room, but not open unless the chest is the primary operative focus. A sternal saw or Lebsche knife should also be available.
- A standard laparotomy set should be open and ready, including a bowel resection set.
- Vascular instruments, including large aortic clamps (Crawford and Satinsky) should be open on the set-up trolley.
- Extra small, medium and large crushing clamps (e.g. Halstead, Crile, Roberts and mosquito) are needed, as there may be many bleeding vessels to clamp.
- Several Babcock forceps should be available for holding or marking a bowel injury.
- A right-angled dissecting forceps such as is used for bile ducts (Lahey, Heiss, Mixter, etc.) should be available.
- A full selection of retractors (e.g. Morris, Army-Navy, Langenbeck, Deaver and copper malleables) as well as some form of a self-retaining system such as a Bookwalter, Omni-Tract or Gray system should be ready for use.
- At least one pair of forceps should be rubber-shod, as retrieval of a bullet will otherwise result in

scratching the round, rendering it inadmissible for forensic evidence, should the case come to court.

Since most major trauma (especially penetrating trauma) affects the abdomen, one must prepare for bowel and solid organ injury:

- Skin staplers can temporize small holes from bullets and lacerations in the stomach (and may be useful on the heart).
- GI-type cutting staplers are handy for the rapid closure of bowel ends during non-reconstructive resection of small bowel or colon.
- TA-type non-cutting staplers can be used to fashion a pyloric exclusion or for distal pancreas resection when the need for rapid resection is present.
- Umbilical tapes or the tapes on large sponges can be used to ligate segments of bowel to control effluent.
- Ligaclips can be useful for controlling bleeding vessels on the liver or spleen or in the mesentery.
- It is useful to keep handy a Sengstaken-Blakemore tube for placing in a bleeding hepatic tract to attempt to tamponade the deep bleeding. A Penrose drain inflated over a 16-gauge nasogastric tube can achieve a similar effect.
- For suspected vascular injury or to control bleeding from non-ligatable vessels, various forms of temporary arterial shunt and similar devices are required.
- The Rumel tourniquet is a useful device made by simply placing a cylindrical plastic tube over a vascular loop and using this to compress a friable vessel once it has been isolated and looped. It may also be used to hold a shunt in place proximally and distally in an injured artery. The tourniquets can be kept in place with either Ligaclips or small artery clamps.
- Proprietary shunts (such as Javid or Barker shunts) should be available; alternatively, one can manufacture them using intravenous tubing, nasogastric tubing or chest drain tubing, depending on the vessel size.
- A selection of vascular grafts should be close at hand.
- A selection of plastic drapes for damage control closure should be available:
  · Opsite (Smith & Nephew, London, UK)
  · Ioban or Steridrape (3M Medical, St. Paul, MN)
- Proprietary vacuum closures:
  · V.A.C. (Kinetic Concepts Inc. [KCI], San Antonio, TX)
- Renasys (Smith & Nephew)

E.3.2 **Special Instruments and Improvised Gadgets**

The next aspect of the damage control procedure is to stop the bleeding and the contamination, while maintaining tissue perfusion. This may require the use of other specific instruments and some improvised or 'home-made' gadgets to achieve the desired result. Again, a useful option is to have this equipment 'pre-selected' and placed for use in a dedicated mobile, multiple-drawer trolley.

A suitable damage control surgery storage cupboard will contain a selection, such as is shown in Table E.1 and Figure E.2.

E.4 **ABDOMINAL CLOSURE**

Closure of the abdomen may be final and definitive, but more likely will involve some form of temporary closure device. The options include a vacuum-assisted closure

(VAC) sandwich (best), plastic silo bags sutured to the skin (Bogota bag) or towel-clip closures (neither of the latter being recommended). Equipment for the VAC-sandwich is described below. The commercial vacuum dressings are not appropriate until definitive closure.

- One sterile adhesive drape (Opsite or Ioban) is placed sticky side up, and one or two sterile towels or swabs are placed on the sticky surface. Note that only one side of the swab is covered in plastic membrane. Placing plastic on *both* sides allows the drape to slide somewhat inside the abdomen and prevents the gauze swabs from effectively 'wicking' any intra-abdominal fluid away into the suction drains but traps the fluid inside the abdominal cavity.
  - Do *not* make slits in the plastic.
  - Do *not* have suction of greater than 24 mm Hg, as this predisposes to fistulae in the hypotensive, cold, damage control patient.
- This is tucked under the fascia over the bowel, with the smooth plastic protecting the bowel, while the

Figure E.2 'Special instrument and consumables' damage control surgery storage.

Table E.1 Damage Control Equipment

Top	Sutures
Tray 1	Surgical drapes
Tray 2	Disposable gowns
Tray 3	Universal instrument set: Babcock right angle forceps, Satinsky clamp
Tray 4	Thoracic instrument set
Tray 5	Abdominal instrument set
Tray 6	Vascular instrument set
Tray 7	Disinfection material; drapes (Steridrape, Opsite, Ioban)
Tray 8	Large gauze, abdominal swabs
Tray 9	Mesh grafts, pledgets; shunts: carotid, Javid; tubes: nasogastric, urinary, chest; silicon loops, Rumel tourniquets
Tray 10	Staplers: Skin/GIA/TA/vascular
Side	Fogarty catheters; list of contents

sponges/swabs prevent evisceration by adhering to the parietal peritoneal surface.

- Two large drains or nasogastric tubes are laid inside the gap between the sheath and the skin, and are tunnelled cranially for about 5–8 cm under the skin to enable an adequate seal of the other adhesive drape over the entire abdomen.
- A second large sterile adhesive drape is then used to close the wound.
- The drains are connected with a Y-connector and may be placed on *low-pressure* wall suction (maximum suction <25 mm Hg). This controls effluent and creates a good seal. It is also easiest to nurse in the ward or ICU.

A commercial VAC device is available, but due to expense, and often the higher suction used, it is *not* recommended for *initial* closure. It is, however, the device of choice for subsequent wound management of the open abdomen.

E.5 INSTRUMENT AND SWAB COUNT

As usual, counts are performed before closure.

However, after *damage control*, a second count is performed *after* the abdominal vacuum dressing has been completed. This allows a count of how many swabs have been left in the abdomen. (Do not forget to count the swabs in the vacuum sandwich.)

An accurate record should be kept of any retained instruments and swabs, as there may be a different scrub team at the time of the re-look laparotomy.

An abdominal X-ray before final closure is advisable, as an extra safeguard to avoid retained swabs or instruments.

E.6 MEDICOLEGAL ASPECTS AND COMMUNICATION SKILLS

- Failing to plan and failing to communicate efficiently are the two major instigators of error, and error avoidance is an important aspect of medicine. The common medicolegal areas of dispute in trauma relate to aspects of consent and management of foreign bodies.
- Consent in emergency in most countries is based on the clinician doing what is in the best interest of the patient and as such the surgery to save a life takes precedence over a piece of paper. Family assent is useful and is of importance with small children, but must not influence against needed surgery unless

there is an advanced directive. Surgical checklists are also of benefit in reducing error prior to surgery.

- Foreign bodies are often present in penetrating trauma. There is a need to remove these and the local procedure for forensic analysis should be well known to the operation suite staff. Bullets should be removed without metal instruments to prevent damage to the markings used for identification of the discharging weapon. Rubber-shod or plastic instruments should be used for removal if they are removed at all, as there are clear indications to leave alone those that are unlikely to cause further harm[6].
- Forensic evidence is also essential in cases of major trauma due to sexual and paediatric abuse. Try to preserve all the evidence as best as possible[7]. Never handle bullets or metal fragments with metal instruments. Use mosquito forceps, the jaws of which are plastic or rubber covered. Wrap the fragment in gauze. Place each fragment in a separate container, marked with the exact site of removal.
- Communication is enhanced by all the members of the trauma team addressing the following aspects:
  · Share information to allow for optimal preparation.
  · Assign roles to each member and ensure each prepares his or her aspect of the care pathway.
  · Think ahead to ensure all possible equipment and patient care aspects are addressed.
- Note that closed-loop communication with feedback to the initial person asking the question/giving the instruction and assignment of actions to named persons reduces risk of error[8].

E.7 CRITICAL INCIDENT STRESS ISSUES

The trauma environment is stressful for all concerned, and time is of the essence – tempers often flare, and one must not take the issues personally.

Occasionally, the patient will not survive, and the risk is that staff may develop post-traumatic stress disorder, especially if major trauma is a rare occurrence for them. The best method for dealing with this situation is via a debriefing session as soon as everyone has cleaned up or first thing the next morning.

E.8 CONCLUSION

The success of trauma surgery depends on a team performing at its peak with effective communication, willing to work outside of the traditional norms and yet with maximal concern for patient safety. This appendix has hopefully provided some ideas to enable the team to prepare effectively for the major trauma patient.

REFERENCES AND RECOMMENDED READING

References

1. Hardcastle TC, Stander M, Kalafatis N, Hodgson E, Gopalan D. External patient temperature control in emergency centres, trauma centres, intensive care units and operating theatres: a multi-society literature review. *S Afr Med J.* 2013;103:609–611.
2. Goslings JC, Haverlag R, Ponsen KJ, Luitse JSK. Facilitating damage control surgery with a dedicated DCS equipment trolley. *Injury.* 2006;37:466–467.
3. Working Party of the Association of Anaesthetists of Great Britain and Ireland. *Infection Control in Anaesthesia.* London, UK: Association of Anaesthetists of Great Britain and Ireland; 2002.
4. Woodhead K, Taylor EW, Bannister G, Chesworth T, Hoffman P, Humphreys H. Behaviours and rituals in the operating theatre: a report from the Hospital Infection Society Working Group on Infection Control in the Operating Theatres; 2002. *J Hosp Infect.* 2002 51(4): 241–55.
5. Ritter MA, French ML, Eitzen HE, Gioe TJ. The antimicrobial effectiveness of operative-site preparative agents: a microbiological and clinical study. *J Bone Joint Surg Am.* 1980;62:826–828.
6. Dienstknecht T, Horst K, Sellei R, Berner A, Nerlich N, Hardcastle T. Indications for bullet removal: overview of the literature and clinical practice guidelines for European trauma surgeons. *Eur J Trauma Emerg Surg.* 2012;38(2):89–93.
7. Wick JM. Don't destroy the evidence, *AORN J.* 2000;72(5):807–827.
8. Firth-Cozens J. Why communication fails in the operating room. *Qual Saf Health Care,* 2004;13:327.

Recommended Reading

Goldman MA. *Pocket Guide to the Operating Room,* 3rd ed. Philadelphia, PA: FA Davis; 2008.

Phillips N, ed. Emergency exploratory laparotomy. In: *Berry and Kohn's Operating Room Technique*, 12th ed. St. Louis, MO: Mosby; 2012.

Saullo DC. Trauma surgery. In: Rothrock JC, ed. *Alexander's Care of the Patient in Surgery*, 14th ed. St. Louis, MO: Mosby; 2003:1182–1223.

Index